Hospice and
Palliative Care
Concepts and Practice

JONES AND BARTLETT SERIES IN ONCOLOGY

SECOND EDITION

Hospice and Palliative Care

Concepts and Practice

WALTER B. FORMAN
JUDITH A. KITZES
ROBERT P. ANDERSON
DENICE KOPCHAK SHEEHAN

JONES AND BARTLETT PUBLISHERS
Sudbury, Massachusetts
BOSTON   TORONTO   LONDON   SINGAPORE

World Headquarters

Jones and Bartlett Publishers
40 Tall Pine Drive
Sudbury, MA 01776
978-443-5000
info@jbpub.com
www.jbpub.com

Jones and Bartlett Publishers Canada
2406 Nikanna Road
Mississauga, ON L5C 2W6
CANADA

Jones and Bartlett Publishers International
Barb House, Barb Mews
London W6 7PA
UK

Library of Congress Cataloging-in-Publication Data
Hospice and palliative care: concepts and practice / [edited by] Denice C. Sheehan,
    Walter B. Forman.—2nd ed.
        p. cm.
    Includes bibliographical references and index.
    ISBN 0-7637-1566-2
1. Hospice care. 2. Palliative care. I. Sheehan, Denice C. II. Forman, Walter B.

R726.8 .H653 2003
362.1'75—dc21

2002034161

Acquisitions Editor: Penny M. Glynn
Production Manager: Amy Rose
Associate Editor: Karen Zuck
Associate Production Editor: Karen C. Ferreira
Production Assistant: Jenny L. McIsaac
Associate Marketing Manager: Joy Stark-Vancs
Marketing Associate: Jennifer Killam-Zambrano
Manufacturing and Inventory Coordinator: Amy Bacus
Composition: AnnMarie Lemoine
Cover Design: Philip Regan
Text Design: Anne's Books
Printing and Binding: Malloy, Inc.
Cover Printing: Malloy, Inc.

Printed in the United States of America
07 06 05 04 03   10 9 8 7 6 5 4 3 2 1

Contributors

Robert P. Anderson, RPh
Oncology Pharmacist
Veterans Affairs Medical Center
Albuquerque, NM

David Barnard, PhD
Professor, Department of Medicine
Director of Palliative Care Education
University of Pittsburgh
Pittsburgh, PA

David A. Bennahum, MD
Professor of Medicine
Department of Geriatrics
University of New Mexico
Albuquerque, NM

Constance M. Dahlin, MSN, RN, CS,
   CHPN
Palliative Care Service
Massachusetts General Hospital
Boston, MA

Carol E. Dixon, RN, MS
Vice President and Chief Operating
   Officer
Hospice of Dayton, Inc.
Dayton, OH

N. Elizabeth Eutsler, MSW, LISW
Oncology Social Worker
Veterans Administration Medical Center
Albuquerque, NM

Walter B. Forman, MD, FACP, CMD
Professor, Department of Medicine
Division of Geriatrics
Medical Director, Delta Hospice
Albuquerque, NM

Judith A. Kitzes, MD, MPH
PDIA Faculty Scholar
Assistant Professor
Division of Geriatrics
Past Chief Medical Officer
Albuquerque Area Indian
   Health Services
Albuquerque, NM

Michelle Lee, MD
Fellow, Department of Medicine
Division of Geriatrics
University of New Mexico
Albuquerque, NM

Marijo Letizia, PhD, RN, CPND
Associate Professor
Loyola University
Chicago, IL

Diane Longeway, MSW
University Hospice
Albuquerque, NM

Jeanne M. Martinez, RN, MPH
Coordinator
The Center for Palliative Medicine
  Education and Research
Northwestern Memorial Hospital
Chicago, IL

Jacqueline Mauk, RN, PhD, CNS
Hospice of the Western Reserve
Cleveland, OH

Polly Mazanac, MSN, RN, AOCN, CS
Hospice of the Western Reserve
Cleveland, OH

Lynn McKeever, JD
Founder, Lynn McKeever and
  Associates, LLC
Grinell, IA

Constance B. McPeak, RN, CHPN
Hospice of the Western Reserve
Cleveland, OH

M. Murray Mayo, PhD, RN
Adjunct Faculty, Palliative Care
The Breen School of Nursing
Ursuline College
Pepper Pike, OH

Dennis Pacl, MD
VistaCare Family Hospice
San Antonio, TX

Diletta M. Renier-Berg, MD
Medical Director, Palliative and
  Extended Care
Assistant Professor
University of New Mexico
Albuquerque, NM

Betty L. Schmoll, RN, MS
President and CEO
Hospice of Dayton, Inc.
Dayton, OH

Robert Schwartz, JD
Professor, Law and Pediatrics
University of New Mexico
Albuquerque, NM

Denice Kopchak Sheehan, MSN, RN
Coordinator, Palliative Care Program
The Breen School of Nursing
Ursuline College
Pepper Pike, OH

Brad Stuart, MD
Medical Director
Sutter VNA and Hospice
Emeryville, CA

Contents

3 **Eligibility and Reimbursement for Hospice and Palliative Care**   **35**

Constance M. Dahlin

4   Hospice/Palliative Care Settings   47

Judith A. Kitzes, Betty L. Schmoll, and Carol E. Dixon

5   Continuous Quality Improvement (CQI) in Hospice   57

Michele Y. Lee

9 **Spiritual Care of the Dying Person**   **119**

10 **General Issues: Fatigue, Dyspnea, and Constipation** 129

11   Principles of Pain Management   143

Marijo Letizia

15 Grief and Bereavement Issues in Hospice/Palliative Care   209

M. Murray Mayo

16 Care of the Patient as Death Approaches in the Hospice/Palliative Care Setting   221

Walter B. Forman and Denice Kopchak Sheehan

17 Death Education and Family Support   229

Diana Longeway

Foreword

Pioneers of hospice and palliative care, including many of the editors and authors of this text, have significantly advanced end-of-life care in the United States over the past 30 years. One might conclude that the basic principles and concepts of hospice and palliative care are "old news," now well integrated into systems of care. This is far from true.

A tragedy of our current health care system is that the philosophy of hospice and palliative care remains relatively isolated in specialized settings. Although remarkable progress has begun, it has only just begun. There is still a tremendous need to integrate key concepts — pain and symptom control, family-centered care, institutional change, bereavement support, cultural consideration at the end of life, and dignified death — across clinical settings and patient populations. The infant whose short life will end in the NICU, the elder dying in long-term care, the patient discontinuing renal analysis, and the grandmother with Alzheimer's cared for at home all deserve quality care at life's end.

There remains a wide gap between how we actually die and how we wish our lives would end. Closing that gap will require a complex bridge with interconnected beams representing professional commitment, institutional support, health policy change, and a public expectation of improved care. The bridge that will close that gap will be built of passion and compassion, competence and commitment. This book is an essential contribution to the "nuts and bolts" needed for the construction. The historical perspective provided and the discussion of essential principles such as interdisciplinary care remind us of the core of our work. Issues of reimbursement and quality improvement must also be included in our plans to bridge the gap.

Much of the past decade of hospice and palliative care has centered on systems issues and professional practice, including certification; the transition in focus from hospice to palliative care; the great challenges involved in managed care; diverse populations; and the intricacies of expanding our scope while retaining basic philosophical tenets.

Amidst the turmoil is the need to remember that at the end of the day there remains one central goal for hospice and palliative care — improving end-of-life care for patients and their families. This text is keenly focused on that goal with content addressing major clinical aspects of care such as communication, symptom management, grief, and spiritual care. The text also addresses the very real and extremely challenging issues of assisted suicide and other ethical dilemmas common at the end of life.

Dame Cicely Saunders, founder of St. Christopher's Hospice and the modern hospice movement, was recently interviewed about her life's work. The final question of the interview asked, "Was there ever an incident that caused you to lose heart in the fight for hospice?"

Dame Saunders replied: "We have nurses who've worked here for 30 years and are still positive and caring. The work can be draining, but it's never depressing. You feel that people have had a better death through what you've done. I was very bereaved here and there, but I've grown through loss. You never forget those who've gone, but I keep reminding myself that we started a movement."[1]

For all of those who have begun the bridge toward more humane care at the end of life, and to those who will join the movement, this text will serve as an excellent travel guide.

Betty R. Ferrell, PhD, FAAN
Research Scientist
City of Hope National Medical Center

1.   *The Education for Physicians on End of Life Project.* American Medical Association, Chicago, IL: 2002.

Preface

Five years ago we undertook the task of preparing a textbook about hospice/palliative care for those starting out in the field or wishing to understand this up-and-coming area in health care. We were aware that much of the activity in this new interdisciplinary field was not occurring in the United States. As we prepared this edition we happily found that the situation had changed. There are now many conferences concerning the various aspects of end-of-life care. Both nurses and physicians can obtain certification in the field. There are active groups of health care (e.g., social work) and non-health care (e.g., spiritual counseling) professionals in all areas of end-of-life care.

In our first edition we even felt the need to define the terms palliative care, family, interdisciplinary team, and hospice care. We refer you to these statements in our first edition if you need to learn some of these basic concepts, which are not as exhaustively discussed in this edition. However, we hope that these terms are now part of the health care vocabulary and will soon be part of yours.

In preparing this edition we thought that it should represent a wider point of view than our first. So, we have expanded the editors to reflect the interdisciplinary nature of this work. Editors include a pharmacist, a nurse, a physician, and a physician involved in the care of a special population. In addition, we have added authors from other disciplines such as law and advanced practice nursing to this edition. We have also included several physicians who are involved as full-time professionals in the care of those for whom a cure is no longer possible. In the first edition, we hoped that the book would represent a shared work. In this edition we are certain that it does. Of course, this philosophy can at times lead to differences of opinion. Please be assured that we recognized this situation and wanted the reader to be aware of some of these differences. Hopefully, if we have the opportunity to undertake a third edition, these differences will have been resolved. Nonetheless, we want to thank all the contributors to this text. They have made it a richer book by being part of the effort to have a textbook that speaks to the needs of the beginner in this field. We hope that schools that undertake the teaching of hospice/palliative care in their curricula will find this text of significant value.

Each of us has special people in our lives who need to be recognized, including teachers, significant others, and colleagues. We wish to thank them, as they are the people that have significantly enriched our lives.

We offer thanks to the many people whom we have attended to as patients, who have taught us how important it is to be able to assist them in the many aspects of care during this part of our living. Hopefully, we have represented their thoughts and wishes that care at the end of life will become as much a part of health care as giving birth is today. Certainly, this passage in living is no less important. It needs to become part of the daily life of every health care professional.

The Historical Development of Hospice and Palliative Care

1

David A. Bennahum

The care of suffering and dying patients is part of human history. In the past quarter of a century, however, we have seen a revolution in the care of terminally ill patients and those in pain. This has been the result of a number of individuals whose critical thinking has reshaped contemporary views of death. In 1963, Jessica Mitford satirized American attitudes toward death in her mordant book (later produced as a film), *The American Way of Death*.[1] Philippe Aries, in his extraordinary 1981 book, *The Hour of Our Death*, examined how Western civilization had come to conceal death in the late nineteenth and twentieth centuries as the Victorians had concealed sexuality in the last century.[2]

As early as 1914, Justice Cardoza asserted the right of individuals to refuse care in a dissenting New York State Appeals Court decision. However, it took a legal and ethical evolution to confirm that patients had the right to be informed about their care, and that physicians and hospitals were accountable for that care. It was this belated recognition that was confirmed by the United States Congress in 1991 in the Danforth Amendment.[3] This law requires that patients admitted to health care facilities receiving federal funds be informed of their right to refuse care and to have advance directives for health care. In addition, a better understanding of pain control and a variety of methods for achieving this end have developed. Despite this landmark legislation, it was the work of two physicians, Elisabeth Kübler-Ross and Dame Cicely Saunders (discussed later in this chapter), perhaps more than anything else, that began to change the way society and health professionals perceived terminal disease, death, and dying.

The Historical Roots of Hospice

Among the Greeks in Homeric times (8th century B.C.), all strangers without exception were regarded as being under the protection of Zeus Xenios, the god of strangers and supplicants. A wanderer would be treated as a guest and offered food, shelter, clothing, and gifts. Violation of the duties of hospitality were likely to provoke the wrath of the gods.

In the Greek world, patients who were not cured by an itinerant physician, the *iatros*, could seek care at a temple to Aesculepius, the god of medicine. Here they would spend the night in the temple precincts, "incubating" with the god. In the morning, the priests of Aesculepius would interpret the patients' dreams. Over time these temples became places where medicine was taught.[4]

In Roman times, the custom of private hospitality was codified and legally defined. *Host* is derived from the root *hospes*. Ties between a guest and a host, meaning the person who receives or entertains, were confirmed by the clasping of hands and the exchange of a written agreement, the *tabula hospitalis*. This sacred contract in the name of Jupiter Hospitalis developed into a practice whereby the Roman state appointed citizens of foreign states, called the Public Hospitium, to protect Romans abroad.[5] *Hospice* derives from the Latin *hospitium*, meaning entertainment, hospitality, lodging, or inn.[6] Thus, the place where a guest was received evolved into the hospital for the temporarily sick and the hospice as a permanent residence for poor, infirm, crippled, insane, and incurable people. Other related words such as hostel, hotel, host, and hostess also were derived from *hospitium*.

The first hospitals appeared on the periphery of the Roman Empire and were military hospitals that served the legions garrisoned on the frontier.[7] By the fourth century, first in Byzantium and later in Rome under the impetus of early Christianity, rudimentary hospitals and hospices began to appear that welcomed travelers and cared for the sick. Dame Cicely Saunders, the founder of St. Christopher's Hospice, points out that, "This was a radically different approach to the Hippocratic tradition in which a doctor did not treat the incurably sick or terminally ill. It was thought unethical to treat a patient with a deadly disease, for in so doing the doctor risked paying the penalty awaiting those mortals who challenged nature and the gods."[8]

In the Middle Ages (476–1453 A.D.), hospices sprang up along routes of commerce and pilgrimage, the most famous being those at alpine passes maintained by the order of St. Bernard. As a response to the Crusades, the order of Knights Hospitalers established hospitals in Europe and the Middle East along the Crusade and pilgrimage routes. Leprosy spread widely during the Middle Ages, but is not found in skeletal remains prior to the fourth century A.D. (The leprosy described in the Bible is probably a group of skin diseases such as psoriasis.[9]) In response to the medieval epidemic of leprosy, houses dedicated to

Lazarus, who is mentioned as healed by Christ in the Roman Book of St. Luke, sprang up near more than 4000 towns and cities in France and Germany.

It is important to remember that both ancient India and Egypt had institutions that possessed some of the attributes of hospitals. As early as 2500 B.C., Egypt had a highly organized system of medical education and health care, as is seen in such documents as the Smith Papyrus. As to Indian health care:

> According to Indian literature in the sixth century B.C., Buddha appointed a physician for every ten villages and built hospitals for the crippled and the poor; his son built shelters for diseased and pregnant women. Hospitals existed in Ceylon as early as 437 B.C. The most outstanding of the early hospitals in India were the 18 built by King Asoka (273–232 B.C.). These are historically significant because of characteristics similar to those of the modern hospital (or hospice). The attendants were ordered to give gentle care to the sick, to furnish them with fresh fruits and vegetables, to prepare medicines, to give massages, and to keep their own persons clean. Hindu physicians . . . were required to take daily baths, keep their hair and nails short, wear white clothes, and promise to respect the confidence of their patients.[10]

Islam also played a prominent role in the institutional care of the sick, particularly the mentally ill, introducing the idea of humane care in special asylums.

As European cities began to grow during the Renaissance (1450–1600 A.D.), the need for care of the indigent, the old, and the insane became essential. Modeled on the leprosaria of the Middle Ages, hospices evolved that provided minimal shelter and food for this population.[11] In addition to leprosaria and hospices, another peculiar institution of the Renaissance was the foundling hospital, which acted as a population control system by accepting unwanted newborns.[12] These institutions evolved into the hospitals of the eighteenth and nineteenth century, whose high rates of infectious diseases resulted in horrendous mortality rates.[13]

The discovery of anesthesia in 1842 and Lord Lister's aseptic surgical technique revolutionized medicine by the end of the nineteenth century.[14] Amputations could be performed and cancers resected without pain and with very little risk of infection. Western medicine had always been heroic; that is, advocating purges, cathartics, emetics, and bleeding to remove noxious humours as advocated by Galenic principles. The Idea of Progress, introduced by Sir Francis Bacon in *The Great Instauration of Knowledge* in 1626, set the tone for the optimistic positivism and meliorism that too often drive the care of patients to this day.[15] It has become difficult not to treat, for to do so is to threaten the almost universally held belief that science can only improve the human condition.

The Modern History of Hospice

Dame Cicely Saunders

The exponential growth of Western medical science in a society that was paradoxically denying the inevitability of death provided the setting for Elisabeth

Kübler-Ross and Cicely Saunders to make their extraordinary contributions to hospice care. A number of institutions had recognized the need for humane care of the dying in the nineteenth century. Saunders, in her introduction to the *Oxford Textbook of Palliative Medicine*, notes that Jeanne Garnier in Lyons, France, founded several hospices or Calvaires as early as 1842.[16] The Irish Sisters of Charity opened Our Lady's Hospice in Dublin in 1879 and St. Joseph's Hospice in East London in 1905, both for incurable or dying patients. Inspired by these examples, Calvary Hospital in New York was opened in 1899. Additionally, three Protestant homes for the dying were open in London by the turn of the century: the Friedenshein Home of Rest, later St. Columbus Hospital, in 1885; the Hostel of God, which became Trinity Hospice, in 1891; and St. Luke's Home for the Dying Poor, established in 1893 to care for those dying of tuberculosis and cancer.[17]

Dame Cicely Saunders entered medical school at St. Thomas Hospital Medical School in London in 1951, after originally training as a nurse at the Nightingale School at St. Thomas Hospital. She had also finished a degree in philosophy, politics, and economics at Oxford and gained a diploma in Public Administration. From the beginning of her work as a nurse, Saunders seems to have recognized that cancer patients challenged the prevailing optimism of medicine. She credits her seven years as a volunteer nurse at St. Luke's, beginning in 1948, and writes that ". . . the reading of its many full and lively reports by Dr. Howard Barrett, its founder, were major influences in the early planning of St. Christopher's Hospice,"[18] which she would help found in 1962. His turn-of-the-century records described patients and the benefits of good pain control. It was at St. Luke's that she came to understand the need for home care, family support, research, and education and that pain and symptom control was crucial. This led her to spend an additional two years of fellowship studying pain control in the Department of Pharmacology at St. Mary's Medical School in London.[19]

Having completed her medical studies in 1957, Saunders began working at St. Joseph's Hospital in Hackney, a working-class section of London. Here she began her work in the use of opioids to control pain in dying patients. On the basis of what she had learned at St. Luke's, she experimented with higher doses of opiates that were given in advance of pain and on a regular schedule. Through this experiment she observed (as Kübler-Ross later would) that patients free of pain were only too eager to talk about their illness and that they benefited from the opportunity.[20] On the basis of her experiences, Saunders wrote a series of insightful articles and developed a personal network of colleagues and friends. By 1967 she was able to raise enough money and persuade the National Health Service to give her sufficient support to design and build St. Christopher's Hospice in Sydenham on the outskirts of London. Her practical, patient-centered approach would have appealed to Thomas Sydenham, a great seventeenth-century physician known as the English Hippocrates, who rebelled against the heroic treatments of his time. On the basis of her remarkable preparation, Saunders was able to understand the complex inter-disciplinary needs of cancer patients and formulate the following principles:

1. Death must be accepted.
2. The patient's total care must be managed by a skilled interdisciplinary team whose members communicate regularly with one another.
3. The common symptoms of terminal disease, especially the palliation of pain in all its aspects, need to be effectively controlled.
4. The patient and family as a single unit of care must be recognized.
5. An active home-care program should be implemented.
6. An active program of bereavement care for the family after the death of the patient must be provided.
7. Research and education should be ongoing.[21]

Elisabeth Kübler-Ross, MD

During the same period in which Saunders was doing her creative work in Great Britain, Elisabeth Kübler-Ross spent time interviewing dying patients. As a psychiatrist, she had found it very hard to find patients to interview because most physicians and nurses thought her interest morbid, if not perverse. After persisting in her inquiry and interviewing more than 500 dying patients, she published *On Death and Dying* in 1969, for the first time creating a theoretical framework that described the psychological stages of dying as she perceived them.[22,23] The impact that Kübler-Ross's work had on the popular and professional environment in the United States was crucial to the acceptance of the hospice concept proposed by Saunders. The taboos and silence erected in the nineteenth and twentieth centuries had to be challenged before the idea of palliative care could be considered. Although some of Kübler-Ross's stages proved to be questionable, thanks to her research the study of the dying process is now acceptable, if not downright fashionable. The prevailing positivism of American medicine continues, but it is now possible to challenge the melioristic assumption that the full thrust of treatment should be to extend life at all cost.

Early Hospice in the United States and Canada

The work at St. Christopher's awakened the interest of physicians and nurses in the United States. As early as 1963, Saunders was invited to lecture at the Yale University School of Medicine. There she met Florence Wald, then dean of the graduate school of nursing. In 1966 Wald would invite Saunders back for a workshop on hospice. This was the beginning of hospice in the United States. Florence Wald opened the New Haven Hospice homecare component in 1974. The inpatient service opened in 1979, with Sylvia Lack as its first medical director. This created a new model that was able to demonstrate that Americans were comfortable with home care. This was confirmed by the Hospice of Marin near San Francisco, which was opened in 1976 and directed by William Lammers, MD. The hospice focused on home care and was largely sponsored and supported by lay workers and volunteers.

Another hospice model, directed by physician Balfour Mount, opened at the Royal Victoria Hospital of McGill University in Montreal. This model demonstrated the value of the presence of a hospital-based palliative care service, especially in terms of research and education on pain control. It was Mount who first used the term *palliative care*. In 1977, the hospices of Marin and Yale sponsored the first major conference on care of the dying, which attracted representatives from seventeen states.

The proponents of another model, that of interdisciplinary palliative care, as developed at St. Luke's in New York, would argue that:

> Hospice care should be part of the mainstream of American Medicine and its institutions. Development of separate facilities for hospice care could be more costly and might result in the public perceiving hospices as another form of nursing home. Furthermore, hospital care should be influenced by the principles of hospice care; that is, caring and curing should be related. A hospice team or consultant in every teaching hospital would enable today's students and tomorrow's health care providers to observe hospice care as an integral part of treatment in the acute care setting.[24]

The Legislative Role in Hospice and Palliative Care

In 1972, the United States Senate's Special Committee on Aging held hearings on "Death with Dignity," at which Dr. Kübler-Ross testified.[25] Although hospice organizers originally sought to separate hospice from traditional hospital care (seeing hospital technology as preventing humane care of the dying), the government now became interested in incorporating hospice care into the work of traditional institutions.

Senators Frank Church and Frank E. Moss introduced the first hospice legislation in 1974, but their proposals were not enacted. That same year, however, the National Cancer Institute funded America's first hospice, the New Haven Hospice, for three years as a national demonstration center. This was followed by additional support to other hospices.

By the late 1970s, interest in the process of dying became widespread in the United States. Kübler-Ross's book had become well known and the subject of innumerable radio, television, and magazine discussions. Also, in the late 1970s, the New Haven Hospice assisted in bringing together hospice advocates in North America. The meeting was held to establish guidelines for operational issues necessary to develop hospice programs. The meeting was successful and the National Hospice Organization was born.

In 1978, the United States Department of Health, Education, and Welfare urged that the hospice movement receive federal support, and in 1979 the Health Care Financing Administration (HCFA) provided support to 26 hospices across the country to test the cost effectiveness of hospice care. This was followed by a grant from the W. K. Kellogg Foundation to the Joint Commission on the Accreditation of Hospitals for the commission to develop standards for hospice accreditation.

In 1983, the National Hospice Organization was able to persuade the U.S. Congress to establish hospice benefits for Medicare beneficiaries. As might have been predicted for the United States, however, enthusiasm for palliative care of terminal illness led to an eclectic mix of hospice programs. The Medicare Hospice Benefit was made permanent in 1986, but payment rates remained low. In 1991, hospice care was authorized for military hospitals and for patients insured by the military (CHAMPUS). That same year, hospice was recommended for the Veteran's Administration, and in 1992 it was recommended for the Indian Health Service. In 1994, HCFA became concerned with questionable certifications of patients with terminal illnesses. Although there has been significant government support for the hospice concept, there has also been concern, as there is for the entire long-term care industry, that palliative care and hospice programs may provide opportunities for unscrupulous individuals to create fraud and abuse. This led to a number of HCFA initiatives in the 1990s that sought to improve data collection and enhance supervision of hospice programs.

The development of the hospice movement paralleled an increasing concern about the unnecessary prolongation of life. The 1976 Quinlan decision, permitting the removal of a ventilator from a comatose young woman, was followed by 15 years of remarkable legal decisions and the evolution of biomedical ethics as a patient care discipline. Most recently, the 1991 Supreme Court decision in the case of Nancy Cruzan affirmed the right of patients to have advance directives and to refuse medical care. Interest in death and dying is now focused on the controversial issues of assisted suicide and euthanasia, with forces polarized between the ideas of the right to die and the right to life. Contemporary palliative care advocates almost universally assert that if pain and suffering are relieved, then requests for assistance in dying are rarely made. Not all commentators agree with this opinion, however, especially when consideration goes beyond the experiences of cancer patients to those of patients with terminal AIDS, end-stage renal disease, and severe, chronic depression.[26,27,28]

Recent Developments in Hospice and Palliative Care

A remarkable development in the past decade has been the interest of a number of foundations in end-of-life care. The George Soros Foundation funded the Death in America Project. The Robert Wood Johnson Foundation has initiated a vast project to improve end-of-life care and has funded many innovative programs. Of enormous help in educating the public has been Bill Moyers's Public Television programs on end-of-life care.

By 2001 there were more than 3000 hospice and palliative care programs in the United States that ranged from home care to hospital care, and from professional, palliative care teams to lay and volunteer workers. Many other countries, including Australia, New Zealand, and much of Western Europe, had developed palliative care and hospice programs, and the World Health Organization under the leadership of Doctor Robert Twycross, the director of the Oxford Hospice in Great Britain, was actively developing programs in India.

The World Health Organization, recognizing the importance of the hospice and palliative care movement, requested a formal definition of palliative care from an expert committee. Their definition is as follows:

> Palliative care is the active, total care of patients whose disease is not responsive to curative treatment. Control of pain, other symptoms, and of psychological, social and spiritual problems is paramount. The goal of palliative care is achievement of the best possible quality of life for patients and their families. Many aspects of palliative care are also applicable earlier in the course of illness, in conjunction with anti-cancer treatment.
> Palliative Care:
>
> • affirms life and regards dying as a normal process;
> • neither hastens nor postpones death;
> • provides relief from pain and other distressing symptoms;
> • integrates the psychological and spiritual aspects of patient care;
> • offers a support system to help patients live as actively as possible until death;
> • offers a support system to help the family cope during the patient's illness . . . and in their own bereavement.[29]

The Contribution of Pharmacological Innovation

The distinguished British medical historian, Roy Porter, in his encyclopedia of the history of medicine published in 1993, points out that,

> Pain is one of the more puzzling, and neglected, topics of the history of medicine . . . it is, however, central to the healer's art. Critics of high-tech modern medicine such as Ivan Illich have deplored this retreat from the head-on confrontation with pain. Such refusal to face reality, they allege, undermines self-management and personal control. He or she who cannot face pain will not be able to face death. Yet, as is amply shown by the liberal policy with morphine dosages followed in British hospices, the signs are that effective pain control can materially enhance the quality of life in the terminally sick. Successful pain management may be one of the more tangible and widespread, if less glamorous, triumphs of modern medicine.[30]

An ancient Egyptian medical document, the Smith Papyrus, dating from 1800 B.C., mentions the "red shepenn," which seems to mean poppy, and small juglets in the form of opium poppies were exported from Cyprus to Egypt as early as 1500 B.C. Before the time of the Greek war against Troy, approximately 1300 to 1200 B.C., there existed a Minoan cult on the island of Crete, dedicated to the goddess of the poppy. There was a "tradition whereby opium was the active principle of Helen's famous Egyptian potion, nepenthes, which relieved the deepest sorrows." Opium was always an ingredient of theriac, the universal panacea first created by King Mithridates as an antidote to poison, and later enhanced by Nero's physician, Andromachus, with up to sixty ingredients. Galen wrote a book on the subject, and theriac was in common use until the end of the nineteenth century. The Chinese called it te-ya-ka, and the great Hindu medical books of Charaka and Sushruta mention similar complex potions, all of which probably contained opium.[31]

For the treatment of pain, the Graeco-Roman physician had opium, wine, and the alkaloids of henbane, belladonna, black nightshade, and mandrake, from which are derived hyoscyamine, atropine, and scopolamine. These were used both as poisons and as analgesics.[32] A number of historians believe that there were other pain relievers—Hippocrates mentions a lost text, *On Drugs*—but these are unknown today. For the treatment of the podagra (pain in the great toe) of gout, the Byzantine physician Alexander of Tralles (525–605 A.D.) recommended the emetic properties of the autumn crocus. In the nineteenth century, colchicine was derived from that flower, and shown to be a specific anti-inflammatory agent for the pain and swelling of gout.[33]

Tea brewed from the bark of the willow tree, *Salix alba*, has been used to treat arthritis for generations. The Doctrine of Signatures states that the cure for many symptoms can be found in the place where the disease occurs.[34] For example, the pain of arthritis is often worse in swampy areas where the willow tree grows. The Reverend Edward Stone published a paper in the *Philosophical Transactions of the Royal Society* in 1763, advocating the use of willow bark in the treatment of arthritis and fever.[35] Eventually the specific, salicin, was isolated from the willow; later, in 1853, acetylsalicylic was synthesized by Charles Gerhardt in Strasbourg. It was introduced into clinical practice by Heinrich Dreser while he was working for the Bayer company in 1899.

The search for analgesic and antipyretic drugs led nineteenth-century German chemists to examine coal tar and its derivatives, leading to the discovery of the analines, so important to the dye industry; phenols, which are antiseptic; and pyrazolines and thus antipyrine, which are anti-inflammatory and analgesic. These researchers would eventually produce acetaminophen. The discovery of ACTH, the corticosteroids, and the nonsteroidal anti-inflammatory drugs (NSAIDs) after the Second World War would in turn enhance the ability of physicians and nurses to control pain.

America's greatest contribution to medicine was Crawford W. Long's demonstration in 1842 of the anesthetic properties of ether (later controversially claimed by Horace Wells and W. T. G. Morton), which introduced painless surgery to the world.[36] A few years later, in 1853, C. G. Pravaz and Alexander Wood introduced the hypodermic syringe. Mid-century physicians would now be able to inject the newly isolated opiates, morphine and heroin, as well as cocaine. The availability of anesthesia and opiates by syringe would soon be tested in the cauldron of the Civil War, initiating the modern era of anesthetic surgery, as well as the plague of intravenous addiction.[37]

Summary

In his recent book, *How We Die*, Sherwin B. Nuland emphasizes the importance of hope to each and every patient:

> Hope lies not only in an expectation of cure or even of the remission of present distress. For dying patients, the hope of cure will always be ultimately false, and even the hope of relief too often turns to ashes. When my time comes, I will seek hope in the knowledge that insofar as possible I will not be allowed to suffer or be subjected to needless attempts to maintain my life; I will seek it in the certainty that I will not be abandoned to die alone; I am seeking it now, in the way I try to live my life, so that those who value what I am will have profited by my time on earth and be left with comforting recollections of what we have meant to each one another.[38]

The hospice movement is grounded in the belief of a few courageous pioneers that dying patients need not suffer alone and without respite. The discipline to study pain, dying, and death did not come easily, and has had to challenge the prevailing view that death is a failure of medicine and something to be hidden and avoided. Emerging from a religious impulse to comfort the sick, the care of the dying was greatly facilitated by research into pain management and a better understanding of the importance of symptom relief, be it thirst, hunger, inflammation, anxiety, depression, or pain. Surprisingly, it has taken, and still takes, rigor, discipline, and objective observation as well as compassion and competence to persuade health professionals, and often patients, that death with dignity is not giving up; rather, it can be the proper completion of an individual life.

References

1. Mitford, J. *The American Way of Death*. New York: Simon & Schuster, 1963.
2. Aries, P. *The Hour of Our Death*. New York: Alfred A. Knopf, 1981.
3. Torrens, P. R. Ed. *Hospice Programs and Public Policy*. Chicago: American Hospital Publishing, American Hospital Association, 1985, pp. 3–29.
4. Edelstein, L. *Ancient Medicine*. Baltimore: Johns Hopkins University Press, 1967, p. 241.
5. *Encyclopedia Britannica*. New York, 1910, p. 791.
6. *Oxford English Dictionary*. Oxford, UK, 1971, 405, p. 1336.
7. Majno, G. *The Healing Hand*. Boston: Harvard University Press, 1975, p. 383.
8. Saunders, C. *Oxford Textbook of Palliative Medicine*. Oxford, UK, 1993, p. vi.
9. Zias, J. E. "Paleopathological Evidence of Leprosy in Palestine During the Talmudic Period." *Koroth*, 9 (1–2), Fall 1985.
10. Cohen, K. P. *Hospice: Prescription for Terminal Care*. Germantown, Md.: Aspen Systems Corporation, 1979, pp. 14–16.
11. Casteglioni, A. *A History of Medicine*. New York: Jason Aronson, Inc., 1969, p. 362.
12. Boswell, J. *The Kindness of Strangers*. New York: Pantheon Books, 1988.
13. Rosenberg, C. *The Care of Strangers*. New York: Basic Books, 1987.

14. Pernick, M.S. *A Calculus of Suffering: Pain, Professionalism, and Anesthesia in Nineteenth-Century America.* New York: Columbia University Press, 1985.
15. Becker, L. C. Ed. *Encyclopedia of Bioethics.* Garland Press, 1992, pp. 848–49.
16. Saunders, p. vi.
17. Ibid.
18. Ibid.
19. Ibid.
20. Torrens, p. 4.
21. Torrens, p. 7.
22. Ibid.
23. Kübler-Ross, E. *On Death and Dying.* New York: Macmillan, 1969.
24. Torrens, p. 14.
25. Paradis, L. F. *The Development of Hospice in America, The Hospice Handbook.* Rockland, Md.: Aspen Publications, 1985, p. 7.
26. Colt, G. H. *The Enigma of Suicide.* New York: Simon & Schuster, 1991.
27. Quill, T. E. *Death and Dignity: Making Choices and Taking Charge.* New York: W. W. Norton & Co., 1993.
28. Rachels, J. *The End of Life.* Oxford: Oxford University Press, 1986.
29. Neigh, J. E. *Hospice: A Historical Perspective.* Adapted by the Hospice Education Institute. See Hospice on the Web. http://www.cp-tel.net/pamnorth/history.htm.
30. Porter, R. *Companion Encyclopedia of the History of Medicine.* Routledge, UK, 1993, pp. 1589–1591.
31. Majno, p. 144.
32. King, H. in *The History of the Management of Pain,* R. D. Mann, Ed. Park Ridge, N.J.: Pantheon Publishing Group, 1988, p. 55.
33. Castiglioni, A., p. 252.
34. Herbalists and medieval alchemists have used the "Doctrine of Signatures" for centuries. During the middle 1600s, the medical community came to embrace the idea. Basically, the doctrine professes that every item created by God is marked with a "signature," indicating what specific purpose the item was created for. By observing the characteristics of the item (e.g., color, shape, place of growth, etc.) the purpose of the item, in God's plan, could be determined. Native American and Oriental cultures have held similar beliefs.
35. Mann, R. D. "The History of the Non-steroidal Anti-inflammatory Agents." In Mann, R. D. Ed. *The History of the Management of Pain.* Park Ridge, N.J.: Pantheon Publishing Group, 1988, pp. 77–125.
36. Castiglioni, p. 723.
37. Pernick, M. S., p. 104.
38. Nuland, S. B. *How We Die.* New York: Alfred A. Knopf, 1994, p. 257.

For Further Reading

Campbell, L. "History of the Hospice Movement." *Cancer Nursing,* 9(6):333–338, 1986.

Dicks, B. "The Contribution of Nursing to Palliative Care." *Palliative Medicine,* 4:197–203, 1990.

Dobratz, M. C. "Hospice Nursing: Present Perspectives and Future Directives." *Cancer Nursing,* 13(2):116–122, 1990.

Stoddard, S. "Hospice in the United States: An Overview." *Journal of Palliative Care,* 5(3):10–19, 1998.

The Interdisciplinary Team

2

N. Elizabeth Eustler

Jeanne M. Martinez

Over the past twenty-five years, hospital-based inpatient care has adopted interdisciplinary care as a preferred model for addressing patients' complex health care needs. This concept followed consumerism and the women's movement, both originating in the 1960s, when consumers identified the need to become more active and assertive in many arenas. This activism affected health care, with a change from a paternalistic view of the physician-patient relationship to one in which the patient was considered a partner and thus a member of the team in prevention, treatment, and healing. This concept also changed the relationship among physicians, nurses, and other health care providers. Each discipline has expertise to contribute to the care of the patient and family. The goal of the interdisciplinary team is to work with patients to identify their specific needs and health goals within a holistic framework. All members contribute from their unique areas of practice rather than focusing on treatment of disease entities or resolution of physical symptoms in isolation. The interdisciplinary team concept varies widely in practice in acute medicine. However, hospice care has been purposely designed to require the initial consultation and necessary follow-up care of an interdisciplinary team.

Staff Characteristics

Regardless of discipline, all hospice practitioners and volunteers should be screened and selected by similar criteria beyond their individual professional expertise. Looking for individuals who balance their lives on a number of levels is essential. For example, interest in working with patients with life-threatening illnesses is obviously required. However, an extremely intense or obsessive interest is a red flag that a candidate may be inappropriate for hospice work.

Hospice caregivers must be empathetic. They should be hardworking but pursue leisure activities outside of work. Home hospice care requires a unique blend of being comfortable with working independently and at times in isolation, yet participating enthusiastically as part of a team. Professional turf issues have no place in hospice care because high-functioning hospice teams often require members to blur their roles with an overlap of responsibilities.

Professionals and volunteers who have worked through their own past grief experience may have much to offer. However, sometimes those with unresolved grief or who are still grieving will seek out hospice work before they are ready. A loss inventory should be part of every hospice screening tool for staff and volunteers.

Other motivations for hospice work should be investigated. As with prospective employees, personal and business references should be obtained on all volunteer candidates before acceptance into hospice volunteer training.

Many hospice programs use communication exercises during volunteer training to further evaluate each candidate's appropriateness and motivation for volunteering. All hospice workers must be good communicators and especially good listeners, and must be trained and evaluated in communication. Staff and volunteers should be made aware of how necessary good communication is for effective functioning of the team. Effective team members are prepared and willing to support their colleagues as needed. Some hospice programs offer staff support groups.

In the interview process, candidates must know that hospice work is often inherently difficult and emotionally draining. They should be taught the responsibility of asking for assistance for themselves when needed, whether that assistance is technical or emotional. Hospice personnel must help each other identify potential or actual emotional issues that may affect individual or group functioning or patient care. Each member of the team must develop his or her own coping strategies. Above all, hospice programs should communicate the value of taking care of oneself as a fundamental ingredient for providing excellent hospice care.

Interview Process for Potential Hospice Employees/Volunteers

A variety of issues should be discussed during the initial interview of prospective candidates, regardless of their potential roles in hospice. The interviewers must determine whether candidates have had a personal loss within the past year, because these candidates may concentrate on their own personal needs rather than on the needs of the patient and his or her family.

Much of the information that is gathered from the potential candidate in the initial interview could become part of the screening process. Discussion of personal interests, reasons for applying for a particular position, communication style, support system, team concept, and ability to work with dying patients is essential for determining whether the person is appropriate for hospice work and how he or she might best serve as a team member. The interview process should also focus on how the candidate receives support, copes, and relieves stress. This discussion is important because the hospice workers must be able to care for themselves before they can provide quality care for the dying.

Discussing conflict resolution and the team approach in the initial interview may assist in the selection of team members who will handle conflict in a constructive, positive manner with direct communication and who will be interactive and cooperative team members. Direct communication and conflict resolution assist in appropriate communication and create effectiveness when working within the team structure.

The hospice team members and the patients and their families often create close bonds. Therefore, the ability to set professional limits is extremely important and should be explored. Failure to set limits is detrimental to the team approach, to the patient and family, and to the team members. Patients and their families may ask the home health aide or volunteer to do things that may be more personal, such as shopping for food. Setting limits allows for open communication and assists in providing a comprehensive approach to hospice care.

Members of the Team

Hospice in the United States began largely as a self-described consumer movement. It is no surprise that the patient and family are identified in hospice standards as the center of the team.

Medicare hospice regulations define the following as core services: physician services, nursing services, medical social services, and counseling services. The patient's attending physician is also a member of the team. Hospice employees must provide these services; that is, the care cannot be provided by contract arrangement except in times of peak patient loads or under extraordinary circumstances.

The Medicare hospice regulations further specify the composition and role of the interdisciplinary team (Table 2-1). The team must be composed of a doctor of medicine or osteopathy, a registered nurse, a social worker, and a

TABLE 2-1   Responsibilities of the Interdisciplinary Hospice Team
Participate in establishing the plan of care.
Provide or supervise hospice care and services.
Review and update the plan of care.
Establish policies governing hospice care and services.

Source: Medicare: Hospice Manual, U.S. Department of Health and Human Services, 2000.

pastoral or other counselor. A patient-care coordinator or team leader facilitates each team.

If the hospice program has more than one interdisciplinary team, it must designate those members responsible for establishing the policies that govern the provision of hospice care and services. Hospice must make nursing services, physician services, medications, and other treatment needs routinely available on a 24-hour basis.

Other covered services must also be available on a 24-hour basis to the extent necessary to meet the specific needs of the persons served in the hospice program. In addition, the following services must be made available to patients as needed (they may be provided on a contract basis): occupational therapy, physical therapy, speech therapy, dietary consultation, homemakers, and home health aides.[1] Some hospices offer additional services that are not outlined in the Medicare hospice regulations. These include music/recreation therapy, art therapy, massage therapy, and financial counseling.

Medical specialists such as surgeons, anesthesiologists, and psychiatrists may also be included as consultants for specific problems. Volunteers are also considered hospice employees. They can provide direct patient care or administrative support in such activities as clerical work in the hospice office.

Because the services provided for each patient are based on the interdisciplinary care plan, the team members are determined by each patient's needs at any given time. The patient may need services provided by only the core team members when he or she enters the hospice program. A home health aide may be needed later to assist with bathing and a music therapist to guide and teach relaxation techniques.

The Core Team

Hospice Medical Director

Each hospice must have at least one physician designated as the medical director. This physician has both administrative and clinical responsibilities. Administratively, the medical director reviews hospice policies and participates in quality assurance studies. Under Medicare regulations, the medical director must determine the medical eligibility of patients for hospice care, and certify (initially, in collaboration with one other physician) that the patient is terminally ill. Second, the medical director must be consulted on each patient's initial plan of care and is responsible for recertifying patients for subsequent benefit periods to continue their hospice benefits under Medicare. Third, the medical director must also be available to provide primary care to the patient if the patient's physician is unable to carry out this role.

Beyond these required administrative functions, the effective medical director must have expertise in pain and symptom management, a strong knowledge base in primary medicine, comfort with difficult emotional issues, and the ability to communicate compassion and empathy. Good communication skills are also required to provide consultation and support to referring physicians and foster cohesive collaboration within the hospice team.

The most common clinical roles for a physician include hospice medical director, attending physician, and team physician. In most hospice programs, the attending and team physicians are members of the core team. The physician must be trained and experienced in assessing the interactions between the various pathophysiologic problems (for example, cancer of the lung, chronic obstructive lung disease, and the use of morphine). With this assessment, the team can assist the patient in choosing among the treatment options. The physician is often most knowledgeable about potentially reversible situations (for example, hypercalcemia as a cause of coma).

Although physical and psychosocial symptoms must be assessed and treated simultaneously, the relief of physical symptoms provides opportunities for patients to explore areas of emotional, social, and spiritual suffering more fully. It is here that the physician serves as one of the key members of the interdisciplinary team.

The role of the medical director varies greatly depending on the degree and scope to which physicians and other interdisciplinary team members collaborate (Tables 2-2, 2-3, and 2-4). The primary role of the medical director is

---

TABLE 2-2 **Factors Affecting the Role of the Medical Director**

Philosophy of the Board of Directors and management

Perceived value of physician involvement

Budgetary considerations

Availability of other physicians with skills, interest, and time to devote to the team

The comfort level of the interdisciplinary team members in working with physicians

---

TABLE 2-3 **Qualifications of a Hospice Medical Director**

Current license in the state of practice

Knowledge and diagnostic skills in a primary care medical discipline

Additional training in oncology, pharmacology, and palliative medicine

Understanding of family counseling and psychological responses to grief and loss

Experience in working with terminally ill patients

Knowledge of local medical community

Ability to communicate effectively with medical peers

Willingness to make home visits

Ability to be supportive and empathize with patients, families, and staff

Ability to work diplomatically with a wide range of personalities and situations

Ability to work within and contribute to an interdisciplinary team

Ability to cope with stress and ambiguity

TABLE 2-4   Responsibilities of a Hospice Medical Director

Medical consultation

Education

Community and professional liaison

Program development

Support and guidance

---

to provide guidance, support, and medical direction in developing interdisciplinary care plans and the ongoing care of patients. The medical director should be available to nurses for collaboration on patient-related problems 24 hours a day. Depending on the culture of the community, the medical director may consult informally with community physicians on occasional patient palliative care needs, or may become more formally involved with the direct care of many terminally ill patients.

When an in-patient unit is a part of the program, direct patient care and supervision will take on an even larger portion of a physician's responsibilities. The attending physician or the medical director will follow the patient in the unit. Guidance on clinical issues goes well beyond symptom-relief issues, often delving deeply into ethical issues and fundamental decisions on pathways of treatment. The medical director may assist in formulating and presenting educational programs to the general and professional communities. This person may also participate in hospice workshops and in-services for staff and volunteers or serve as a professional and community liaison.

As hospice and palliative care is integrated more and more into mainstream medicine, the hospice physician plays a paramount role in promoting and facilitating healthy dialogue between palliative care teams and the physician community at large. The medical director is in a key position to represent hospice services to the medical community, often through one-to-one dialogue. Persons on either side of the treat-to-cure and treat-for-comfort spectrum of care often need tactful and skillful assistance in understanding each other's point of view and how it translates best into appropriate patient care. The literature is increasingly calling for a tighter integration of palliative medicine into the medical system and cancer centers. In fact, the World Health Organization suggests that many aspects of palliative care may be applied in conjunction with anticancer treatment earlier in the course of the illness.[2]

The medical director must be a good liaison with the general community to help dispel the potential negative connotations of hospice. The medical director also plays a role in program development by working with the managing leadership of a hospice program in the development of policies and procedures involving all the clinical aspects of the program. Many of the policies are required by certifying bodies or agencies and require ongoing physician attention. The Medicare hospice certification process is one example. Important aspects of a medical director's duties are utilization review, quality assurance activities, and involvement in clinical research. The medical director can also be an important source of support to the members of the interdisciplinary team and to patients and their families. In collaboration with the hospice team, he or she may provide reassurance that what is being done is right for that patient. The qualifications of the medical director are listed in Table 2-3; the responsibilities are listed in Table 2-4.

Hospice Team Physician

One or more team physicians possessing special interest and experience in palliative medicine may be available to an interdisciplinary team and attending physician. They can assist the medical director with clinical issues or administrative duties. Some large hospice programs employ physicians specifically for this role.

Attending Physician

The patient's primary physician remains an integral part of the patient's care team and is designated as the patient's attending physician.[3] The physician can bring information regarding the patient's medical history and its effect on the patient's life to the team. He or she may also be a stable and trusted resource to the patient and family, a relationship that often develops only over time. The attending physician collaborates primarily with the patient's hospice nurse and may also interact with the hospice team physician or medical director on complex symptom management or ethics and philosophy of care issues.

Registered Nurse

Many of the qualities that attract people to nursing are also the qualities so finely suited to the practice of hospice nursing. Nursing practice has always brought together multiple components of health care delivery in its approach to patient care: clinical issues, nurturing spiritual concerns, teaching, and patient advocacy. All of these elements are a part of the continuum of nursing practice. Hospice offers nurses the opportunity and the responsibility to engage in the many issues facing patients and their families. These elements become particularly important when advanced diseases alter lifestyle and self-image. Here the full spectrum of nursing practice comes into play by going beyond physical assessment and delivery of prescribed treatment to include the psychological aspects of disease and the impact that such stressors impart on overall function.[4]

Hospice nursing requires special knowledge, training, and skills. Dobratz describes four categories that define and describe the hospice nurse (Table 2-5).[5]

In developing the interdisciplinary plan of care, the nurse assists the patient and family members to identify their needs. The plan of care should assist a

TABLE 2-5   Attributes of a Hospice Nurse

Capacity to manage physical, psychological, social, and spiritual problems of dying patients and their families

Ability to coordinate the extended and expanded components of hospice services

Acquisition of counseling, managing, instructing, caring, and communicating skills/knowledge

Ability to balance the nurse's self-care needs with the complexities and intensities of repeated encounters with death

Source: Source: Dobratz, M. C. "Hospice Nursing: Present Perspectives and Future Directives." *Cancer Nursing,* 13(2):116–122, 1990.

patient and family with optimum adaptation to illness as well as promotion of comfort and independence. The hospice nurse is a principal figure in assessing coping mechanisms that address the patient's need for information concerning his or her disease and symptoms. He or she helps insure an open and honest dialogue while helping the family retain as much control as they desire within the plan of care.[6]

Physical symptoms must be accurately assessed and interventions must be initiated quickly and proceed in a logical sequence. The nurse must have the knowledge and skill to modify the plan of care as the disease progresses. The experienced hospice nurse can communicate the needs of the patient and family to the members of the interdisciplinary team. In hospice, nurses gain experience essential to maximizing their ability to provide holistic care.

In 1990, the Hospice Nurses Association (HNA), with the support of other hospice nursing organizations across the country, including the Academy of Hospice Nurses, began working on a certification process for hospice nurses in the United States.[7,8] An examination was developed by the National Board for Certification of Hospice Nurses (NBCHN) and was offered for the first time in March 1994. Successfully passing the examination were 482 hospice nurses, who earned the credentials CRNH (Certified Registered Nurse Hospice).

Primary Care Nurse

Most hospices use registered nurses as the primary care nurse for a specific number of patients. They are responsible for the nursing care of those patients and supervising the home health aides working with the patient. These nurses may have several roles, including assessment, on-call, and administrative duties.

Assessment Nurse

Some of the larger hospice programs use registered nurses specifically to make the first home visit to admit the patient into the hospice program. The goal of the visit is to begin to develop a holistic picture of the patient and family and begin the interdisciplinary plan of care. This visit may include a description of the program and a discussion of the expectations of the patient and family. The assessment nurse should discuss hospice philosophy and come to an agreement concerning the expectations of the family about what the hospice program can provide. The assessment nurse may also complete a medical history, physical examination, and brief psychosocial assessment. Sometimes the social worker may make a joint visit with the assessment nurse.

On-Call Nurse

The on-call nurse responds to the needs of hospice patients and their families either by telephone or by home visits during off hours (Table 2-6). This role meets the requirement for 24-hour availability of nursing services outlined in the Medicare hospice regulations.[1]

The structure of the on-call system is defined by the hospice program. The on-call nurse provides assistance consistent with the plan of care. They visit the patient in cases of emergency or death and are available for any other contingencies. In some programs the primary care nurses rotate through the on-call position. In others, the on-call position is separate, and one or more nurses are used for this role. Large hospices often employ some nurses to triage telephone calls and other nurses to make home visits, in which case, home health aides and social workers may also make home visits, as decided by the triage nurse. Nurses may also work in the referral office or hold positions in management, human resources, public relations, or education.

Social Worker

The philosophy of social work encompasses the values and principles embodied in hospice. Social workers have long been involved with organizing and

---

TABLE 2-6 Qualifications of a Hospice Nurse

Current licensure in the state of practice

Minimum of one year of clinical practice in nursing. Oncology, psychiatry, and home care experience are preferred

Knowledge of pathophysiology and disease progression

Understanding of pain and symptom management

Excellent assessment communication skills

Ability to work within and contribute to an interdisciplinary team

Ability to assist the patient and family in coping with emotional stress

Understanding of and aptitude for organization and communication with patient, family, and team members

TABLE 2-7   Qualifications of a Social Worker

Masters degree in Social Work (MSW) or a Masters of Science/Arts in Marriage and Family Counseling (recommendation of NHO)

At least one to three years of supervised experience in the health care field

Ability to work within and contribute to an interdisciplinary team

Understanding of and compassion toward patients and families

Knowledge of community resources available to patients and their families

---

leading interdisciplinary teams, and will often be the team leader. The social worker identifies family needs and community systems and makes the referrals to appropriate community resources that may not be offered by the hospice organization (for example, transportation, financial assistance, and assistance with locating and negotiating funeral details). The social worker may also counsel the patient and family on financial issues, advance directives, or psychosocial issues. They may also provide support and direction to team members faced with interfamily or interteam conflict. The social worker is expected to prepare a comprehensive psychosocial assessment and organize a strategy to approach the problems that may include appropriateness of caring for the patient at home. The qualifications vary depending on licensure and certification to a particular state, most requiring a master's degree in social work (Table 2-7).

Counselor

The Medicare hospice regulations require a counselor to be a member of the interdisciplinary team.[1] Usually this role is occupied by a chaplain or other spiritual counselor. However, social workers, nurses, and physicians may also counsel patients and family members. In some hospices, one of these people might have special qualifications in bereavement counseling.

Ancillary Team Members

Chaplain

The chaplain may be the spiritual advisor for patients, families, and the interdisciplinary team (Table 2-8). This person must be a skilled listener and meet patients where they are in their own spiritual belief system. The chaplain should be able to elicit and respond to questions of meaning, guilt, disappointment, loss, the mystery of life, and fears about the future. They must be concerned with the fundamental emotional and activating principles of a person. These principles may include the patient's deepest relationships with themselves, others, and perhaps a higher being. A chaplain may also assist the interdisciplinary team to deal with issues of meaning as they care for patients and

TABLE 2-8	Qualifications of a Chaplain

Graduate of accredited seminary or school of theology, or appropriate certification in clinical pastoral education

Mature in own belief system; ability to be open and flexible, ecumenical but not evangelistic in ministry

Experience working with patients and families facing life-threatening illness

Knowledge of spiritual effects of terminal illness, grief, and loss

Ability to respond compassionately and sensitively to patient and family members

Ability to work within and contribute to an interdisciplinary team

their families. Education encompassing spiritual issues is part of the hospice chaplainry. As a nonmedical person, a chaplain brings an important community/consumer perspective to the interdisciplinary team.[9]

Bereavement Counselor

Most hospice programs have a health care professional as a bereavement counselor (Table 2-9). This person may be a nurse, counselor, or social worker. The Medicare hospice regulations require an organized bereavement program under the supervision of qualified personnel.[1] Bereavement services are provided up to one year after the death of the patient.

Bereavement is a process that occurs following the death of a person with whom one has shared a significant relationship. Grief is the emotional response to bereavement, and mourning is the physical statement of grief. A psychosocial transition follows bereavement in which a person's place in their world is suddenly altered. During this transition period a bereavement counselor is of great value in assisting the family members through their phases of grief.[9] It is essential to recognize individuals and families at risk for complicated bereavement, such as unresolved emotional entanglements.

Bereavement outcomes in the first few months after a death must encompass a continuum of experiences, which include physical, emotional, social,

TABLE 2-9	Functions of a Bereavement Counselor

Assist team members in identifying family members at risk for complicated bereavement by developing assessment tools, interventions, and referral patterns

Assist the interdisciplinary team members with bereavement issues

Develop and facilitate bereavement support groups

Coordinate and facilitate memorial services for bereaved families

Establish training goals for interdisciplinary team members concerning grief issues

Work within and contribute to an interdisciplinary team

and spiritual components.[10] The counselor will often encourage bereaved family members to attend bereavement support groups in which statements of grief and loss can be safely expressed and in which support and acknowledgement may be received. Bereavement groups are not designed to function as therapy groups; discussion of deep inner issues is not encouraged. If possible, it is best to run groups that bring together people with similar experiences, for example, parents who have lost a child. Many hospices use volunteer bereavement counselors to lead the group. Although this practice has certainly proven helpful, licensed staff should consistently monitor the group to provide guidance and support.

Memorial services are often arranged as quarterly or annual events. Hospice staff and bereaved families join together to commemorate the dead. Symbolic ritual can often assist the process of closure.

Educational and training programs are available to bereavement counselors, specifically, certification in death education is offered through the Association for Death Education and Counseling (ADEC).

Home Health Aide/Homemaker

A survey conducted by the Foundation for Hospice and Home Care (1986) found twelve different commonly used names in the United States for describing paraprofessionals who provide health and supportive services.[11] The most appropriate names to describe these persons in hospice are homemaker or home health aide (Table 2-10). Home health aides play a vital role in the care of the dying patient because they are the team members who are in the patient's home most frequently and who usually experience the home situation most intensely. Creating an intensive selection, orientation, support, and evaluation process for home health aides assists in their retention and success.[12] During the selection process, it is necessary to consider candidates with home health aide experience, preferably hospice home care. A home health aide may have personal experience caring for a dying patient or family member, which may give the candidate the ability to understand the hospice philosophy and approach to care.

The responsibilities of the home health aide include providing personal care to patients and respite to caregivers. They may assist the patient in administering their medications and preparing healthy meals. The home health aide does light housekeeping to provide a safe environment, and reports changes in the patient's status promptly to the primary nurse.

The home health aide must attend interdisciplinary team meetings to communicate regularly with all team members. The orientation, support, and evaluation processes are vital to the success of the home health aide.[13] Orientation and support begin on the first day. Expectations should be clearly outlined in the job description and discussed in the context of hospice philosophy and care. The importance of communication and team interaction should be emphasized. Discussion should include the roles of all team members, the hos-

TABLE 2-10 **Job Description: Home Health Aide/Homemaker**

Qualifications

Empathetic communication skills

Flexibility

Respect for the patient's privacy and property

A positive attitude

Dependable techniques in personal hygiene

Good observation skills

Understanding of team approach

High school diploma or equivalent

One year homemaker or hospice experience

Ability to work within and contribute to an interdisciplinary team

Reliability

Responsibilities

Observe, report, and document patient status and care promptly

Maintain clean, safe environment

Read and record temperature, pulse, and respiration

Perform safe transfer techniques

Perform normal range of motion and positioning

Assist in healthy meal preparation

Assist patients to self-administer medications

Perform appropriate and safe techniques in personal hygiene and grooming

Light housekeeping

pice mission statement, history, funding, and organizational culture in an effort to assist new employees in understanding their roles within the organization. The home health aide must also understand what occurs during the initial referral, case opening, initiation of the interdisciplinary plan of care, interdisciplinary team meetings, role of each team member in the home, and bereavement process. With this knowledge, the home health aide can comprehend the hospice concept and their own role in the program.

Proficiency of skills is often evaluated during the orientation process. The supervisor demonstrates a specific skill and then observes a return demonstration by the aide (Table 2-11). A specific skill may need to be reviewed before proficiency can be documented. The skills test should be repeated at least every twelve months. Medicare hospice regulations require the primary nurse to supervise the home health aide. The home health aide's first home visit alone is sometimes stressful, but appropriate information, support, and guidance can help ease the stress.

TABLE 2-11 **Home Health Aide Skills**

Complete bed, bath, and linen change

Bowel and bladder care (for example, digital rectal examination to check for fecal impaction, ostomy care, Foley catheter care)

Skin care (for example, simple dressings, decubitus ulcer care)

Back rub

Active and passive range of motion

Transfer techniques

Personal grooming (for example, shaving, shampooing, oral hygiene)

Safety measures (for example, oxygen safety, safety during seizures, environmental safety)

Before the first visit, the primary nurse should prepare a written plan of care for the home health aide and must discuss the patient's physical needs and home situation with all the team members involved in the case. Entering a difficult situation in the home without prior knowledge of it can be overwhelming for the home health aide.

Home health aides provide intimate personal care to their patients. This service may be provided during a time when patients reveal their deepest feelings. During the orientation process, it is important to teach the home health aide basic communication skills, encourage open communication between team members, and assist the aide in meeting the patient's needs.

The role of the home health aide can be very challenging. A typical day may include a meeting in the office, followed by three to four home visits to assist in personal care. Some of the patients may be actively dying and need personal care as well as emotional support. The family may need support and guidance in providing comfort measures. The personal care for hospice patients is very involved, with most patients requiring total care. The home health aide may share a special bond with patients and their families because of the amount of time spent in their homes. Moreover, because the aide spends less time in the office and more time in the patient's home, other members of the team must be aware of their level of stress and provide support. The information that the home health aide shares with the team is integral to a comprehensive plan of care. As a member of the interdisciplinary team, the aide can participate in team conferences, mini-team conferences, and support groups. They receive informal support from other team members and give support when needed.

Pharmacist

The pharmacist is specially trained, holds a Bachelor of Science or Pharm. D. degree in pharmacy, and is registered with the state board of pharmacy or the boards in several states. Just as each patient comes to hospice with his or her own attending physician, the patient may also choose a pharmacist. If the patient is enrolled in one of the managed care options (for example, Medicare hospice benefit), the choice must be made from a list of pharmacies with which the hospice has contracts. It is important for one pharmacy to fill all of the patient's prescriptions so that polypharmacy can be monitored and minimized. The pharmacist also monitors the patient's medication profile for allergies and drug/drug and food/drug interactions. The pharmacist is a valuable resource for the nurse, physician, patient, and family.

Volunteer

Volunteers are vital members of the team. Briggs suggests that most hospice organizations rely heavily on volunteers to provide many hospice services.[14] Patients, families, and the interdisciplinary team have a variety of needs. People have many reasons for volunteering. It has been shown that the most important reasons people volunteer are to help others, to repay others for their own good fortune, and religious beliefs.

Many people become hospice volunteers because they had a good experience with hospice, or someone close to them died alone in pain. Hospice programs employ volunteer coordinators to facilitate volunteer recruitment, orientation, and assignments. The coordinator may represent the volunteers in the interdisciplinary team meeting, although volunteers are encouraged to attend meetings when their patients are present. The volunteer coordinator is a source of support and guidance for the volunteers.

Hospice volunteers share many characteristics. The first is empathy, putting oneself in another's place in order to understand them better. A second characteristic is being comfortable with dying patients and their families. Paradis and Usui, however, state that these characteristics, combined with minimal anxiety and caring, will not predict success in a volunteer. They suggest that a volunteer's success is predicted by traits such as comfortableness with death, motivation, involvement in other community activities, and availability.[15]

Volunteers care for individuals and their families in a variety of ways, including direct personal care through bed baths, toileting, shampoos, and exercise. Volunteers provide support by reassuring, consoling, listening, and assisting in life review. The volunteer may entertain the patient and family by sharing jokes, playing music, working together on hobbies, and reading. Spiritual support is also very important in the role of spiritual care volunteer. The volunteer may discuss spiritual issues, assist in prayer, and listen to fears of death and dying. Many volunteers do housekeeping, vacuuming, and laundry, and run errands. Volunteers provide respite to the caregivers.

Volunteers may also work in the hospice office. They can assist with filing and billing, answer the telephone, enter data into the computer, help with correspondence, and order and organize medical and office supplies. Volunteers may serve as fundraisers, board members, and consultants.[13]

Many hospice programs include volunteer training sessions in the orientation of all new hospice employees, paid staff, and volunteers. These sessions include presentations on the hospice philosophy and mission, the interdisciplinary team concept, and the roles of the team members. Pain and symptom management issues are presented in basic terms to assist the volunteer in understanding the disease process. Personal care may be provided by some volunteers and is therefore a part of the training program. Discussions regarding family dynamics, alcohol and substance abuse, and therapeutic communication provide the volunteer with the knowledge needed to identify situations that may potentially affect the safety of the patient. New hospice workers are presented with procedures for communicating their concerns to other team members.

Other Consultants

The list of possible consultants is endless. The Medicare hospice regulations mandate an ongoing program for the training of hospice employees. Staff and volunteers have many options for in-services and workshops, including pain and symptom management, team building, developing a quality assurance program, and cultural diversity. Hospices may hire consultants to develop and provide educational programs. Other consultants may include proposal writers, experts in computer program development, public relations consultants, and community leaders.

Expressive Therapists

Expressive therapies are also known as creative arts. They include music, art, drama, dance, poetry, and writing. These therapies focus on personal contact and the value of the individual as a creative person.[16] A patient may use the arts as a vehicle to discuss memories and associations that arise from the creative process. Life review may encompass places, friends, work experiences, and meaningful life events. The arts stimulate the senses. Music and the spoken word provide auditory stimulation. Paintings, photographs, or a vase full of flowers provides visual stimulation. Tactile stimulation may be found in petting a dog, receiving a back rub, or holding a person's hand. Fragrant flowers, seasonal greens, or familiar cooking smells may stimulate the olfactory sense. Patients may express themselves artistically through painting, sculpture, designing masks, jewelry, or collages.

Therapists in music, art, and recreation may be employed by the hospice agency. These therapists may offer a more comfortable, less threatening mode of statement than verbal communication.[17] The opportunities are as endless as the imagination.

The art therapist is specially trained. Some colleges and universities in the United States offer a Master of Arts degree in art therapy. The individual may become a registered art therapist (ATR) after 1000 hours of supervised clinical work. Currently, there is no third-party reimbursement for art therapy.

The Office Staff as Team Members

Hospice Managers

The executive director is responsible for the vision and direction of the hospice program. The management staff works together to develop goals and objectives for the program. They must define what is needed and who will be involved in the work. The managers involve their staff in the planning and implementation phases of the work. Staff involvement is integral to the success of any hospice program.

Office Staff

The members of the office staff play a vital role in the daily operations of the hospice program. The three most common roles are medical records clerk, clerical, and receptionist. To perform successfully, the office staff should meet the following minimum requirements: holding a high school diploma, knowledge of medical terms, word processing skills, experience in a medical office setting, and basic understanding of the hospice concept. These roles are vital because they provide continuity of record keeping and communication between the hospice staff, family, and patients. Finally, the staff is a resource for the information necessary to successfully carry out the mission of the hospice program.

The Team in Action

For those who care for patients in their homes, the only time the entire team can physically work together is at team conferences (Table 2-12). As one mechanism for assuring interdisciplinary care, Medicare hospice regulations require

---

TABLE 2-12   A Structure for a Hospice Team Conference

Bereavement Report	Current Patient Report	New Patients
Bereavement coordinator reports on family follow-up.	Patient care coordinator facilitates the team conference.	Patients who are new to the program since the last team conference are presented by the assessment nurse, patient care coordinator, or primary nurse.
Primary or on-call nurse reports on deaths that have occurred since the last team conference.	Primary nurse begins with patient demographics and asks team for new information.	
	Team members add their comments, including identification of additional problems and interventions. Team members may ask questions or give input.	

---

that a formal team conference be conducted to review each patient every two weeks.[1] For most programs, patient acuity and short-term patient stays make weekly team conferences a necessity.

Medicare also requires written evidence of care-planning at these team meetings. Meeting minutes are not sufficient to meet this written requirement. Each involved team member must document updates on a care plan summary form for each patient reviewed.

Aside from meeting regulatory requirements, the size of the program often dictates the formality, content, and length of team conferences. Some programs incorporate a strict format for patient review. Others allow an informal format, recognizing staff members' needs to tell their stories, support one another, and enjoy the social aspects of conferences. Team conferences can also serve as mini in-services to discuss issues such as pain and symptom management or spiritual distress.

When reviewing patients who require particularly complex problem solving and interventions, team conferences can model the best of interdisciplinary care. In addition, team conferences may be the ideal or only time that most hospice members can come together to hear a bereavement report. Often the most positive feedback from families comes after the patient death during bereavement follow-up visits or telephone calls. Staff may use this feedback as a mechanism to evaluate their patient care. By actually hearing in the bereavement period how supported family members felt, staff members may gain a different perspective in situations in which they felt they were ineffective.

Each program must develop its own structure and philosophy about team conference. The structure and purpose of the conferences then must be clarified for the staff. Because most interdisciplinary care occurs outside of the formal team conference, team members must be able to trust each other to provide appropriate assessment and timely intervention. When this does not happen, team members must confront these issues with each other, and when necessary, with supervisory staff. When conflicts are ignored, team process will be impaired.

Family Conferences

Hospice care commonly begins with a family conference that usually involves discussion of difficult emotional issues and decisions. The patient identifies the important friends and family members who will be involved in caretaking and decision making.

Because patients and family members commonly try to protect each other from emotionally painful information, a family conference is most helpful in facilitating communication between all persons involved in the care of the patient (Table 2-13). Initial contact with the patient and family together helps identify communication and coping styles, and current areas of conflict among

TABLE 2-13   Components of Family Conference

Clarification that both patient and family understand the terminal nature of the illness

Current concerns of the patient and each family member

Expectations of the patients and family members of the hospice program

Specific services the hospice can provide

Identifying the patient's and family members' goals for care and how the hospice can help to meet them

Expectations the hospice program has of the patient and family

family members. The conference is most helpful in beginning to break down communication barriers when they exist.

The initial conference should include written materials about the program's services, including specifics about the Medicare or other insurance benefits available to the patient. Generally, consent forms are also reviewed. Some programs use a primary caregiver consent form that defines this person's responsibilities in working with the hospice team in caring for the patient. Subsequent family conferences generally occur because there are problems in the care of the patient at home or because many family members are involved, requiring communication to be focused. These conferences must be carefully arranged so that all appropriate parties can attend.

To emphasize the concept of team care, more than one hospice team member should attend a family conference. Ideally this should include the patient's physician, primary hospice nurse, and social worker or hospice counselor. The focus of the conference often determines which specific team members should be present. When family conferences are necessary after the initial meeting, the topics can range from bathing to exhaustion of the caregivers. Family conferences are effective means of problem solving, redirecting care, and clarifying issues concerning barriers to patient care.

Office Space and Equipment

The size and general scope of the program determine the space needs. Some programs may develop a community bereavement or educational focus; others may decide to provide their own durable medical equipment (DME), effectively becoming a DME vendor. The small volunteer program common in the early days of hospice is rare. Most current programs are competitive and run with the efficiency common in the world of business.

Computerized data management is a necessity for all but the very smallest of programs. Programs should plan for the computerization of clinical records because this technology is fast becoming available; laptop computers and cellular phones are optional but strongly recommended for home-care staff.

Independent programs must be able to store medical records and some medical supplies. Nursing bags, stocked according to regulations, should be provided. An adequately sized conference room and the usual office paraphernalia are necessities. Finally, private space should be provided for counseling patients and families and other work that requires a closed door.

Summary

Hospice care has been designed to provide holistic care by an interdisciplinary health care team that includes lay volunteers and professional caregivers. The patient, family members, and patient's attending physician are also part of this team. Hospice staff and volunteers must balance the ability to work independently with the responsibility of being part of the team. In addition to the office space and supplies required by most home care agencies, adequate conference room space for team meetings and private counseling space are necessary for hospice care. New technology such as computerized medical records and cellular phones can further enhance effective hospice work in the community. Hospice programs must screen, select, and prepare staff for the emotional and technical aspects of care. Volunteers also require careful screening and training for the rewarding and intensely emotional work of caring for the dying and their families. Interdependence and collaboration are the cornerstones to a strong interdisciplinary team. As the team works together by learning from one another and supporting and encouraging each other, a sense of competence and self-confidence will develop to provide a creative team and individual growth.[18]

References

1. *Medicare: Hospice Manual.* U.S. Department of Health and Human Services, U.S. Department of Commerce National Technical Information Service. Washington, D.C., 2000.
2. World Health Organization. *Cancer Pain Relief and Palliative Care.* Geneva, Switzerland: World Health Organization, 1990.
3. Eng, M. A. "The Hospice Interdisciplinary Team: A Synergistic Approach to the Care of Dying Patients and Their Families." *Holistic Nursing Practice,* 7(6):49–56, 1993.
4. Johanson, C. A. *Physician's Handbook of Symptom Relief in Terminal Care.* Santa Rosa, Calif.: Sonoma County Academic Foundation for Excellence in Medicine, 1988.
5. Dobratz, M. C. "Hospice Nursing: Present Perspectives and Future Directives." *Cancer Nursing,* 13(2):116–122, 1990.
6. Nichols, G., Rice, R. The Hospice and Palliative Care Patient. In *Home Care Nursing Practice: Concepts and Application,* Rice, R., ed., Chapter 24, pp. 434–35. St. Louis, Mo.: Mosby, Inc., 2001.
7. Knight, C. F., and Knight, P. F. "Developing a Certificate Course for Hospice Nurses: A Delphi Survey of Subject Areas." *Hospice Journal,* 8(3):43–57, 1992.
8. Amenta, M. "Certification for Hospice Nurses? Assessment of Need." *Hospice Journal,* 8(3):73–87, 1992.

9. Dunlop, R. J., and Hockley, J. M. *Terminal Care Support Teams.* Oxford, England: Oxford University Press, 1990.
10. Billings, J. A. *Outpatient Management of Advanced Cancer.* Philadelphia: Lippincott Co., 1985.
11. Foundation for Hospice and Homemaker and National Association for Home Care. "Training and Certification of Homemaker-Home Health Aides." *Caring,* 9 (4):31–38, 1990.
12. Tomczyk, M. "Preparing Homemaker-Home Health Aides to Care for Hospice Clients." *Caring,* 9(11):18–21, 1990.
13. Stephany, T. "Hospice Home Health Aides." *Home Healthcare Nurse,* 2:71, 1993.
14. Briggs, J. "Volunteer Qualities: A Survey of Hospice Volunteers." *Oncology Nursing Forum,* 14(1):27–31, 1987.
15. Paradis, L., and Usui, W. "Hospice Volunteers: The Impact of Personality Characteristics on Retention and Job Performance." *Hospice Journal,* 3(1):3–30, 1987.
16. Aldridge, D. "Hope, Meaning and the Creative Art Therapies in the Treatment of AIDS." *The Arts in Psychotherapy,* 20:285–297, 1993.
17. Krug, C. *Art Therapy with the Terminally Ill in a Hospice Setting.* Pepper Pike, Ohio: Ursuline College, 1993.
18. Dunlop, R. J., and Hockley, J. M. *Terminal Care Support Teams.* Oxford, England: Oxford University Press, 1990.

For Further Reading

Bunn, E. "Volunteers as the Backbone . . ." *Caring,* 4(2):19–20, 1985

Cassell, E. J. "The Nature of Suffering and the Goals of Medicine." *New England Journal of Medicine,* 306:639–645, 1982.

Levy, M. H. "Integration of Pain Management into Comprehensive Cancer Care." *Cancer,* 63:2328–2335, 1989.

MacDonald, N. "Oncology and Palliative Care: The Case for Co-ordination." *Cancer Treatment Reviews,* 19(Supplement A):29–41, 1993.

Mor, V., Greer, D. S., and Kastembaum. R., eds. *The Hospice Experiment.* Baltimore: Johns Hopkins University Press, 1988.

Orser, A. M. "The Creative Arts in the Hospice Setting." *Thanotas,* 9:9–15, Fall 1991.

Porchet-Munro, S. "Music-Therapy." In *Oxford Textbook of Palliative Medicine.* D. Doyle, C. W. C. Hanks, and N. MacDonald, eds. Oxford, England: Oxford University Press, 1993.

Ryan, K. *Personal Communication.* Hospice of the Western Reserve, Cleveland, Ohio, 1993.

Stephany, T., "Identifying Roles of Hospice Volunteers." *Home Healthcare Nurse,* 7(3):51–52, 1989.

Eligibility and Reimbursement for Hospice and Palliative Care

3

Constance M. Dahlin

In the United States for the year 2000, approximately 75% of deaths occurred in some sort of medical facility, either a hospital or a nursing facility. Twenty-five percent of patients chose to die at home. Just 57% of those patients who died at home had cancer; the other 43% had noncancer diagnoses.[1] These figures are important in weaving the tapestry of end-of-life care. First, it is clear that end-of-life care takes place in a variety of settings outside the home. Second, home-care deaths now account for a higher percentage of noncancer deaths. Enhancing the care that can take place in these settings requires knowledge about funding and reimbursement. This chapter will review reimbursement sources for both hospice and palliative care.

In 2001, the National Hospice and Palliative Care Organization (NHPCO) reported that there are approximately 3100 hospice programs. Of these programs, 42% are freestanding entities, 42% are affiliated with hospitals or hospital systems, and 22% are affiliated with home health agencies. Further, 91% of hospice programs are Medicare-certified programs.[1] Research on the exact number of palliative care programs is unavailable because there is no clearinghouse for the collection of these data. However, the Center to Advance Palliative Care (CAPC) has collected data on palliative care programs or people interested in forming some sort of palliative program. As of December 26, 2001, there were some 310 hospitals that were either interested in starting some sort of hospital-based initiative or had an existing palliative care program. There were also 26 home health/hospice programs and 48 Veteran's Administration systems forming some sort of end-of-life care programs.[2]

Insurance

When the Health Care Financing Administration (HCFA) discontinued the required cost report from hospices in 1992, a centralized statistical and financial database was lost. Therefore, data on cost savings and cost expenditures concerning direct insurance and reimbursement is not available.[3,4] Nonetheless, reimbursement for hospice is more clearly delineated than is reimbursement for palliative care (Table 3-1). Currently, hospices are in large part defined by Medicare guidelines, whereas palliative care programs are more nebulous and encompass a broader scope in philosophy of care. In addition to Medicare, other types of insurance cover health costs, including Medicaid, commercial insurance products, and Veteran's Administration benefits.

Medicare and Veteran's Administration benefits have fairly consistent rules on a national level. HCFA, now known as the Center for Medicare and Medicaid Services (CMS), is an agent for the federal government that defines and interprets Medicare law. It does not manage billing; rather, CMS awards contracts to agencies to receive Medicare benefits. However, reimbursement rates vary by state, location (urban vs. rural), and institution. Medicare is handled by contracts on a state and regional basis.[5]

Medicare Part A benefits are managed by regional intermediaries from nine different regions of the country. Medicare Part B benefits are managed by local carriers that are determined at an individual state level. Currently, there are approximately 20 carriers managing the Medicare benefits of the 50 states and the American territories.[5]

Medicaid benefits vary substantially from state to state. Again, the federal government contracts with the states to administer Medicaid benefits. Commercial products include health maintenance organizations (HMOs), preferred provider organizations (PPOs), and indemnity plans. Uninsured payers include both people who choose to self-pay and those not covered by insurance due to lack of qualifying employment status or low income.[4,5]

Eligibility for Hospice

Eligibility for hospice and thus reimbursement is defined by the Medicare guidelines. The Hospice Medicare Benefit is under Part A. Home Health Guidelines, which state that patients must be homebound and have specific skilled needs that differ from hospice eligibility criteria, as noted in Table 3-2.

TABLE 3-1   Reimbursement Sources
Medicare—Part A for hospice and Parts A and B for palliative care
Medicaid
Commercial products—HMOs, PPOs
VA benefits
Uninsured—private pay[3,5]

TABLE 3-2 **Hospice Admission Criteria**

1. The individual is certified as being terminal, which is having a life expectancy of six months or less if the illness runs its course. This certification is given from both the individual's attending physician and the hospice medical director.
2. The individual wants hospice care.
3. The individual has a physician willing to provide medical care and consultation.[3,4,6]

Eligibility for Palliative Care

Eligibility for palliative care differs from hospice care in that there are no federal guidelines. Rather, palliative care programs have many slightly differing interpretations. Some programs may use the Medicare definition of hospice as a guideline; others may not. The following is a commonly accepted definition of palliative care as it differs from hospice care developed by the Last Acts Task Force:

> Palliative Care refers to the comprehensive management of the physical, psychological, social, spiritual, and existential needs of patients. It is especially suited to the care of people with incurable, progressive illnesses.[7]

Thus, with palliative care, there is usually a diagnosis of a life-limiting illness with no specific prognosis. In most palliative care programs there is a holistic perspective of the patient. However, the palliative care team can be consulted while curative options are pursued to assist with pain and symptom management and offer support. As a patient becomes more debilitated, the palliative care team can then provide care more focused on the end stage treatment of the disease, including the terminal phase.

Hospice Reimbursement

Medicare

The Medicare Hospice Benefit was established in 1983 for terminally ill patients. HCFA created regulations and eligibility requirements. This reimbursement, which is under Part A, covers intermittent nursing, home health aide, social work, chaplain, and occupational/physical therapy as well as medications and durable medical equipment related to the terminal illness. To receive Medicare reimbursement, a hospice must provide care under the U.S. Department of Health and Human Services guidelines. That is, the hospice agrees to meet the conditions of participation (Table 3-3).

After a hospice is certified, Medicare conducts surveys to monitor that the hospice is indeed complying with government regulations. Conditions not related to the terminal illness can still be treated under Medicare Part A.[3,5,8]

TABLE 3-3   Conditions of Participation

1. Interdisciplinary with core services including medical care, nursing, home health aides, and counseling. Other services include pastoral care and volunteer services.
2. Coverage of medicines and biologicals related to care of terminal illness.
3. Radiology and radiation therapy related to care of terminal illness.
4. Emergency services.
5. Ambulance and transport services.
6. Bereavement support for 13 months after death.[8]

For example, a patient with lung cancer who has kidney failure can continue to receive treatment for the kidney. The lung cancer care would be covered under the Medicare Hospice Benefit and the kidney care would be covered under Medicare A.

Because Medicare is usually for care of the elderly, and the population of Americans over 64 is growing exponentially, the Hospice Benefit has become the major source of reimbursement for hospice care. Payment rates for Medicare increased as of April 1, 2001 (Table 3-4).

Medicaid

In 1986, the Consolidated Omnibus Budget Reconciliation Act gave states the option to add hospice services to their Medicaid programs. Because Medicaid is a means-tested entitlement program jointly administered and funded by state and federal governments, there are dramatic differences in eligibility, benefits, and payments.[3,4,6] The challenge is understanding each state's Medicaid hospice benefit. Most states with a Medicaid hospice benefit use the Medicare hospice eligibility requirements, as well as the stipulation that the hospice must comply with the Medicare Conditions of Participation requiring core services.[3,4,8] Medicaid also has the four types of hospice care listed earlier in Table 3-4. States without Medicaid hospice benefit include Connecticut, Nebraska, New Hampshire, Oklahoma, and South Dakota.[1,10]

Because Medicaid hospice care can be an aid to low income persons, some Medicaid programs require the person to give up other Medicaid services.

TABLE 3-4   Hospice Levels of Care and Their Medicare Rates

Routine home care—Per diem rate of $110

Continuous care—Must be greater than 8 hrs/day with 51% RN time—$644 for 24 hours divided by an hourly rate for number of hours above 8

Respite care—Per diem of $120

General inpatient care—Per diem of $491[9]

This can be problematic to pediatric patients or HIV/AIDS patients who may need continuous nursing or high levels of home health aide time.[10]

Commercial Insurance

Commercial insurance varies in its coverage in regards to hospice. Some insurances have hospice benefits that mirror the Medicare benefit. Others with a hospice benefit may only have home hospice and no inpatient benefits. Some insurances have benefits that are more home health focused without the holistic function. Some have no hospice benefits at all. It is important for the patient to ascertain the full extent of benefits from case managers because they are the ones who allocate services.

Veteran's Administration Benefits

Veteran's Administration (VA) programs are administered on a national budget. VA programs include VA hospitals and integrated systems. Often, a VA hospital works within an integrated system. The goal is to organize care across the continuum. Because services are prepaid, hospices must be careful about what is seen as double billing. Services were formerly delivered under CHAMPUS, now known as TRICARE. This is a new program initiated by the Department of Defense.[3,5] Care is coordinated by VA case managers to serve patients across the continuum of care with contracted agencies.

Palliative Care Reimbursement

Medicare

Palliative care, like hospice services, can be delivered in a multiplicity of sites, including in a hospital, an outpatient clinic, a home, a rehabilitation setting, or a nursing home. Because it may be administered directly by inpatient health care providers or in a home setting, Medicare Parts A and B may both be utilized.

Under home health benefits, Part A is utilized. However, care must be skilled and usually encompasses pain and symptom management or monitoring of current, active treatments. Specifically, a patient must be homebound, need intermittent skilled nursing, physical therapy, speech language pathology, be under the care of a physician, and receive services from a Medicare certified home health agency. Home health agencies were paid in the past either by actual costs, median costs, or a complex equation based on the agency's individual Medicare population. However the 2000 guidelines have heralded a new program. Now home health agencies are paid by prospective payment, a diagnosis related group (DRG) for home care.[10]

Likewise, Medicare skilled nursing facilities (SNF) also began a prospective payment based on facility rates. This is to assure that the Medicare SNF benefit is only for brief post-acute care to shorten hospital length of stay.

In the hospital, physicians and advanced practice nurses utilize Part B for billing. See the sections on physician and advanced practice nurse billing later in this chapter for more specifics.

Medicaid

Medicaid does not specifically recognize palliative care. However, the care for the management of the disease would be included in hospital care and home health care. The issue usually is medications, because some state Medicaid benefits may not cover the wide variety of medications and technology for pain and symptom control. In addition, psychological support may need to be provided under state mental health benefits.

Commercial Insurance

Commercial insurance may not cover "palliative services" per se. However, creativity may be used to get reimbursement under other benefits such as home care, hospice, and site-specific benefits. Usually, it is most beneficial to request a designated case manager to discuss the overall picture of care, so that goals can be specified and care delivered appropriately to the patient's needs.

Physician Services Reimbursement

Medicare

Generally, physicians use the same technique for care whether the patient is in hospice or palliative care. However, there are specifics in how the billing must be done.

Hospice   Physician services under hospice care are reimbursed at 100% of the usual and customary fee schedule for care related to the terminal illness.[11,12] However, billing is complicated depending on the employment status of the physician. If the attending physician designated by the patient is neither the hospice medical director nor an employee of the hospice, the physician continues to bill under Medicare B. The attending physician or consultant fees do not affect the daily rate paid to the hospice. However, if both the attending physician and the hospice physician are employed by the hospice, the hospice physician or attending physician does not submit bills directly to Medicare. Rather, they submit them to the hospice agency for processing and the agency reimburses the physician. Care unrelated to the terminal illness indicated on the certificate of terminal illness is reimbursed by standard Medicare mechanisms.[10,11,12]

Medical services provided by either a medical director or a hospice-employed physician can be reimbursed in two ways. The first is "General

Supervisory Services," which is oversight by way of team meeting, supervising care and services, and review of care plans. This care is potentially partially reimbursed from the hospice daily rate, paid to the medical director at a negotiated amount or through an annual salary. The second, "Direct Patient Care," is billed under Medicare A under the hospice benefit. The hospice is reimbursed separately for the physician's services, which in turn may also be negotiated as part of the medical director's salary.[10,11,12]

Procedures, laboratory tests, and medications related to the terminal illness are covered under the Hospice Medicare Benefit. Therefore, care should be collaborative between the attending physician and the hospice. Any procedures, tests, and medications should be coordinated and planned within the goals of comfort care. These charges must be submitted to the hospice, which then will reimburse the vendor.[10,11,12]

Palliative Care   Palliative care reimbursement is based on both the *International Classification of Diseases*, 9th edition (ICD-9)™ diagnosis codes and the procedure/service codes from the Current Procedural Terminology (CPT)™ codes, established by the American Medical Association. In palliative care, the most frequently utilized procedure/service code is the evaluation and management (EM) codes. They are therefore billing under a procedure or service code and a diagnosis code.[11,12] HCFA, now known as CMS, promotes extensive documentation to support EM codes. Particularly in palliative care, the provision of time is important in billing, because the care demands extensive communication. Therefore, when a visit is composed of more than 50% counseling, time may be the factor that determines which evaluation and management code to use.[11]

Medicaid

Coding for Medicaid patients is similar to the federal guidelines. However, each state may vary in specifics. It is important for the practitioner to understand and become familiar with the guidelines within his or her specific state. Again, hospice may be better recognized in billing than palliative care.

Commercial Insurance

Although some commercial insurance products recognize terminal care, many do not. They may have some hospice coverage, often modeled after the Medicare Benefit. However, physician's services are separate and billed according to the previously established system. Palliative care, however, is not commonly recognized. Some companies are looking into the broader umbrella of end-of-life care to explore expanded hospice and palliative care coverage.

Advanced Practice Nurse (APN) Services Reimbursement

In 1989, nurse practitioners (NPs) were granted limited reimbursement potential. However, billing was only possible for nurse practitioners under the direct supervision of a physician and was restricted by rural location and outpatient practice site. The only possibility to bill in this setting was known as "incident to" billing, which means the NP provided care under a physician's direct supervision and had to have notes co-signed.[5] This is still possible; however, now both Clinical Nurse Specialists (CNSs) and nurse practitioners can practice and bill in an independent practice. The Balanced Budget Act (BBA) of 1997 stated that APNs were eligible to practice under their own scope of practice and bill independently.[13]

> As long as the services the nonphysician practitioners furnish are medically reasonable and necessary, and fall within the scope of service that they are licensed to perform, the Medicare program covers these.[14]

Thus, with Medicare reform and some progressive state nurse practice acts, there are more possibilities for reimbursement for both CNS and NP. The challenge is understanding the guidelines, interpreting how they relate to a particular setting, and then implementing a reimbursement process.

The BBA of 1997 allows for reimbursement of both the CNS and NP subject to certain criteria (Table 3-5). It clarifies the prerequisites for being able to bill. First, beginning in 2003, the APN must have a master's degree. Prior to this year, an APN without a master's degree, but who met all the other requirements, was certified. Second, the APN must practice in a state that recognizes the advanced practice role and allows autonomous practice. The intent of the BBA of 1997 was to extend the scope of the APN as defined by a given state's nurse practice act and its rules and regulations.[16] The APN should investigate his or her state advanced practice act to see if it allows autonomous practice, or if he or she must practice under a physician. Third, a nationally credible certifying body must certify the nurse. Finally, the APN must have a collaborating physician, as defined by Medicare.

Collaboration with a physician has always been an area of debate among APNs. However, HCFA defined collaboration in the following manner, and even made provision for nurses who lived in states where collaboration was undefined in the APN guidelines:

> The process in which the nurse practitioner works with one or more physicians to deliver health care services within the scope of the practitioner's knowledge with medical direction and suitable supervision as

TABLE 3-5   Eligibility Criteria for Reimbursement

Master's degree after 2003; grandmothered in before that

APN and autonomous practice recognized by state nursing practice act

Certified by national body in area of specialty

Work in collaboration with MD[5,14,15]

provided for in the jointly developed guidelines and or other mechanism as provided by the law of the state in which services are delivered.

The collaborating physician does not have to be in attendance with the APN when the services are furnished or to construct an independent evaluation of each patient who is seen.

In the absence of state law governing collaboration, it is a process in which the APN has an association with one or more physicians to deliver health services. This can be evidenced by APNs documenting their scope of practice and indicating they have a relationship with physicians to deal outside that scope.[14,15]

To actually bill, APNs must meet these eligibility requirements as well as some other criteria, including being an RN in the state where they are providing the service. This is important for nurses who live on the border of two states and who may provide care in both states. They must meet the APN requirements for both states, which can vary in terms of educational requirements, insurance, and paperwork. In addition, the APN must apply for a practice number (UPIN) from the Medicare intermediary.[15] The APN must also be clear about salary source. A physician's group, and not the hospital, must pay the APN's salary. If an APN comes under a nursing department in a hospital, he or she cannot bill because the APN's salary is bundled in the Medicare payment and billing separately for nursing services would constitute fraud. If an APN is paid from a physician's group or department of a hospital a bill can be generated.[15] The APN would then need to follow the same techniques as physicians in terms of using CPT procedure codes (Table 3-6).

APN billing does not currently occur universally in our health care system. A cultural shift needs to occur for some hospitals to set up independent billing for APNs. The barriers to APN billing include changing billing paperwork, lack of understanding of the Medicare guidelines for inclusion of independent APN billing, discounting the payment to 85% of the physician rate for similar services, and not valuing the APN role.

Changing paperwork is difficult, but there might be a great deal of APN work that could be billed but is not because there is no structure to do so. More efficient time utilization can justify the difference in rate. The APN saves money by not having to have the MD see each patient at the end of each visit. Therefore, money is saved (because of less down time of duplicative documen-

---

TABLE 3-6   Requirements to Bill

Master's degree

RN in state where providing service

Meet state advanced practice statutes

Certified by national credentialing body

Medicare provider number

Source of salary[5,14,15,16]

tation), and the NP and the physician can see more patients, each without being interrupted. Thus, both the APN and the physician can be more productive and generate more revenue.

Hospice Care

With hospice, APN billing is more complicated. The federal hospice guidelines make no mention of NPs or CNPs as primary providers of care to make prognosis or certification. Therefore, many hospices and home health agencies will not accept medical care directed by an APN. However, an APN could provide consultation to a hospice. It may be best to be hired by a hospital/institution and be available on a consultative basis with the hospice. Then the APN could bill separately. If the APN is hired by the hospice, there is no mechanism to bill.

Palliative Care

APN billing in palliative care is subject to the same criteria as APN in general care. If the nurse is in independent practice, billing can be done separately. However, she or he must meet the conditions of participation by Medicare in having a collaborating physician.

Summary

Reimbursement continues to challenge hospice and palliative care providers. Hospice care has more readily accessible funding. Hospice providers can be recognized within Medicare, which allows for a steady funding source. Medicaid is also a steady source of income in most states. In addition, there is acceptance by some commercial insurance products, which also allows for funding. Finally, philanthropy to hospice has been one of the hallmarks of community support. However, the challenge for hospice is providing care within the per diem as health care costs rise.

Palliative care providers must be creative in potential funding sources. Medicare utilization is the best source of funding. Much work needs to be done to have Medicare and commercial insurance providers recognize the specialty of palliative care. Using both physician and advanced practice nurse billing will increase the maximization of funding.

References

1. *NHPCO Facts and Figures.* Accessed from NHPCO.org on Dec 26, 2001.
2. CAPC National Directory. Accessed from CAPC.mssm.org on Dec 25, 2001.
3. Spragens, L. H. "National Overview of Health Care Financing." On CAPC.mssm.org. Accessed December 26, 2001.

4. Balsano, A. E., and Cella, P. M. "The Changing Role of Hospice and Its Fit in an Integrated Delivery System." *AHA Hospital Technology Series Special Report*, Vol 15(8):1–28, 1996.

5. Buppert, C. "Reimbursement for Nurse Practitioners." *The Nurse Practitioner*, (1):67–81, 1998.

6. Tilly, J., and Wiener, J. "Medicaid and End-of-Life Care." *Last Acts National Program Office*. 1–44, 2001.

7. Task Force on Palliative Care, Last Acts Campaign, Robert Wood Johnson Foundation. "Precepts of Palliative Care." *Journal of Palliative Medicine*, 1(2):109–112, 1998.

8. *Medicare: Hospice Manual, U.S. Department of Health and Human Services*. U.S. Department of Commerce National Technical Information Service. Washington, D.C., 1992.

9. Hogan and Hartsen. "Hospice Care and the Medicare Hospice Benefit." *National Hospice and Palliative Care Organization*. Available at the NHPCO website: http://www.nhpco.org. Accessed on December 21, 2001.

10. Fowler N. M., and Lynn, J. "Potential Medicare Reimbursements for Services to Patients with Chronic Fatal Illness." *Journal of Palliative Medicine*, 3(2):165–180, 2000.

11. Von Gunton C. F., Ferris, F. D., Kirschner, C., and Emanual, L. L. "Coding and Reimbursement Mechanisms for Physicians Services in Hospice and Palliative Care." *Journal of Palliative Medicine*, 3(2):157–164, 2000.

12. McKeen, E., and Billings, J. A. "Reimbursement for Physician Services Under the Medicare Benefit." *Academy of Hospice Physicians Hospice Update Newsletter*, December 1991.

13. "Balanced Budget Act of 1997." Medicare and Medicaid. Subchapter B—Other Health Care Professionals. 42 USC 4511, 4512 (1997). Pub L No. 105.

14. Richmond, T. S., Thompson, H. J., and Sullivan-Marx, E. M. "Reimbursement for Acute Care Nurse Practitioner Services." *American Journal of Critical Care*, 9(1):52–61, 2000.

15. Iris, M. "A Review of Third-Party Reimbursement Issues for Advanced Practice Nurses." *Journal of Psychosocial Nursing*, 37(1):36–40, 1999.

16. Towers, J. "Medicare Reimbursement for Nurse Practitioners." *Journal of the American Academy of Nurse Practitioners*, 11(7):289–292, 1999.

For Further Reading

Emanual, L. L., Von Gunton, C. F., and Ferris, F. D. "Procedure/Diagnosis Coding and Reimbursement Mechanisms for Physician Services in Palliative Care." *The Education for Physicians on End of Life Care (EPEC) Curriculum*. EPEC Project. The Robert Wood Johnson Foundation, 1999.

"HCFA Rules Concerning Medicare Reimbursement to NPs." *American Journal for Nurse Practitioners*, 2(11):32, 1998.

Lindeke L. L., and Chesney, M. L. "Reimbursement Realities of Advanced Nursing Practice." *Nursing Outlook*, 47(6):248–251, 1999.

Price, L. C., and Minarik, P. A. "Update on Federal Medicare Rules Affecting Advanced Practice Nurses." *Clinical Nurse Specialist*, 3(2):90–92, 1999.

Hospice/Palliative Care Settings

4

Judith A. Kitzes

Betty L. Sehmoll

Carol E. Dixon

Palliative care/hospice care is a model for quality, compassionate care at the end of life. The current definition of palliative/hospice care includes a distinct, comprehensive cluster of services for terminally ill individuals and their families, which are provided on a continuum of intensity (levels of care) in a variety of settings. All hospice and palliative care includes access to and availability of appropriate and necessary services to meet the identified needs and choices for care made by the patient and family. The Medicare Hospice Benefit conditions of participation define a distinctive cluster of services that the hospice must provide regardless of the care setting.[2] They also establish guidelines for how hospice care is provided by hospice personnel.

Levels of Care

Four levels of care are identified in the Medicare hospice regulations.[2] They are listed in Table 4-1.

TABLE 4-1 Levels of Care
Routine home care
Continuous home care
Respite care
Inpatient care

Routine home care, the most common level of care, is the heart of hospice care. The hospice team provides the full scope of hospice services, most often in the patient's personal residence. Care begins with an admission process, which includes an assessment and evaluation of the patient's status and appropriateness for hospice care. During the initial visit, the focus is on discovering the concerns and issues that are troubling the patient and family and in helping them understand what hospice care is and how it can help them.

Frequently, care during the first few visits is directed toward relieving specific problems such as pain, symptoms of the disease, or anxiety. From the assessment visit on, the patient and family are evaluated for the need of specific services, supplies, equipment, and community resources. This initial attention to the needs of the patient and family is a pattern for continuing reevaluation. Patient and family needs and concerns are continually being reappraised to ensure that support and comfort-oriented services, appropriate and necessary for the palliation and support of the patient and family, are offered in a timely manner. In routine home care, there is usually significant involvement of family or primary care support persons providing direct, hands-on care for the patient. This care can be quite complex, and teaching and support for the caregiver are important parts of hospice care. By meeting the comfort needs of the patient and the support needs of the family, many patients are able to die, as they prefer, at home.

Continuous home care is an expanded level of care in the home. It allows up to twenty-four hours a day of skilled nursing to ease patients through periods of crisis and to prevent hospitalization for management of acute symptoms. Although the chief reason for this level of care is management of acute physical symptoms, it may also be used when the burden of caregiving for families is greater than their resources. Usually this occurs because care of the patient is complex, difficult, or extensive. There are no limits to the number of hours or days allowed at this level, but care must be primarily skilled nursing for at least 8 hours out of 24 to qualify. Hours need not be consecutive, nor does all of the care need to be provided by a registered nurse. However, a registered nurse or licensed practical nurse must provide a minimum of at least one hour more than half the total continuous home care hours. Continuous home care provides an invaluable resource for helping patients to stay at home—and die at home.

Respite care supports the patient's family and caregivers. They need time away from the intensity of caring for a terminally ill individual. Families can plan a mini-vacation, attend special events, or simply get much-needed rest and recreation at home while the patient is cared for in an inpatient setting. Hospices in either their own facilities or contracted beds in nursing homes or hospitals provide respite care for five-day periods. Care is very similar to home care except that room and board and assistance with basic activities of living by nurses and nursing assistants are provided in an inpatient setting to replace the care usually provided by the family and caregivers. Respite care must be provided in a Medicare-certified facility. The episodes of respite care must be intermittent, relatively infrequent, and limited to five-day periods. These patients are often very ill or have significant need for assistance with activities of daily living (ADL), which is often the precipitating factor in the family's need for respite care. The typical needs of the patient who requires respite care are expensive due to the intensity of care. The staffing and support required for this level of care usually far exceed the reimbursement for the service.

Inpatient care or acute symptom management is a short term admission to a Medicare certified facility for medical problems requiring nursing and medical management. Typical problems that may prompt inpatient care are outlined in Table 4-2. In general, any patient whose care is so complex or demanding that the family can no longer continue to provide home care is a candidate for inpatient care. The most noticeable similarity between acute hospitalization and palliative inpatient care is the skilled nursing and medical management of the patient. The major differences are the focus on palliation of symptoms, the complexity of hospice team services provided, the attention to the family, and the psychosocial and spiritual support that are prevalent in hospice care. Palliative care is designed to provide comfort and support rather than cure of the illness or the problem. There is a limit to the number of inpatient care days a hospice can provide under the Medicare hospice benefit.[2] At least 80% of all patient care days must be home care days, and no more than 20% of days can be spent in the combination of respite and regular inpatient care.

The limitation on inpatient days has created a problem for small rural hospices, and amendments to the Medicare hospice program have been suggested to waive the 80/20 rule.

TABLE 4-2	**Triggers for Inpatient Palliative Care Admissions**

Imminent death under specific conditions

Bleeding—active and potential

Sepsis

Seizures

Impending delirium tremens

Uncontrolled pain

Any uncontrolled symptom

Central nervous system dysfunction—delirium, coma, dementia

Fractures of weight-bearing bones

Management of complex medications

Acute cardiac symptoms—myocardial infarction, arrhythmias

Complex treatment schedule requiring frequent dressing changes or procedures that require the time, skill, and observations of a professional nurse

Terminal agitation

In 2000, according to the National Hospice and Palliative Care Organization, 96% of the days of hospice service were routine care, 3% of the days were inpatient, 0.3% was respite care, and 0.3% was continuous home care.[1]

Additional Non-Medicare Levels of Care

Not included in the Medicare hospice benefit are three separate levels of specialized care—residential care, day care, and extended caregiver programs (in-home respite). These levels of care are being provided to expand services to meet identified patient care needs. There are patient/family charges for these services, usually based on a sliding scale. Charges are frequently waived for indigent patients. Some hospices/palliative care programs operate these optional services with grant money from foundations or from special fund-raising projects.

Residential care is provided in hospice/palliative inpatient settings for patients who require supportive care related to safety needs, weakness, or the inability to perform self-care. It was developed in response to the Medicare hospice benefit's limit on regular inpatient care and the need to provide inpatient care for patients without caregivers or for those whose caregivers are frail, elderly, or fatigued by the intensity of care. Other patients who utilize residential care have caregivers who must work to ensure continued health insurance coverage and family income. Residential care also provides a way to offer better continuity for those patients who are no longer appropriate for regular inpatient care status. In defining criteria for residential care admission, the norm is patients whose care can safely be provided by a nursing assistant with minimal supervision. This helps to differentiate between regular inpatient and residential care patients. If the patient's condition changes so that a more intensive level of care is needed, the hospice can transfer the patient to a regular inpatient or continuous home care level to meet the care needs.

Residential care is provided in hospice facilities or in contracted beds in hospitals or nursing homes. In either case, the hospice is responsible for ensuring that care and services meet hospice standards.

Day care is relatively new to hospice in the United States. It is designed to provide relief to the caregiver and diverse activities for the patient. It is similar to other adult day care programs for patients with specific health care problems. Patients are transported to the day care site by family or by the hospice. There are planned activities, meals, and observation and assistance as needed. Severely ill or very debilitated patients should not use this portion of the program. This has tended to slow the development of day care programs in hospice settings. Recently, some hospice programs have extended hospice day care to "pre-hospice" patients and their families as a way to familiarize them with hospice care.

Extended caregiver services or in-home respite care is a new level of care that is growing in popularity in hospice programs. The term describes a program that offers shifts of nursing assistants to a patient to supplement or substitute for family caregivers. The goal is to keep the patient at home. Extended caregiver service is needed and used by working families, frail caregivers, and in situations where the physical demands for caregiving are beyond the strength of the caregiver. It is also a way to supplement care when residential care beds are not immediately available. It is possible to use extended caregiver programs, where extra help in the home is offered to supplement the family's care for patients whose temporary needs cannot easily or appropriately be satisfied through regular home-care or inpatient services. This is an optional service some hospices provide when they are able to fund the care through special fund-raising projects, community support, or foundation grants. Although extended caregiver service is not a mandated level of care, it is important to remember that other required levels of care must be available to hospice patients.

There are financial and staffing limitations to hospices' ability to provide these new services. However, these added levels of care have become a valuable extension to hospice services.

Service Settings

Hospice care is defined not only by services and levels of care provided, but also by the settings in which these services are delivered. Care in the patient's personal residence is always considered either routine home care or continuous home care. Care in a facility can include any of the levels of care provided by hospice: routine home care, continuous home care, residential care, day care, respite care, and inpatient care.[2]

Home

What is home? The National Hospice Organization, in its Standards of a Hospice Program of Care, simply defines home as "a person's place of residence."[4] This definition includes a variety of settings that, at first glance, do not seem to be "home." Hospice home care is being provided in the following settings— adult foster care homes, congregate living and group homes, AIDS housing, hospice residences, tents, homeless shelters, jails, nursing homes, and many other kinds of personal residences. The commonality in this care is the services provided by hospice, and the responsibility that hospice has to ensure the safety and comfort of the patient, the patient's family, and the hospice staff.

Facility-Based Care

When care is provided in a facility, regardless of the level of care provided, hospice has a professional management responsibility for the safety and comfort of the patient. This may be a more significant responsibility than in the patient's home because care is being provided by paid caretakers rather than family. Currently there are few rules for residential or nursing home care to ensure quality care and appropriate services. The National Hospice Organization's Standards of a Hospice Program of Care and the Medicare Hospice Regulations provide basic guidelines for this care.[4] Currently, the basic requirements include hospice's responsibility for ensuring that the scope of services is adequate to meet the needs of the patient. The services must be of the same quality and volume to ensure comfort and safety.

Hospice staffs are expected to meet with the facility's staff to ensure that care is congruent with the hospice plan of care. The hospice retains management oversight responsibility for the patient, and there are some distinct expectations for the care setting that have been established as part of the Medicare hospice benefit guidelines. These reflect hospice values related to facility-based care and include adapting the environment and modifying facility rules to meet the needs of the patient. Table 4-3 lists the adaptations required of the facility.

Common Service Sites Hospital

Hospital settings are the most common sites for regular inpatient care, and the most frequent method for providing that care is a "scatter bed" approach. In this model, a hospice contracts with a number of different hospitals in its service area to admit hospice patients for symptom management. The hospice trains hospital staff, develops the plan of care, approves care provided, and pays the hospital for the care. All the usual hospice services are provided, with an emphasis on palliation and support for the patient and family.

A less common model is the dedicated unit. This is a contracted arrangement with the hospital in which a specific unit or number of beds are reserved for hospice patients. The unit is usually staffed by the hospital, but sometimes the hospice simply rents the space and services of the hospital and staff and operate the unit. It is somewhat easier to control the services provided and ensure appropriate care in this model than in the scatter bed approach

---

TABLE 4-3   Required Facility Adaptation

Ensure privacy and space for family gathering

Allow 24-hour visiting and overnight stays

Provide for religious and spiritual worship

Provide flexibility in scheduling care, accommodating individual needs

Permit family to prepare meals

Allow patient choice in food and timing of meals

Provide a comfortable, homelike atmosphere

Ensure access to services required by plan of care

Ensure safety, comfort, and patient satisfaction

Maintain coordination of care by hospice team member

because hospice staff are in more direct contact with the patient and better able to control the care provided.

A disadvantage of the hospital setting for hospice care is the difficulty in controlling the care provided in a setting owned and operated by another health care provider. In the hospital environment it is easy to access invasive, curative interventions; this availability can create a problem for the hospice in ensuring palliative and comfort-oriented care. A patient may refuse to use a particular hospital for various reasons such as convenience, family preference, religious or philosophical perspectives, or because of their physician's privileges or preferences. However, the financial and logistical advantages of the hospital setting more than offset the disadvantages, and the hospital setting continues to be the dominant inpatient service setting. Occasionally, hospices also provide respite care in hospitals, but this is rare because the reimbursement level for respite care is too low to be appealing to many hospitals.

Long-Term Care Facility

Nursing homes are used as sites for regular inpatient care, respite care, and routine home care. Reimbursement and the ability to offer expanded care for residents are inducements to the nursing home to contract with the hospice. The favorable surroundings, lower cost of contracting for regular inpatient and respite care, and ability to increase their patient census are benefits for the hospice.

The differences between long-term care regulations and hospice regulations require careful negotiation and ongoing cooperation between nursing home and hospice staff. The nursing home must be Medicare certified, and the hospice requirement that a registered nurse be on the premises and available to provide hands-on care 24 hours a day can create a problem for the nursing facility.

It is a growing trend for hospices to provide care in extended care facilities. Dedicated beds or dedicated units for regular inpatient and respite care are a familiar part of hospice inpatient care. Routine home care offered in nursing homes is a more recent and growing part of hospice care. It requires the same level and mix of services provided to other hospice home care patients, and it can be an equally valuable resource to terminally ill patients in nursing homes. Specific guidelines have not been established for routine home care in nursing home settings; there is a growing concern that some way to ensure the quality of hospice care in nursing homes needs to be developed. It is quite probable that Medicare will develop some measurable guidelines in the near future.

Hospice Facilities

In the early days of hospice, there was no reimbursement or licensure for hospice care. As a result, the first hospice facilities were licensed as specialty hospital hospices, nursing homes, or extended care facilities, and the level of care they could offer was limited to regular inpatient care. The difficulty with this classification was that the licensure requirements, which applied specifically to those facilities, were inappropriate for hospice care. In addition, the cost of meeting those requirements increased the cost to hospices for providing inpatient care. When the Medicare hospice benefit was enacted, the reimbursement level for inpatient care was much less than the actual cost, and hospices were continually forced to employ fundraising events in order to keep the facilities operating.

The same difficulties have been encountered with the development of hospice residences. These facilities are primarily designed to care for home-care patients who needed a sheltered "home" setting. Obtaining licensure for the facility is frequently a long and arduous task, and there is typically no reimbursement for the room and board cost of residential care. Because many hospice patients have very diminished resources to pay for care, fund-raising to support the facility once again has become a way of life for hospices. However, enactment of the Medicare hospice benefit influenced licensure laws and created a reimbursement source for hospice care.

The mandate that hospice control the inpatient setting for hospice patient care led to a greater awareness of what quality inpatient care should be and created an incentive for developing a freestanding hospice facility. The broad but clear requirements for freestanding hospice facilities meant that hospices could design cost-effective settings to provide acute, residential, and respite care and justify licensure of the facility as a hospice. There are clear advantages to this model. For one thing, it allows for expeditious transfer of patients from one level of care to another. Because care is provided in the same facility, continuity is enhanced and the need for patients and their families to adapt to new caregivers and new settings is reduced. It also ensures both hospice control of the care setting and a consistent pattern of care that meets the hospice's policies and procedures for care. A freestanding hospice facility that provides all levels of care becomes a valuable and important community resource that enhances the hospice's public image and increases access to those who need a variety of levels of care.

Specialized Residences

Certain populations of patients with terminal illness are spurring the development of specialized hospice/palliative care settings. These include patients with the diagnosis of AIDS, Alzheimer's dementia, and all pediatric terminal illness. Although nearly 10,000 children die of conditions such as cancer each year, fewer than 10% of the 3100 hospice programs provide end-of-life care and fewer are geared specifically toward kids.[5]

Advocacy for holistic hospice services, tailored to the needs of an individual's diagnosis and age-specific developmental skills and requirements, is increasing. The settings include community-based homes, residences owned by hospices, and designated inpatient wards.

Summary

Hospice and palliative care is a complex mix of interrelationships between services, levels of care, and sites of service. This complex mix of services that are patient-centered and patient-driven will continue to be the impetus for dynamic changes in the settings and levels of care for terminally ill patients.

References

1. National Hospice and Palliative Care Organization, NHPCO Facts and Figures, 2001, www.nhpco.org.
2. U.S. Department of Health and Human Services. *Interpretive Guidelines—Hospices.* Washington, D.C.: U.S. Department of Health and Human Services, 1992.
3. U.S. Department of Health and Human Services. *Medicare: Hospice Manual.* Washington, D.C.: U.S. Department of Commerce National Technical Information Service, 1994.
4. National Hospice and Palliative Care Organization. *Standards of a Hospice Program of Care.* Arlington, Va.: National Hospice Organization, 1997.
5. PBS Healthweek Report, January 11, 2002. www.pbs.org/healthweek.

Continuous Quality Improvement (CQI) in Hospice

5

Michele Y. Lee

Continuous Quality Improvement (CQI) or Total Quality Management (TQM) is an industrial concept that many hope will provide significant improvement for the quality, productivity, and outcomes of medical care. CQI programs strive for a comprehensive and cycling evaluation of an organization that includes analyses of the impact of any improvements. New suggestions are generated to maintain gains and positive outcomes, or to improve on them. Therefore, each CQI project has specific goals, and when these are met, new goals are generated.

To set goals for a hospice, a definition of quality must be made. Unlike the automobile industry, where quality can be measured by concrete outcomes of an automobile in a certain time frame, it is more difficult to assess outcome measures for health care that accurately reflect quality. In general, quality is a value and a discipline of knowledge, skills, and practices to achieve excellence in products, services, and environment based on the requirements, perceptions, and future needs of our customers.[1] This definition has been applied to health care in different ways. Quality in health care can be thought of in terms of the technical aspects, such as the skills and knowledge that clinicians apply, communication between doctors and patients, or good access to care in an equitable manner.[2] Quality in health care can also be described as the sum total of all dimensions of health care—to achieve the highest quality care at the best possible price.[3] Note that both definitions combine system and outcome. The effectiveness and appropriateness of the service is hoped to have a positive effect on the health status of the client. Thus, service is just as important as costs in the definition of quality heath care.

What does quality mean at the end of life? The Institute of Medicine Committee on Care at the End of Life defined a good death as "one free from avoidable distress and suffering for patients, family and caregivers; in general accord with patients' and families' wishes; and reasonably consistent with clinical, cultural, and ethical standards."[4] The Ethics Committee of the American Geriatrics Society (AGS) proposed 10 areas in which quality could be measured[5] (Table 5-1). Singer et al. identified five quality measurements as:

- having adequate pain management;
- avoiding inappropriate prolongation of dying;
- achieving a sense of control;
- relieving burden; and
- strengthening relationships with loved ones.[6]

Ideally, humane and effective end-of-life efforts include an assessment of psychological, social, and financial needs of the patient and family, and an individualized multidimensional combination of health care, social services, and caregiver support is created. When using definitions of quality in hospice, the CQI team needs to determine what the modifiable aspects of the patient's experience are at the end of life. Once identified, these aspects can be the foci of the CQI program. However, attention to these individual issues should not supercede the mission or the overall ideals of quality end-of-life care for driving the CQI process.

During the CQI process, the hospice team needs to keep in mind its definition of quality hospice care. If the focus of the CQI measures become survival rather than caring for dying patients, the process could degenerate to cost-

TABLE 5-1 Ten Areas for Quality Assessment in the Health Care of the Dying Patient
Physical and emotional symptoms
Support function and autonomy
Advance care planning
Aggressiveness of care near death
Patient and family satisfaction
Global quality of life
Family burden
Survival time
Provider continuity and skill
Bereavement

From The American Geriatrics Society Ethics Committee. "The Care of Dying Patients: A Position Statement from the American Geriatrics Society." *Journal of the American Geriatric Society* 43:577–578, 1995.

cutting and service restrictions.[7] For example, to cut costs, a hospice places restrictions on services. The more restrictions on service that occur, the fewer services the patient receives. The patients and families may then go to another hospice that will provide more services. As the number of patients drops, the income to the hospice decreases. This may induce more cost-cutting measures and fewer services. In another case, other measures are done to encourage patients to enter and stay in the hospice program. With good services, patients have high satisfaction and more patients may want to enroll in this hospice rather than in another. The importance of the patient as a client has become one of the common characteristics of current CQI programs.[8] If all staff understand and support the mission statement of the hospice, the CQI process can produce quality hospice care without an excess of restrictive policies.

Assessment of Quality

Donabedian presented a seminal paper in 1966 that described a conceptual framework for measuring quality in health care.[9] The framework refers to dimensions of structure (where the care is provided), process (how the care occurs), and outcomes. In hospice, structure can be thought of as the resources available to the hospice, such as inpatient beds, staff, and services.[10] Process measurements can be identified as advance directives documentation, symptom assessments, and aggressive interventions. Outcome measurements for hospice are such indicators as cost of care, spiritual well-being, and family satisfaction (Table 5-2). A comprehensive CQI program includes improvements of structure, process, and outcome.

Who does the assessment? A team approach is utilized for CQI programs. The CQI team is responsible for setting the goals for the project, brainstorming regarding improvements, collecting and analyzing data during the improvements, and making suggestions to maintain the gains or further improvements. With so many tasks, CQI teams need to be interdisciplinary. Quality assessment and improvement involve not only the board members and administrators of the hospice, but also physicians, staff, and volunteers. Including members of the hospice team in the CQI process not only helps the hospice team gain ownership of the process, but also gives the CQI team some practical input during the planning and implementation phases. CQI teams should be small and each team should work on a specific outcome or process. It is important to identify leaders, who will work with different teams during the assessment and improvement processes.

Because family caregivers are often providers as well as customers, their input and involvement are welcome. Also, hospice services need to include support for family caregivers. Many of the current standards acknowledge the dual role of the family member and have requirements written into their standards.

Goals and Standards

Although each individual hospice program should determine its own goals for quality, various organizations have published standards for hospice

TABLE 5-2 Measures of the Quality of End-of-Life Care	
	Type of Indicator
Medical director	Structure
Staff (nurses, social workers, etc.)	Structure
Volunteers	Structure
Inpatient hospice beds	Structure
Administrative staff	Structure
Outpatient office	Structure
Self Determination	
Advance directives documentation	Process
Advance directives completion	Process
Reference documentation	Process
MD understanding of patient preferences	Process
Care concordance with preferences	Outcome
Symptom Control	
Symptom assessment	Process
Symptom management	Process
Symptom outcome	Outcome
Quality of life	Outcome
Spiritual well-being	Outcome
Patient satisfaction	Outcome
Family satisfaction	Outcome
Family support	Outcome
Care Decisions	
DNR orders	Process
Timing of DNR orders	Process
Aggressive care interventions	Process
Hospital days	Outcome
Venue of care (hospital, home)	Outcome
ICU days	Outcome
Cost of care	Outcome
Survival duration	Outcome

MD = physician, DNR = do not resuscitate

Modified from Rosenfeld, K., and Wenger, N. S. "Measuring Quality in End-of-Life Care." *Clinics in Geriatric Medicine,* 16(2):387–400, 2000.

services. The National Hospice and Palliative Care Organization (NHPCO) Standards provide a comprehensive description and objective of each facet of a hospice program from the home program to the respite program to the inpatient program.[11,12] The NHPCO guidelines also provide job descriptions for physicians and staff, including recommended percentages of full time employees (FTEs). NHPCO defines services for family support and bereavement and describes required documentation. The NHPCO Standards document has an accompanying tool, which can help assess hospice services.

The Joint Commission on Accreditation of Healthcare Organizations (JCAHO) and Medicare also have guidelines and rules. Some managed care payors require JCAHO accreditation for referrals to a hospice.[13] An application is submitted to JCAHO and, when the application is accepted, a JCAHO survey of the hospice occurs. A consultant may be helpful in assessing the current state of readiness and preparing the hospice to meet JCAHO's standards.

Solomon et al published recommendations involving access to care, accountability, and payment.[14] The twelve recommendations are:

- Provide managed care insurance products that cover humane and effective end-of-life care for patients and families.
- Create specific programs for patients dying of chronic, degenerative conditions and their family caregivers.
- Base access to hospice care on severity of need, not estimated life expectancy.
- Ensure continuity of care for patients and families across different providers and settings.
- Focus continuous quality improvement efforts on end-of-life care.
- Design valid, standardized measures to assess the quality of end-of-life care.
- Report on quality of care to Medicare, Medicaid, commercial purchasers, and consumers.
- Improve the clinical competence of physicians, nurses, and other health care professionals providing care to patients near the end of life.
- Reach out to patients and families as partners in end-of-life care.
- Test new methods for aligning financial incentives with the provision of humane and effective care.
- Ensure access by developing risk adjustment strategies or other payment methods that properly compensate managed care providers and plans for costs of caring for patients near the end of life.
- Develop and study the effects of alternative reimbursement methods capable of enhancing coordination between managed care organizations and hospice programs.

For each of the above recommendations, the task force suggests action steps to managed care leaders, policy makers, and purchasers to implement the recommendations.

If a specific problem has been identified, guidelines may exist for that problem. For example, the American Pain Society (APS) set forth guidelines that were incorporated into a CQI project at Baylor University Medical Center.[15,16] The CQI team used these guidelines to improve the pain management process.

The CQI Process

A systematic approach is needed to implement the CQI process. One method is to use a framework, such as the FOCUS/PDSA (Figure 5-1). After the CQI team identifies an improvement and plans for its implementation, data collection occurs for the process as well as for the outcome. This data is studied for improvement in both the process and the outcome. Then, the process contin-

---

FIGURE 5-1   **Focus/PDSA Process**

F	Find process improvement opportunity
O	Organize team that knows the process
C	Clarify current knowledge of the process
U	Understand causes of process variation
S	Select process improvement plan

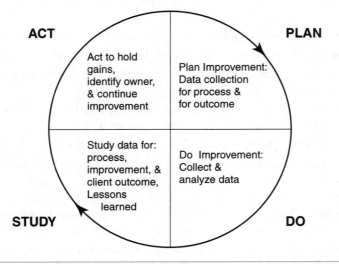

From Comley, A. L., and DeMeyer, E. "Assessing Patient Satisfaction with Pain Management through a Continuous Improvement Effort." *Journal of Pain and Symptom Management*, 21:27–40, 2001.

ues again. The CQI team looks at the results, maybe suggests an improvement, and starts to plan for its implementation and evaluation. Flowcharts and cause-effect diagrams may assist in the overall conceptualization of the plan and enable the CQI team to identify problems in the process.

For example, a hospice may have evaluated data from patients who have died, needs of the current patients and families, or staff and volunteer assessments. The hospice may want to improve its clinical programs. Using the FOCUS/PDSA framework, the hospice may find opportunities to improve the efficiency and effectiveness of the volunteer program or develop and implement a pediatric hospice program. "F" would have us focus on an opportunity, such as the volunteer program. "O" would be to organize a team that knows the process, being sure to include volunteers on the CQI team. "C" would have the team look at the problem, make a flow chart to see how the process flows from admitting the patient through the bereavement of the family. Barriers to the volunteers' involvement and places for improvement can be placed on these charts. Places where the volunteers are effective must also be identified. "U" means understanding the causes. "S" is to select a process improvement plan, such as to develop an improved volunteer orientation program. Also, an assessment tool, such as a questionnaire about patient satisfaction or to track volunteer hours and activities, may be chosen and placed in the hospice administration's computers. After a plan is made, it can be implemented, and the data collected and analyzed. The data then needs to be studied for problems and gains. The hospice volunteers may like the improved orientation program, but would like it given at a different time. Finally, the team needs to act to hold these gains, continue improvement, and modify the improvement as necessary.

Benchmarking is another management tool to be used after the hospice services have been ranked in the community of your peers and issues that need improvement have been identified.[17] The goal of benchmarking is to measure against the "best." For example, after a JCAHO survey, recommendations are made to the organization to be addressed before the next JCAHO survey. The four phases of the benchmarking process are: 1) Planning, 2) Data collection and analysis, 3) Integration, and 4) Action. Planning determines what your organization is addressing, who will lead the teams, what data will be collected, and what the requirements are for success. Data collection can include administering a questionnaire, identifying best practices, and doing site visits. In the integration phase, the information is communicated and goals are established. Finally, a plan of action is determined and implemented along with a way to monitor the results.

Data Collection and Analysis

In order to gather data, questionnaires and surveys are needed. Besides the assessment tool developed by the NHPCO, other organizations have developed ways to monitor the effectiveness of an improvement or new protocol.[11]

Teno has compiled several measurement techniques and survey items for carrying out quality-of-life assessment (www.chcr.brown.edu/pcoc/tool.htm).[10] An individual CQI team can make its own assessment tools to address specific issues that need to be addressed. Patient satisfaction and family outcome measures must be included in the evaluation of any new procedure.

The CQI team's job is not done after it chooses quality indicators and tools. It needs to monitor protocols and procedures and make necessary changes based on the data. Statisticians or computer consultants can provide advice on database design and data analysis. After data is generated, data systems store the data, and members of the CQI team use programs to analyze data. The CQI team reviews the results and makes suggestions to maintain or change the procedures or protocols. The cycle then begins again.

Barriers to Implementation

Problems with applying CQI in medical practice stem from the inherent complexity of medical care processes, as well as physicians' understanding and support of the process.[18] Barriers to CQI implementation include a lack of leadership and motivation, the absence of explicit plans, competing priorities, physicians' sensitivities, poor or nonexistent data, and unclear roles and responsibilities. When changes are suggested, the "but we've always done it that way" attitude may be the response.

Overcoming barriers requires support for the CQI team from the organization.[2] Education for physicians, staff, and volunteers may be necessary so they can understand the CQI process. It is important that everyone understands that the changes for CQI are not just for management, but also for good patient care. The CQI team needs to keep all members of the hospice team informed regarding CQI activities within the hospice, such as the results of CQI improvements, even if they are not on the CQI team.

Summary

Quality in hospice is important. By setting clearly defined goals and designing new procedures and protocols to meet those goals, a CQI program can be successfully applied to a hospice. CQI programs need to look at all aspects of the hospice—structure, process, and outcomes—while always remembering the mission of the organization. Improved end-of-life care will result through teamwork and communication using this systematic approach.

References

1. Morath, J. M. *The Quality Advantage: A Strategic Guide for Health Care Providers.* Chicago: American Hospital Association Co., 1998.
2. Schattner, P, and Markey, P. "Divisions, General Practice, and Continuous Quality Improvement." *Australian Family Physician,* 30(7):725–728, 2001.
3. Nash, D. B. *The Managed Care Manual.* Boston, Mass.: TLC Medical Publishing, 1997.

4. Field, M. J., and Cassell, C. D. (eds.). *For the Institute of Medicine, Approaching Death: Improving Care at the End of Life.* Washington, D.C.: National Academy Press, 1997.

5. The American Geriatrics Society Ethics Committee. "The Care of Dying Patients: A Position Statement from the American Geriatrics Society." *Journal of the American Geriatric Society,* 43:577–578, 1995.

6. Singer, P. A., Martin, D. K., and Kelner, M. "Quality End-of-Life Care: Patients' Perspective." *JAMA,* 281:163–168, 1999.

7. Herbst, L. H. and Cetti, J. "Management Strategies for Palliative Care: Promoting Quality, Growth, and Opportunity." *American Journal of Hospice and Palliative Care,* 18(5):327–333, 2001.

8. Enck, R. E. "Performance Improvement in Hospice Care." *American Journal of Hospice and Palliative Care,* 18(4):222–223, 2001.

9. Donabedian, A. "Evaluating the Quality of Medical Care." *Millbank Mem Fund Q.* 44(supp):166–206.

10. Rosenfeld, K., and Wenger, N. S. "Measuring Quality in End-of-Life Care." *Clinics in Geriatric Medicine,* 16(2):387–400, 2000.

11. The National Hospice Organization. *Standards of a Hospice Program of Care and the Self-Assessment Tool.* Arlington, Va.: The National Hospice Organization, 1993.

12. The National Hospice Organization. *Hospice Service Guidelines.* Arlington, Va.: The National Hospice Organization, 1994.

13. Groves, L. E. "Preparing for an Initial JCAHO Survey: One Hospice's Experience." *American Journal of Hospice and Palliative Care,* 18(5):299–302, 2001.

14. Solomon, M. Z., Romer, A., and Sellers, D. *Meeting the Challenge. Twelve Recommendations for Improving End-of-Life Care in Managed Care.* Newton, Mass.: Center for Applied Ethics and Professional Practice, 1999.

15. Braveman, C., and Rodrigues, C. "Performance Improvement in Pain Management for Home Care and Hospice Programs." *American Journal of Hospice and Palliative Care,* 18(4):257–263, 2001.

16. Comley, A. L., and DeMeyer, E. "Assessing Patient Satisfaction with Pain Management through a Continuous Improvement Effort." *Journal of Pain and Symptom Management,* 21:27–40, 2001.

17. Tweet, A. G., and Gavin, K. *The Guide to Benchmarking in Health Care.* New York: Quality Resources, 1998.

18. Shortell, S. M. "Physicians' Involvement in Quality Improvement." *Improving Clinical Practice, Total Quality Management and the Physician.* D. Blumenthal and A. C. Scheck (eds). San Francisco, Calif.: Jossey-Bass Publishers, 1995.

Communication at the End of Life

Jacqueline Mauk, RN, PhD, CNS, CHPN

In 1949, famed journalist John Gunther wrote, *Death Be Not Proud.*[1] In this poignant memoir, he describes his teenage son's wit, courage, and cheerfulness throughout an ultimately unsuccessful 15-month struggle with a malignant brain tumor. Gunther tells the story of a desperate search for a cure and great attempts to keep hope alive by not talking with John Jr. about the seriousness of his illness. At the end Gunther writes:

> It was only after his death, from his brief simple diaries . . . that we learned he had known all along how grave was his illness, and that even as we had gaily pretended with him that all was well and he was completely recovering, he was pretending with us, and bearing our burden with the spirit, the élan, of a singing soldier or a laughing saint. (p. 189)

Gunther wrote in a time when conventional wisdom maintained that to suffer alone and in silence was heroic. Although current attitudes toward death have not entirely evolved past this point of view, much more is known about the cost to inner resources of all involved when patients die in silence. More than any other group in health care, the dying need good communication with those around them.[2] Open and honest communication at the end of life can bring meaning out of suffering, growth out of decline, and joy out of sadness. Dying patients, their loved ones, and their health care providers all derive great benefit when end-of-life care is based on the acknowledgement that life does not last forever, and, indeed, the end is coming near.

To give voice to the importance of effective communication at the end of life, this chapter presents an overview of principles of human communication, highlights the value of good communication at the end of life, and reviews practical approaches that enhance such exchanges. The reader who wishes to delve more deeply into communication concepts and techniques is referred to the many excellent texts on this topic, such as van Servellen or Ivey and Ivey.[3,4]

Principles of Human Communication

Communication is the essential process by which individuals share something of themselves, whether it is thoughts, feelings, opinions, ideas, values, or goals. What life would be like without communication is unimaginable. Interpersonal communication is woven into the basic fabric of human life and social order. As ubiquitous as human communication is, there are some situations that require more than rudimentary skills. Health care professionals, in general, require effective communication skills, but good end-of-life care calls for excellence in interpersonal communication.

Communication is an art as well as a science. For a few gifted persons, good communication skills are inherent. These individuals have a special sensitivity to and adeptness with the multiple dimensions involved in this fundamental life skill. Most people, however, are unaware of the tacit rules of communication. An understanding of some basic principles of communication can enhance relationships between health care providers and dying patients and their families. Communications experts affirm, however, that a health care provider's own natural approach and style should be valued as a strength, and that new approaches to interpersonal communication should be adopted only if they seem to fit naturally.[4]

Communication is multidimensional. Nothing is more important to understanding human communication than to appreciate the complexity of how information is sent and received. In every message, there is the *content* of the message sent, the *feelings* that modify the message, and a *relationship level.*[3] More specifically, the content is the primary message the sender thinks is being sent, whether true or false, sensible or nonsense, or even undecipherable. In short, content is the words spoken. The feeling aspect of a message describes the emotional content embedded by the sender in the communication. A message can be sent with any feeling included in the human emotional repertoire: grief, anger, joy, confidence, peace, boredom, and so on. It is sometimes intentionally chosen, but more often the sender is not aware of the full emotional information that is being sent. The relationship aspect of communication refers to how a message is received given the perceived social positions of the communicants. This is often intertwined with the feeling component of communication. An illustration of this principle is when a patient defers to a physician because of the physician's social role. In the health care setting, a physician is typically viewed as the foremost authority figure, and one whose opinions regarding illness concerns are recognized as superior and authoritative. Patients typically believe their own ideas about health matters are less significant, and this is communicated in their interactions with physicians.

Overarching the three dimensions listed above is the fact that communication is sent in both verbal and nonverbal ways.[3] Verbal communication describes the content level of a message and refers to what is actually said in words. Nonverbal parts of communication include facial expression, body positioning, and gestures. Tone of voice, voice inflections, and sequence and rhythm of words are also part of nonverbal communication. Feeling and relational dimensions are typically at the nonverbal level. Awareness of both verbal and nonverbal aspects of communication is of utmost importance. For example, support given fleetingly by a health care provider at the doorway of a bed-bound patient's room is likely to ring falsely to that patient. This mismatch between the verbal message and the nonverbal body language is not likely to be missed. Indeed, it is only when there is congruence between verbal and nonverbal messages that trust between a provider and a patient can be established and maintained.

Perception is selective. A second principle of communication is that perceptual abilities are selective.[3] People, in the best of circumstances, perceive only a part of the information sent to them. When significant stressors are added, only a fraction of this amount is perceived. This is particularly relevant in providing care for people in stressful circumstances such as end-of-life settings. It is common for vital information to go unperceived because an anxious person is overwhelmed and cannot discern what is relevant and what is irrelevant. Furthermore, people typically, but incorrectly, assume that they perceive complete, correct information about what is going on around them. In short, people do not know what they are missing. The idea that what is perceived is not precisely what actually is, is a critical principle of human communication.

Communication is an interactive and continuous process. Communication is a circular process in which one person sends an idea by putting thoughts and feelings into words and gestures. Sight, sound, and movement are used to transmit the message. The listener simultaneously responds to the message being sent, and the sender receives these responses as messages from the listener. In other words, the sender is also a receiver of information during the sending, and the listener is at the same time a sender of information as the incoming messages are processed.[3]

Communication is inevitable. It is impossible not to communicate.[3] Communication is always occurring whether words are being spoken or not. Sitting silently and peacefully at someone's bedside can communicate one thing, such as the worthiness of the person with whom one is sitting. Sitting silently, but glancing frequently at a wristwatch, can communicate something quite different, such as a preoccupation with the march of time. It is essential for health care providers to be aware that even when words are not used, communication is occurring.

Related to the inevitability of communication is the regularity with which messages are sent unintentionally.[3] Much of what is communicated is neither planned nor realized. Shadows of thoughts not put to words are frequently evident in nonverbal behavior. If thoughts are incongruent with the conversation at hand, a mixed message will be sent. Confusion and mistrust can be the results. A health care provider who seeks to be trustworthy always sends verbal and nonverbal messages that are congruent. Serious words should be paired with somber behavior. In practice, when a patient displays nonverbal behavior that does not match the words spoken, a provider may want to pursue the discrepancy for the source of some possible conflict.[5]

Culture influences communication patterns. Culture involves customs, beliefs, values, relationship patterns, prescribed behaviors (such as dress, food preferences, and time consciousness), and communication rules. It is critical for health care providers to recognize their own cultural conditioning in order to explore the impact it has on their communication with those of another cultural background.[3] Acknowledging the tacit rules of one's own culture can minimize narrow-mindedness when faced with the effects of another cultural system. Culturally competent providers have knowledge of and respect for the various cultures they encounter, and their communication patterns reflect these values. On the other hand, a lack of cultural knowledge should not prevent a provider from offering care. Too much attention to cultural differences can result in unnecessary distancing. Indeed, a dying patient from another culture will frequently welcome opportunities to talk if the conversation is carried on with sensitivity, regardless of cultural differences.[6]

The Importance of Good Communication at the End of Life

What terminally ill patients fear most are isolation and abandonment by significant others and health care providers.[7,8] Poor communication creates this separation of patients from those they need most. Indeed, most dying patients know they are dying and the need for communication with loved ones is of overwhelming importance.[9] Dying patients value being able to express feelings to loved ones, saying goodbye to people closest to them, and talking to their physicians truthfully.[10] Keeping up a front that all is well bars dying patients from speaking the truth and sharing the weight of impending death, including the burden of having to make treatment decisions alone.[11] Honest communication increases the likelihood that the dying experience will be one through which all participants can grow emotionally and spiritually.[12]

For families, when the reality of a terminal diagnosis is not acknowledged, there is more guilt, avoidance, and pretence. Relationships are more strained, and grief is more complicated. On the other hand, when what is happening is openly acknowledged, family members have more honest relationships and easier interactions with their dying loved one. They have better communication experiences with health care providers. Families are better prepared for the final death event and have better bereavement experiences.[13]

Health care providers have a responsibility to facilitate open communication with dying patients and their families. Although death is a natural, ultimately unavoidable event, many people have never experienced the death of a close friend or relative. Many people do not know how to talk about death. One of the important tasks for providers in an end-of-life setting is to identify obstacles to open communications. Some of the common barriers are discussed next.

Barriers to Good Communication

Problems in communication are common in end-of-life settings due to the stressful nature of death and dying for all involved. According to some authorities, poor communication during terminal illness causes more suffering than any other problem with the exception of uncontrolled pain.[14] Intentionally or unintentionally, barriers to honest communication about death and dying can be erected by patients and families, by health care providers, and by the structure of the health care system.

Patients and Families

Although some patients with a terminal diagnosis want to talk about life, death, and what happens after death, many find this difficult. Ideally, open discussions about thoughts and beliefs about death should occur long before a terminal illness is diagnosed.[15] However, with the fragmentation of the American family and the frequency of institutionalization of elderly persons, many people reach adulthood without ever being exposed to the practical issues surrounding the end of life. As a topic for discussion, death is often considered a taboo subject.

Dying is frequently a time of great stress. A wide variety of uncomfortable feelings, such as embarrassment, guilt, anger, and fear, can arise and inhibit open communication.[16] For some families, recalling past horrible experiences with a death can affect responses to a current situation. Common reactions are withdrawal from the patient or situation, denial of the reality of a terminal diagnosis, or avoidance behavior, such as telling jokes or changing the subject. Denial masked as hope for a cure is often used to circumvent an honest discussion of end-of-life issues.[17]

People in crisis frequently have limited abilities to express ideas, thoughts, and emotions, and often simply cannot hear what is being said to them because of the overwhelming stress of their situation. Poor sleep, fatigue, poor nutrition, and impaired concentration only exacerbate these limitations. Dying often threatens cherished beliefs, and a common protective reaction is to freeze communication.[18]

Communication can be hindered when patients or family members have a lack of understanding of what is being communicated.[19] When patients and families are not sure what they know and do not know, a sense of uncertainty can prevent them from asking clarifying questions.

Dysfunctional family patterns are as common in families dealing with a death as they are in society at large. Conflict within families can make honest communication very difficult. Also, longstanding problems with decision-making and memory, which are frequent in all health care settings, only complicate efforts at good communication.

Hierarchical role definitions can interfere with honest communication. Some patients and families are intimidated by the social position of health care providers, particularly physicians, and rather than engaging in an active conversation, may retreat inappropriately.[18] Others, sensitive to the distress of the provider in difficult conversations, may strive to avoid adding discomfort and disappointment by minimizing the display of their own emotional reactions. They may even reverse roles and struggle to meet the needs of the provider by encouraging brevity in interactions or changing the subject.[20]

Health Care Providers

Health care providers are not untouched by the general discomfort most people have when facing death. Terminal illness is seen by many as a failure, either a physician's failure or the failure of the patient or family to heed warning signs in a timely manner. Thus, guilt can impair honest communication. Fear of causing additional pain to a patient and family can also contribute to a provider choosing to avoid the topic altogether.[16]

Health care providers bring their own personal fears, anxieties, and experiences into their relationship with a dying person.[21] Being pulled out of one's own area of competence and fearing one's own emotional responses to dying can cause providers to avoid dying patients and their families. Distracting personal thoughts and feelings, frequently referred to as *personal baggage*, can intrude into a therapeutic relationship.[22]

Health care providers can become preoccupied by technology and focus all conversation and efforts on the technical aspects of care.[20] Patients and families often follow this lead, becoming very engaged in technical concerns, and avoid discussing the emotional and existential issues altogether. Legal concerns can also result in avoidance behaviors.[16]

A lack of confidence in one's own communication skills is a barrier to information sharing between health care providers and their patients.[23] Providers are more likely to initiate end-of-life discussions when they feel competent in the necessary interpersonal skills, yet many believe they have inadequate training in this area. They often feel unprepared to guide the discussion or manage the strong emotions that may emerge.[24] Providers can find themselves compensating by avoiding patients or indulging in excessive concern with maintaining routines. These behaviors close channels of communication.[17]

Health Care System

The pace of the modern health care delivery system is fast. Health care providers often feel they have inadequate time to thoughtfully engage in a profound discussion of important matters. Indeed, there may be no provider who has had a long enough relationship with a patient to feel qualified to engage in conversation about end-of-life issues.[16] In complex health settings with many providers involved, it is often unclear who is responsible for initiating and providing follow-up end-of-life conversations.

Other factors that can place a wedge in communication between health care providers and patients and families include cultural differences, as well as sometimes inexplicable interpersonal conflict.[16] Awareness of these barriers is essential, even though they are frequently not amenable to change. Structuring the sharing of information with consideration of these obstacles is the only appropriate response.

Finally, situational and physical conditions may not always be ideal for serious conversations, but attempts must be made to modify the environment as optimally as possible.[22] More will be said on this topic later.

Practical Aspects of Communicating at the End of Life

The single most important approach to good communication at the end of life is for health care providers to listen and to come to understand the patient and family.[25] Some guidelines may be helpful to achieve this end.

Understand oneself and speak honestly. For a health care provider, it is important to know oneself. Providers should acknowledge and strive to understand their own feelings, especially as they percolate up during communication with those facing death. Indeed, an increased self-awareness is a benefit of working with the dying, and is the basis for being able to speak honestly and be oneself in communication with others. It is vital to know one's own fears about death and dying, but to remember that one's own fears may not be issues for a dying patient. The key to talking with dying persons is to focus on their needs, rather than one's own.[26]

Consider the timing of communication. It is important to surrender one's own idea of what is timely.[27] Truth can be discussed openly only when individuals are ready to do so.[20] "Is this a good time to talk?" is a simple and straightforward way to determine if a patient or family member is ready to converse. Timing conversations in relation to verbal and nonverbal cues of readiness or withdrawal is important.

Provide a setting for open communication. When talking with dying persons and their families, it is important for health care providers to consider both how to arrange the environment and how to adapt their own behavior to facilitate conversation. No physical objects, such as IV stands or tables, should be located between communicants. Being seated at eye level, at about a 90-degree angle, and within hand's reach so a comforting touch can be offered are the optimal positions for serious conversations.[7,19,28] Although leaning back with arms spread out may seem to imply relaxation, it is more likely to communicate a sense of arrogance, and should be avoided. Leaning forward toward the patient or family member, with arms close to sides, is a position of attentiveness and should be adopted.[29]

Eye contact is crucial because it provides important information about the effectiveness of communication. The face will usually show quite clearly whether what has been said is being understood.[28] If possible, when talking with a dying person, a health care provider's head should at times be positioned below the patient's, so that the provider is looking up into the patient's face. Kneeling or taking a low chair next to the patient indicates that one wishes to be of service. If standing seems the only option, then positions of power, such as standing with a widespread stance, should be avoided.[29] Arms should be held close to sides, feet should be together, and chin should be down. Signs of inattention or distraction, such as glancing away, must be avoided. Using body language thoughtfully can tell others that they will not have to hurry in their communication. In reality, of course, time is a precious resource and most providers do not have large amounts of unclaimed time. Nevertheless, really important conversations can take place over very little time, often less than 15 minutes.[25]

Allow the patient to guide the communication process. As much as possible, a patient's personal autonomy and control should be preserved.[30] Using open-ended questions allows the patient to steer the discussion by offering information that they believe is most relevant. There should be no anticipation of what is to be said, but rather a sincere openness to the words being stated and emotions being revealed.[3]

Make no assumptions about what the patient knows. A patient may know much more or much less than a health care provider expects. Even patients who have not been formally told of their diagnosis may be aware that they are dying through the nonverbal behavior of others or by an inner knowledge that is hard to define.[7] On the other hand, patients may have been given vital pieces of information at times when they were unable to completely process messages, such as when they were recovering from anesthesia or after they were given pain medication.[31]

There may be times when a patient who was presumed to be informed of a terminal diagnosis seems to be unaware of it. When it is uncertain whether denial is at play, or whether a patient really does not know the implications of the illness, a patient may be asked "What did your doctor tell you about your illness?"[9,29] It is not uncommon for some patients to truly misunderstand what was told to them. All correct knowledge should be affirmed with a statement such as "That is how I see it also." Understanding a patient's perspective increases effectiveness of all communication efforts.

Ask and listen. Listen and ask. In the end-of-life setting, the most important general rule is to listen more and talk less.[25] Attentive listening requires focusing entirely on the other person and minimizing concerns about whether one is doing everything correctly. *Being with* the patient takes precedence over *doing for* the patient.

Health care providers should strive to learn about coping skills and communication styles of the patient and family. This early assessment usually involves asking a few straightforward questions, attending thoughtfully to verbal and nonverbal responses, and phrasing follow-up inquiries carefully. Yes-or-no questions are often helpful initially to broach a difficult subject.[32] Simple questions, such as "Have you ever experienced the death of a loved one before?" or "What is the most difficult thing you had to face before you became ill?", can be followed with "Can you tell me what that was like for you?" A probing and sincere "How are you feeling?" may work, but this can also elicit the perfunctory "Fine, thank you." Careful phrasing, such as "Do you feel like talking about what it is like to be seriously ill?", can facilitate conversation by both giving information and asking a question.[33] In this example the listener is invited to talk and is also made aware that they are not alone in the knowledge of a diagnosis.[34]

When it appears a patient wants to talk about death, but beginning the conversation seems difficult, describing what is observable and asking for clarification is often helpful.[26] A statement, such as, "You are very quiet. I'd like to understand what's going on with you a little better, not just physically, but on the inside too," acknowledges the possibility of inner processes occurring, and offers an opening for conversation. When nonverbal behavior indicates emotional strains, "Is this getting a bit rough on you?" is a simple question that may be followed with "Can you tell me about what is hardest for you right now?" Stating an observation, such as "I can see this is a very difficult time for you," also expresses empathy and may lead to a discussion of the profound issues at hand.[30,35]

When the patient communicates that they are ready to talk about deeper issues "What are you most proud of?" and "Who and what have you loved?" are questions that can be used to encourage the patient to look deeply into their life experience.[36] A question such as "What do you think happens to people after they die?" may reveal strong faith or great fear.

Verbalization should be encouraged by nodding the head or by affirming comments such as "Oh, I see" or "Tell me more." Attentiveness is shown with the restatement of key phrases such as "You were shocked when you heard the word cancer." Another skill, reflection, can be used to summarize what has been said, and to restate it in a way that includes the feeling aspect of the message. "So, as I am listening to you, I sense that you are very afraid that the pain will get out of control" is an example of reflecting the content of the spoken words as well as the emotional component of the message. Reflection is particularly beneficial in reducing the experience of isolation and loneliness that is common in end-of-life experiences.[3]

Attentive listening involves not interrupting others, but listening patiently until there is a pause in the conversation before speaking.[5] Interruptions have a significant impact on communication. They are a disruption of a person's speech and generally have the effect of cutting short the expression of the person's ideas. When interruptions and overtalk (the circumstance in which two people in conversation are speaking simultaneously) impair communication, the primary corrective measure is a conscious and deliberate use of silence to alter the nature of the exchange.[3]

Use understandable terms. It is very important for health care providers to translate technical medical information into understandable terms.[3,19,37] To do otherwise undermines honest communication. Many people are reluctant to admit a lack of knowledge of terminology when it is used with great ease by others. Asking patients and families "Is this making sense to you?" or "Are some things I am talking about confusing to you?" can elicit whether understanding is occurring.

Ask patients what they want. At the end of life, as much as possible, the wishes of the dying should be discerned and used to guide care. Human beings know what is best for them right up to the moment of death.[38] When a dying patient is asked "What do you wish for?", the reply may be "I wish to be well again." This should not be a stumbling block to honest communication because health care providers can respond with a statement such as "I wish you would get well again too, but now that doesn't seem likely." This response is honest and acknowledges the wishful thinking.[39]

The use of the word *now* can be helpful in identifying achievable desires. A statement such as "Tell me, is there anything you want now? I'd like to help you regain some control over your life" provides focus. The patient may want to go fishing one more time, or see a favorite relative. Dying people usually know their limitations and rarely ask for the unattainable.[39]

Use silence liberally. Silence is a valuable communication tool. Being comfortable with silence is a way of demonstrating that the patient is worthwhile whether conversation is occurring or not.[3,40] To remain nearby and relaxed, yet attentive, is a powerful statement of the value of the other person and their needs.

Silence encourages a patient to speak. It provides the opportunity for a patient to collect and organize thoughts and think through what to say next. Conversation in end-of-life settings should not be hurried. A terminal diagnosis has profound implications; time is needed to contemplate its depth and to put thoughts and feelings into words. To assume that silence means that a conversation is at its end is a rejection of the thought-processing needs of the other.

Silence communicates empathy. It indicates a willingness to hear what a patient has to say. It gives a health care provider the opportunity to enter the world of the patient and to understand it more fully. Hurried providers are often perceived as incapable of full understanding. Silent presence can offer more comfort than words; it is a sign of true caring. A sincere smile, a touch on the arm, or a moment of hand-holding can transmit great comfort and a sense of connection. Rich communication can occur in silence.

Silence also allows for assessment of the patient's condition. Both verbal and nonverbal behaviors can be thoughtfully assessed during periods of silence. Inconsistencies between verbal and nonverbal language or evidence of uncomfortable emotions can be noted.

Silence permits time for self-reflection. It allows one to observe oneself in the context of patient encounters, especially when the use of silence becomes a standard part of a health care provider's communication style. Providers have the opportunity to ask themselves "How do I feel about what is being said?", "How am I reacting to what this patient is saying?", and "What is the most important thing for me to communicate right now?" Such use of silence goes a long way to improving the quality of interpersonal communication between providers and patients.[3]

Support varying emotional responses. Patients and families will vary in their emotional responses to the end of life. Much of this has to do with culture, family history, and individual personality characteristics.[19] It is important to provide reassurance that people react differently to the end-of-life experience and that feelings being experienced are neither wrong nor abnormal. Emotions may be intensely expressed or equally suppressed. They can range from numbness and depression to anger and frustration. Acceptance of feelings and a continuing presence provide affirmation of the validity of the emotions being felt.[31]

When a patient expresses fear of pain and suffering at the end of life, it is very important to emphasize how vigilant and active the health care team will be in managing uncomfortable symptoms throughout the dying process. Many questions about death are unanswerable, and dying patients do not expect a health care provider to have all the answers. Dying patients do, however, require honest communication and support and, above all, a willingness to listen and help when possible.[26]

Accept denial, usually. Denial is a very powerful coping mechanism that shields people from terrifying or painful information until they can better deal with it.[26] Health care providers may have to balance what is known to be true about a patient's illness with what the patient is ready to accept.[20] Denial is indicated when there is incongruence between verbal and nonverbal behavior. Repeating back cue words, such as *only* or *a little*, communicates to a patient that the provider is detecting a mixed message.[5] Support can be given to patients in denial by acknowledging the validity of their feelings. If a cancer patient talks about hiking in the mountains to regain their strength, for example, a provider can respond, "Yes, the mountains are so wonderful. I can tell that hiking in them is very special for you." Sometimes this simple affirmation is all that is needed. At other times, it may be appropriate to respond with an informative comment that the disease process will likely not be reversible and that increasing weakness is going to be the rule.

Some patients live with denial as their main defense from reality, yet this denial prevents them from being able to share their burdens. Denial can become dysfunctional, such as when it interferes with determining patient wishes and values at a critical time. When clinical decisions must be made, the advantages of maintaining denial are often outweighed by the information needs of the decision-makers. For example, whether CPR is desired or not requires honest communication. Does the patient value a peaceful death, or is CPR, a procedure typically incompatible with a peaceful death, desired?[41] Sometimes a patient's denial forces upon relatives the painful responsibility of making end-of-life decisions without knowing what the patient wants.[15] Furthermore, denial deprives patients of the opportunity to work on issues of life closure, a process most people value highly. Nevertheless, if denial is in place it should be respected unless there is clear evidence of the advantages of breaking down this defense mechanism. Indeed, in certain circumstances, a person may have a legitimate need to deny death to the very end.[42]

Accept symbolic language. Often, as the end of life draws near, a patient's communications become less literal and more symbolic.[43] A person may speak about death veiled in such terms as an anticipated journey. A deep but otherwise unspoken need may be asked for with symbolic words such as "Do you have the keys? I need the keys to heaven." Trains, boats, maps, and doorways are common images dying persons use in describing the next stage of their life journey.[44] A patient may recognize every person in the room, but may also refer to events, objects, or people that are clearly imaginary to everyone else in the room. Dreams are often experienced as real external events, and patients often go into great detail with descriptions of unusual people and places.

This increase in symbolic communication can cause discomfort in family members and sometimes even health care providers. Even a strongly supportive family environment can weaken when a patient begins to speak in terms that make no sense to others.[43] Relatives and others should be told that such dream images and visionary activity are common at the end of life. Providers should model appropriate supportive behavior toward the patient.

Providing emotional support to dying patients who are communicating symbolically requires the assumption that the symbolic communications are meaningful.[43] Logical responses are usually unhelpful, but the emotional content of the communication should receive attention. For example, when a patient reports having unique but pleasant visitors in the room, health care providers can model supportive communication skills by referring to the characteristics of the unseen visitors, as described by the patient, and the feelings with which the patient describes the encounter. A reflection such as "Those ladies with long gloves and leather hats are making you smile" is appropriate. Maintaining contact through presence, continued listening, and affirmation of the patient's experiences are ways to provide effective emotional support.[43] Providers can encourage loved ones to share in some of the mystery seen at the end of life.

A dying person may want to have a deep conversation in metaphorical terms. In such situations, sensitive health care providers listen with the ear of metaphor and speak with metaphor.[44] Asking, "The keys you speak about, can you tell me about these keys?", invites the patient to reveal the meaning of the symbolism. Acceptance of what the patient says is important, but providers should not be afraid to admit when they do not understand. Statements such as "I think you are telling me something important, but I am not understanding. Can you help me understand?" can encourage the patient to progress into a discussion of something less abstract, although patients often prefer to remain safe behind the veil of mysterious images.[45]

Encourage patients to tell their life stories. People telling their own life stories are transformed into active interpreters of their lives.[18] Reflecting on and telling one's life story to loved ones have therapeutic and integrative effects, especially among those who are dying. Some maintain that encouraging life review and storytelling are among the most important services that family members or health care providers can offer a dying person.[26] Feelings of satisfaction often arise when a dying person reminisces about their life. Remembering accomplishments and significant events, sharing family stories, reflecting on important friendships, and even reflecting on significant losses and failures, all help the dying person attain perspective and sometimes relieve emotional pain that has been stored for years. Communicating stories with family members can build bridges of healing and increase a sense of belonging, of being loved by others, and of loving oneself at the end of life. Emotional well-being may be enhanced, and loneliness and sadness, which often accompany the dying process, may be diminished. Inner peace may be attained if life has been well lived. On the other hand, the dying process can be filled with utter anguish if life has been lived with selfish and abusive actions. In circumstances such as these, it may be helpful, if possible, for the individual to acknowledge mistakes made along the way and to ask forgiveness from those who were injured. Some way to take care of unfinished business may be discovered.

Tell people what to expect. Many people have an inadequate knowledge of the dying process.[15] End-of-life care includes communicating factual information about the signs of approaching death. Patients and loved ones both may have questions. Interested persons should be told, in as much detail as they desire, the common signs of approaching death, such as decreased need for food and drink, increased time spent sleeping, increasing confusion, cooling and darkening of arms and legs, urine and bowel incontinence, and irregular and moist-sounding breathing. Written materials supplementing the discussion of the dying process can be helpful and are often appreciated by families.

At the very end of life, assume hearing is still intact. The practice of continuing to converse with a dying individual after they have entered an unconscious state assumes that an unconscious person remains available as an experiencing being, although their world is now an inner world unknown to others.[43] Families should be told that the sense of hearing usually remains intact the longest in the dying process. Words such as "I love you," "I forgive you," and "Goodbye" can still be spoken. Friends and relatives should be encouraged to communicate at this precious time.

Breaking Bad News

All of the communication skills discussed above apply to the very difficult task of breaking bad news.[23] Simply stated, there is no easy way of telling a person that their life is coming to an end. No matter how skillful a health care provider is, the news will almost certainly cause sadness for patients and their significant others.[33] For the health care provider who must break the bad news, factors that add to the distress of the situation include fear of being blamed for the bad news, fear of not knowing all the answers, fear of showing emotion, and fear of being reminded of one's own mortality.[23]

Although it has traditionally been the physician's responsibility to share with the patient the implications of a fatal diagnosis, it is advantageous for all health care providers to have an understanding of how to share bad news. Nurses and other health care providers are frequently in the position of explaining, clarifying, and reinforcing the physician's message.[23] It is helpful to be present when the bad news is initially shared, but this is only occasionally possible. The next best arrangement is the interdisciplinary team setting where the various health care team members can share information and thereby offer consistency in their communications with patients, families, and others.[46]

When bad news is to be shared, a meeting should be scheduled without delay and at a time when important support persons are available. Ideally, all parties should be rested so that fatigue is not a factor. All participants should be known to each other, but if not, introductions should be provided and relationships identified. The issue of confidentiality is crucial and the patient should be asked explicitly if there are specific individuals who should be present to share information about condition and prognosis at this time.[31] The patient has the right to change who is included at any time.

The physical setting should be quiet and private. Televisions, radios, cell phones, and pagers should be turned off. As mentioned previously, eye contact is crucial and is more likely to be maintained if all parties are seated at the same level. Physical barriers such as tables or beds should not separate communicants. Seating arrangements should be close enough so that the bearer of the news can extend a comforting touch to the patient's shoulder or hand.

"I'm afraid I have bad news" is a simple but effective way to begin the job of giving painful information.[19] This approach gives the listener a moment to prepare for the distressing information. Next, the purpose of the interview should be explained with a statement such as "I have received the report of your most recent tests, and the results don't show what we had hoped." Using the word *we* is intentional; it transmits the message that the patient is not unaccompanied in their situation. Following up with "How much do you want to know?" allows the patient to have some control.[47] No assumptions should be made about the reply. Although there are overwhelming benefits of an open awareness of the meaning of a terminal diagnosis, it must also be recognized that not all patients will want full information. Some people want to know everything, and others will have difficulty with just minimal information.

Being sensitive to how much detailed information can be understood is essential. Often people are unable to hear anything more after a first piece of bad news is uttered. The stress they are feeling simply limits their comprehension. The listener's face can be revealing. A glazed look usually means the patient is no longer listening.[28] It may be helpful to say "It is common for people to say that after being told bad news, they hardly hear another word. How are you doing?" Information frequently needs to be repeated. Affirmation that one is being understood should be sought by asking "Am I making sense to you?" or "Can I rephrase something to make it more understandable?"[31]

The scene should avoid seeming to be rushed or routine. Nonverbal responses should be continually assessed, and emotional support provided.

Simple gestures, such as offering a cup of water or a box of tissues, provide comfort. The promise not to abandon the patient, but to continue to provide service, or to arrange for service by others as appropriate, should be made. The patient and family must be given time to listen, reflect, and ask questions. If necessary, a break in the discussion may be offered with the assurance that the conversation will be continued.[9,21]

There are times when keeping the truth of a terminal diagnosis from a patient may seem to be protective, but this initial benefit usually dissipates in light of the long-term consequences, which can be devastating. The progressive nature of terminal illnesses almost inevitably leads to an increased awareness of decline on the part of the patient. When the patient uncovers deceit, the loss of trust can never be fully restored. Purposefully withholding information ultimately points to an underlying intent to manipulate a patient. It takes away a patient's autonomy and, once the practice of collusion begins, the withholders of information must continue on an endless path of fabrication and lies.[33]

According to legal precedents, competent patients must be informed of the nature of their illness.[23,31] Although the interests of the patient are primary, health care providers cannot simply disregard other family members involved. It is not uncommon for relatives to have powerful needs (emotional, legal, or otherwise) that influence what information they want given to a patient. When a family requests that a terminal diagnosis be withheld from a patient, the implications and likely effects of failing to be open and honest should be described for the family. The call to collude with a family should be challenged.[30]

There are many uncertainties with every patient's prognosis. Life is a mystery, and no one knows precisely what the next hour will bring. Yet these uncertainties should not prevent health care providers from communicating honestly. When a patient asks "How long do I have to live?" or "What will happen next?", the provider can reply "I can't tell you for certain what will happen to you, but I can tell you what has happened in the lives of others who had the same diagnosis as you have." It is not dishonest to have incomplete knowledge and to communicate these limitations.[26]

Emotional reactions should be recognized and validated. Denial is often the first stage in the process of adjusting to a loss, and it should be respected, especially in the short term.[5] If emotions are openly hostile, a supportive reply, such as "I know this news can make you angry, but I want to help," can be useful.[19] If the news is taken very calmly, it may have been anticipated. The patient and family may be prepared for it, or even feel relieved of the distress of uncertainty. Others may be very calm because they are shocked into passivity or do not understand the implications of what has been said. A statement, such as "You are taking this very calmly, but people are different in how they respond to bad news," may elicit an explanatory comment.[19] Of course, emotional displays that run the whole gamut of human behavior are possible.

A frequent complaint by those who have been given bad news is that it is often done in such a way that it leaves them without any sense of hope.[23] In almost any conversation that gives bad news there should be at least a glimmer of a smile at some point.[28] A sincere smile is supportive and friendly and provides a sense of warmth, concern, and empathy that is vital at this time. Helpful resources for emotional and spiritual care should be recommended. As the conversation winds down, patient and family strengths should be identified. It is important to not underestimate inner resources.[33]

Ideally the bearer of bad news should sit with a patient or family for these purposes, although this is not always possible. For example, when a patient dies without a relative at the bedside, it is standard practice for a health care provider, usually a nurse, to notify the significant other by telephone as soon as possible. When bad news must be given by telephone, the caller should initially give their name and state their professional role. The relationship of the person answering the telephone should be determined next because the appropriate person must be notified first. The provider should describe his or her relationship to the patient. Speaking slowly and carefully is essential, especially when the hour is late and fatigue is a factor. A forewarning of the news to come, such as "I am saddened to bring you bad news," should be spoken. This gives the listener a moment to prepare. In sharing the news of a death, the phrase *has died* is gentler than *is dead*.[31] The provider should offer to contact other family members or another supportive person so the listener does not have to move into action immediately, especially if the news has shocked or numbed. Sometimes in a panic the listener will hang up the telephone abruptly after the first words of the message are given. In this case, the caller should wait a few minutes before another call is attempted. This gives the significant other a few moments to adjust. Because observation of nonverbal behavior is not possible during a telephone call, a provider is limited in what can be perceived and what can be done to support the listener. For this reason, breaking bad news by way of the telephone is not the preferred approach. Nevertheless when it must be done, planning what is to be said and careful wording of the message can minimize the trauma of the experience.

Assessing for Suicide Potential

Among the skills requisite for end-of-life care is the ability to identify depression and assess for suicide potential. Depression is common in terminal illness, and some authorities maintain that the worst part of a terminal illness, even harder than fighting the disease, is depression.[10] A heightened suicide risk is associated with a terminal diagnosis.[7]

The patient who is thinking about suicide may express this in a verbal way, a nonverbal way, or a combination of both. A depressed, suicidal patient may say "I just don't see any point in prolonging my life" or "Everyone would be better off with me dead anyway." The general appearance of depression is typically one of sadness, resignation, apathy, and hopelessness.[7] Sometimes, however, when the act of suicide has been decided on, a depressed patient will suddenly appear cheerful for having made a decision to end the suffering. Health care providers are encouraged to talk about suicide with someone whom they suspect may be thinking about ending their life.[48] Talking about suicide does not encourage commitment of the act. In some cases a patient may obtain relief through the acknowledgement of the depth of anguish being experienced.[7]

A simple question, "Are you depressed most of the day, nearly every day?", is the best predictor of a clinical diagnosis of depression.[49] Likewise, for assessment of suicide potential, a direct approach is recommended. Asking "Have things gotten so bad that you are thinking about killing yourself?" gives the patient permission to talk openly.[48] If the patient answers affirmatively, encouraging the patient to speak further can reveal sources of depression and suicidal thoughts, such as uncontrolled pain or fear of abandonment. In response, discussion of alternatives to improve quality of life and acquisition of supportive physical, emotional, and spiritual care are imperative. If it is determined through direct questioning that an actual plan for carrying out the suicide is made, then there is a higher likelihood that suicide will occur. An immediate call for additional support is warranted.[48]

Summary

The value of open and honest communication at the end of life is hard to overestimate. Everyone engaged in such communication benefits. Effective communication in end-of-life care can be achieved through thoughtful application of universal principles of interpersonal communication: that communication is multidimensional, continuous, and inevitable, and that perception is selective and varies widely depending on personal, cultural, and situational variables. The practical skills of communication in end-of-life settings have been discussed in this chapter, including special attention to the difficult task of breaking bad news and assessing for suicide potential.

The reader is encouraged to enter into the rewarding realm of effective communication with dying patients. The personal growth that can occur at the end of life is experienced not only by dying patients and their loved ones, but by health care providers, too. Although there is a responsibility to communicate effectively, providers soon discover that communicating with dying patients is also a privilege.

References

1. Gunther, J. *Death Be Not Proud.* New York: HarperCollins, 1949.
2. Llewelyn, S., and Fielding, G. "Am I Dying, Nurse? Care of the Terminally Ill Patient." *Nursing Mirror,* 156(16):30–31, 1983.

3. van Servellen, G. *Communication Skills for the Health Care Professional: Concepts and Techniques.* Gaithersburg, Md.: Aspen Publishers, Inc., 1997.
4. Ivey, A., and Ivey, M. *Intentional Interviewing & Counseling: Facilitating Client Development in a Multicultural Society.* Pacific Grove, Calif.: Brooks/Cole, 1999.
5. Davidhizar, R.. and Giger, J. "Patients' Use of Denial: Coping with the Unacceptable." *Nursing Standard,* 12(43):44–46, 1998.
6. Becker, R. "Teaching Communication with the Dying Across Cultural Boundaries." *British Journal of Nursing,* 8(14):938–942, 1999.
7. Braverman, G. "Eliciting Assessment Data from the Patient Who Is Difficult to Interview." *Nursing Clinics of North America,* 25(4):743–750, 1990.
8. Tucker, P. "Communication Improves Care for Terminally Ill Residents." *Provider,* 18(2):42, 1992.
9. Farrar, A. "How Much Do They Want to Know?: Communicating with Dying Patients" *Professional Nurse,* 7(9):606–610, 1992.
10. Greisinger, A., Lorimor, R., Aday, L., Winn, R., and Baile, W. "Terminally Ill Cancer Patients: Their Most Important Concerns." *Cancer Practice,* 5(3):147–154, 1997.
11. Singer, P., Martin, D., and Kelner, M. "Quality End-of-Life: Patients' Perspectives." *JAMA,* 281(2):163–168, 1999.
12. Durham, E., and Weiss, L. "How Patients Die." *American Journal of Nursing,* 97(12):41–46, 1997.
13. Field, D., and Copp, G. "Communication and Awareness About Dying in the 1990s." *Palliative Medicine,* 13(6):459–468, 1999.
14. Wist, E. "Teaching Communication with Cancer Patients and Terminally Ill Patients to Medical Students." *Journal of Cancer Education,* 8(2):119–122, 1993.
15. Herbst, L., Lynn, J., Mermann, A., and Rhymes, J. "What Do Dying Patients Want and Need?" *Patient Care,* 29(4):27–35, 1995.
16. Larson, D., and Tobin, D. "End-of-Life Conversations: Evolving Practice and Theory." *JAMA,* 284(12):1573–1578, 2000.
17. Parry, J. "The Significance of Open Communication in Working with Terminally Ill Clients." *The Hospice Journal,* 3(4):33–49, 1987.
18. Attig, T. "Can We Talk? On the Elusiveness of Dialogue." *Death Studies,* 19(1):1–19, 1995.
19. Campbell, M. "Breaking Bad News to Patients." *JAMA,* 271(13):1052, 1994.
20. Zerwekh, J. "The Truth-Tellers: How Hospice Nurses Help Patients Confront Death." *American Journal of Nursing,* 94(2):31–34, 1994.
21. Lloyd, A. "Stop, Look and Listen." *Nursing Times,* 87(12):30–32, 1991.
22. Stevens, R., and Katsekas, B. "Being with People in Difficult Times." *Home Healthcare Nurse,* 17(8):504–509, 1999.
23. Farrell, M. "The Challenge of Breaking Bad News." *Intensive and Critical Care Nursing,* 15(2):101–110, 1999.
24. McGrath, P., Yates, P., Clinton, M., and Hart, G. "'What Should I Say?': Qualitative Findings on Dilemmas in Palliative Care Nursing." *The Hospice Journal,* 14(2):17–33, 1999.
25. Lynn, J. "An 88-Year-Old Woman Facing the End of Life." *JAMA,* 277(20):1633–1640, 1997.
26. Brady, E. "Stories at the Hour of Our Death." *Home Healthcare Nurse,* 17(3):176–180, 1999.
26. Callanan, M. "Breaking the Silence." *American Journal of Nursing,* 94(1):22–23, 1994.
27. Hinshaw, S. "All in Good Time." *Nursing,* 29(9):88, 1999.
28. Brewin, T. "Three Ways of Giving Bad News." *Lancet,* 337:1207–1209, 1991.

29. Ray, M. "Seven Ways to Empower Dying Patients." *American Journal of Nursing,* 96(5):56–57, 1996.

30. Woods, S. "Ethics and Communication: Developing Reflective Practice." *Nursing Standard,* 12(18):44–47, 1998.

31. Creagan, E. "How to Break Bad News: And Not Devastate the Patient." *Mayo Clinic Proceedings,* 69(10):1015–1017, 1994.

32. Brown, M. "Lifting the Burden of Silence." *American Journal of Nursing,* 94(9):62–63, 1994.

33. Kendrick, D., and Kinsella, M. "Beyond the Veil: Truth Telling in Palliative Care." *Journal of Cancer Care,* 3(4):211–214, 1994.

34. Ufema, J. "Death and Dying. Keep on Scrappin'." *Nursing,* 29(12):26, 1999.

35. Ufema, J. "Insights on Death and Dying. Communication: Collections of a Lifetime." *Nursing,* 31(2):22, 2001.

36. Ufema, J. "Insights on Death and Dying. Communication: Favorite Things." *Nursing,* 29(3):26, 1999.

37. Puopolo, A. "Gaining Confidence to Talk About End-of-Life Care." *Nursing,* 29(7):49–51, 1999.

38. Ufema, J. "Reflections on Death and Dying." *Nursing,* 29(6):56-59, 1999.

39. Ufema, J. "Insights on Death and Dying. Patients' Requests. Afraid to Ask." *Nursing,* 26(12):31, 1996.

40. Donaldson, D. "Effective Ways to Communicate with the Dying." *Caring,* 18(2):18, 1999.

41. Quill, T. "Initiating End-of-Life Discussions with Seriously Ill Patients: Addressing the 'Elephant in the Room.'" *JAMA,* 284(19):2502–2507, 2000.

42. Smith, D. "The Terminally Ill Patient's Right to Be in Denial." *Omega,* 27(2):115–121, 1993.

43. Dugan, D. "Symbolic Expressions of Dying Patients: Communications, Not Hallucinations." *Nursing Forum,* 24(2):18–27, 1989

44. Hutchings, D. "Communicating with Metaphors: A Dance with Many Veils." *American Journal of Hospice and Palliative Care,* 15(5):282–284, 1998.

45. Callanan, M. "Farewell Messages." *American Journal of Nursing,* 94(5):19–20, 1994.

46. Linkewich, B., Setliff, A., Poling, M., Bailey, S., Sellick, S., and Kelley, M. "Communicating at Life's End." *Canadian Nurse,* 95(5):41–44, 1999.

47. Ufema, J. "Insights on Death and Dying. Truth Telling: I Don't Want to Know!" *Nursing,* 28(3):22, 1998.

48. Ferdinand, R. "I'd Rather Die Than Live This Way." *American Journal of Nursing,* 95(12):42–47, 1995.

49. News in Mental Health Nursing. "Just Ask!" *Journal of Psychosocial Nursing,* 35(7):10, 1997.

Ethical Issues in Hospice Care

7

David Barnard

Health care is essentially a moral enterprise. Every clinical encounter is influenced by the personal and cultural values of both the patient and the provider, the moral traditions of the health professions, and the social and political contexts of the health care system. Many of the ethical issues that arise in the care of the dying, therefore, are similar to issues that arise in many other areas of health care: truthfulness and confidentiality, decision-making authority in the professional-patient relationship, and the appropriate use and allocation of technology and other health care resources. Other issues are more commonly associated with the care of the terminally ill, although they are not absent from other arenas—decisions to withhold or withdraw life-sustaining treatment; decision making for patients who have lost their own decision-making capacity; requests for assistance in suicide or active euthanasia.

Two other factors assure the need for moral reflection in palliative care. First, most professionals who enter the field do so because they want to help people die well. But what does it mean to "die well"? What is a "good death"? There is no single, universal answer to these questions. Even with respect to elements of a "good death" on which most people could probably agree—freedom from pain, resolution of personal affairs, the supportive presence of loved ones—there is room for considerable personal variation. People differ in how they balance pain relief against alertness; in their willingness to face the reality of their imminent death; in their desire to talk about their feelings to friends, family, or caregivers; and in their willingness to tolerate increasing weakness, dependency, and uncertainty rather than trying to control the timing and manner of their death through an act of suicide or euthanasia. This variability requires health professionals to approach patients and families as individuals, and attempt to provide care that is consistent both with patient and family values and with their own conscience.[1] Second, the approach of death and loss is profoundly stressful for patients, families, and caregivers. And yet, in this atmosphere of stress, anxiety, fear, and grief, decisions must continually be made about complex matters of pain and symptom control, the use of diagnostic tests, how much to tell whom about what, and so on. Clarity about the moral dimensions of these decisions, and about the factors one ought to take into account, can be of great help to all involved.

In addition to the volume by Randall and Downie cited above, the *Journal of Palliative Care* devoted two special thematic issues to ethics in palliative care, in Volume 10, Numbers 2 and 3, 1994. A chapter of this size cannot address all of these topics. Rather, it emphasizes issues that are most likely to arise in everyday practice. Discussion of these topics will emphasize ethical and clinical considerations that apply to other issues as well.

Expectations of Patients, Family, and Team

Palliative care is appropriate when a patient's disease is no longer amenable to cure, when the burdens of life-prolonging treatments appear to outweigh their benefits, and when maximizing the patient's comfort and quality of life takes precedence over other objectives. Ideally, a patient's or family's decision to enter hospice care is the result of an open, deliberate decision-making process in which the goals and expectations of patient, family, and professional team are closely matched. Unfortunately, this is not always the case. Some patients may be referred to hospice without adequate preparation by the referring physician. Sometimes the referring physician will have provided a full explanation of the limitations of curative treatment and the options for palliative care, but the patient's or family's denial will have prevented the physician's message from getting through. Sometimes expectations are unclear because the patient's clinical status is unclear. The distinction between acute, curative care, and palliative care is not always obvious. The transition from curative to palliative goals is often a gradual process, full of clinical uncertainty and ambivalence on both sides of the professional-patient relationship.[2]

For all of these reasons, it is important to assess and clarify goals and expectations from the very beginning of the relationship between the patient, family, and hospice team. The team needs to know as much as possible about the patient's previous clinical course, and equally important, *what the patient and family have been told*, and *what they appear to understand* about that course. Medical records are often seriously deficient in recording the details and nuances of a patient's understanding of his or her disease. The cursory notation, "Patient and family educated about the situation," can mask a host of ambiguities and distortions. These problems are less likely to occur if the hospice team has been following the patient on a consultative basis for a period of time before taking full clinical responsibility for the patient, but this situation is relatively rare. More often the team will need to familiarize itself with the patient's situation on short notice, and clear communication with the referring physician is essential. The new relationship between the hospice team and the patient and family is most likely to get off on the right foot when ambiguities in the patient's understanding are identified and clarified as soon as possible.

Even when the philosophy and goals of hospice and palliative care are generally understood and accepted, however, divergent expectations can emerge in interactions with the patient or family around a number of specific issues. Two of the most common are the communication of information about the patient's condition—to the family or to the patient him- or herself—and the management of pain, especially with narcotic analgesics.

Communication of Information

Open and forthright communication about diagnostic and prognostic information has become a widely accepted norm in health care over the past thirty years. This contrasts with a more paternalistic past in which communication about "bad news" was routinely avoided in order to protect patients from the distressing impact of such information. There is now a greater understanding that deception and the "conspiracy of silence" are likely to cause more harm to the patient and family than the information itself. As a result, discussions of truth telling in health care have shifted from the question of *whether* to disclose bad news to the questions of *how, when, to whom,* and *how often* to disclose it.[3,4]

Nevertheless, even in the hospice and palliative care setting, where open acknowledgment of dying, death, and grief is regarded as a cardinal virtue, the team is occasionally faced with conflicts over the issue of truthfulness and information control. They may encounter families who insist that information regarding diagnosis or prognosis be withheld from the patient, or, conversely, patients who demand that their relatives not be told the truth about their condition.[5] The latter situation has become more common in the case of patients who are dying of AIDS.

In responding to patients or family members who insist that information be withheld from others who, in the judgment of the team, ought to have that information, it is important to remember the *individuality* of patients and families. Pat answers or doctrinaire moralizing are inappropriate. Each request or demand should be treated sympathetically and with respect, but each should also be assessed thoroughly. Why does the family member, for example, believe that the patient should not be given more information about her or his situation? What *specific harms* does the family member foresee as consequences of more open communication? Is there any evidence from the past that supports the family member's concerns? Questions such as these, asked in a sympathetic and understanding manner, may elicit valuable information, including greater awareness of cultural factors that should indeed be taken into account in communicating with the patient. More commonly, these questions will give the team the opportunity to allay the family members' own anxieties and open the way to freer communication with the patient.

The team can recount that in their wide experience, patients typically understand more of the truth of their situation than family members suspect; that restricted communication and conspiracies of silence tend to increase the patient's sense of isolation at the very time connectedness and intimacy are most important; and that the relief that comes from mutual recognition of the patient's situation can lead to very meaningful family interactions, and can contribute to the family's ability to make the most of the time they have left together.[6,7,8] Finally, the team can offer to help with communication by being present at key moments, or by taking the lead in introducing a difficult topic. A similar, individualized approach should be taken with patients who request that information about their condition be withheld from family members.

Communication of information about illness and prognosis is a *process.* It is not a once and done event. Patients and families move in and out of direct awareness of threatening information. Periods of denial can be protective, allowing threatening information to be absorbed gradually.[9,10,11] Conversations will likely have to be repeated several times. Similarly, a family member or a patient who initially insists that information be withheld may change his or her position as time goes by. This is another reason not to respond confrontationally to the initial request: to preserve a supportive relationship that can facilitate change over time.

Pain Management

Particularly in the management of patients at home, patient or family attitudes toward the use of narcotic analgesics can be a source of frustration and ethical concern for the hospice team. Patient stoicism, fears of addiction, fear that admitting to pain means admitting that the disease has progressed, or reluctance to tolerate side effects can all lead patients or families to resist analgesic medications, leaving the patient in pain. As in the case of communication of information, a sympathetic assessment of patient and family concerns is the best course to follow at the outset.

The team can address misconceptions about addiction. Medication, dosage, or route of administration can be adjusted to minimize side effects.[12] It is important to ascertain the patient's own preferences regarding the trade-off between drowsiness and pain relief—a common issue in the use of opioids. Although the goal is maximum pain control *and* maximum alertness, some balancing is usually necessary, and the patient is the person who should—if he or she is able—strike the balance for him- or herself.

More difficult problems arise in cases where patients depend on family members to receive their pain medications, and the family is withholding the medication for reasons of their own. Such patients may be excellent candidates for continuous subcutaneous analgesia—via a portable syringe driver—

to obviate the need for family member involvement in the administration of the medication. Yet some family members may refuse to allow the syringe driver to be applied, again out of fear that this would be a sign of advancing disease, or out of frustration at losing control of yet one more aspect of the patient's care.

In these situations, which fortunately are infrequent, the family members' anxieties and concerns need to be addressed sympathetically and directly. Often, simply giving the family member an opportunity to ventilate fears and frustrations leads to a greater spirit of cooperation in the management of the patient's pain. In other cases it may be useful to admit the patient for a period of inpatient care (if appropriate facilities are available). This can serve at least two important purposes. First, it allows the team more direct observation and control of the patient's experience of pain. Second, it provides the family with respite from the heavy demands of caregiving. This may be crucial in allowing the family to face the patient's situation more realistically, and help them participate more constructively in the patient's care, when and if he or she returns home.

There are rare and extreme situations in which the hospice team believes a nonautonomous, dependent patient is suffering extreme pain because of family members' inability or unwillingness to cooperate in pain management. In such situations more drastic and forceful interventions may have to be considered. These may include invoking abuse and neglect statutes under state law, institutionalization of the patient, and judicial appointment of a guardian for the purposes of accepting recommended medical treatment. Because such measures are so intrusive and adversarial, however, and introduce the impersonal mechanisms of the court system into the deeply personal and intimate context of a family's encounter with death, they should be considered a last, desperate resort. They may have a limited role, but only when all other measures have failed, and the risks of grave harm to the patient seem otherwise unavoidable.

General Considerations in Managing Conflicting Expectations among Patients, Families, and Team

Communication and pain management are but two of a variety of issues around which patients, families, and hospice and palliative care teams can experience conflicting expectations. Other important issues that cannot be thoroughly discussed for reasons of space include expectations regarding how aggressively to diagnose or treat problems that arise in the terminal phase (e.g., dyspnea, dysphagia, anorexia, renal insufficiency, bowel obstruction, or fever). Even where all agree that the patient's comfort is the chief concern, rather than prolongation of life, there is room for uncertainty about the appropriate response to these problems in particular situations. As in each of the preceding sections, a sympathetic, individualized approach is indicated in response to patient or family inquiries about available interventions. It is important to avoid simply falling back on sweeping statements such as, "We don't do that in palliative care," or "That would be inconsistent with the goals of hospice," without a careful assessment of the individual circumstances and the motivations behind the inquiry.[13,14]

Individualized care and sympathetic responses to patients and families are the most important general considerations in managing and minimizing conflicting expectations. There are several other points to keep in mind as well.

First, in evaluating and responding to family expectations, it is essential to remember the family's crucial roles in the patient's care. The family provides emotional support, participates in shared decision making, performs much of the concrete caretaking, absorbs social and financial costs associated with the care of a dying family member, and works hard to maintain a sense of stability in the midst of change.[15] This list reveals how much the team depends on the family in achieving its own professional goals, and thus how important it is to maintain strong and positive relationships between the family and the team.

Second, when confronting expectations on the part of patients or family members that appear to conflict with the goals of palliative care, it is important to ask, *what are the origins of these expectations?* Are they, for example, indicators of patient or family denial, or have the patient and family been misled or confused by their care providers? Are seemingly inappropriate expectations the result of misunderstandings that are amenable to educational efforts, or signs of severe family stress or psychopathology that require more intensive psychological intervention?

Third, in the face of seemingly intractable conflict, there are often additional resources that can be brought to bear. For example, friends, other family members, or clergy can frequently play significant roles in resolving apparent impasses between family, patient, and team. In institutional settings, a hospital ethics committee can play a useful role in clarifying medical facts, permitting the ventilation of strong feelings, and exploring a range of options.

In summary, whatever the issue, setting, or combination of team members, family, and patient who are involved, open communication and mutual respect are the hallmarks of successful resolution of conflicting expectations in hospice and palliative care. This has been well expressed by Lederberg, who writes:

> When all is said and done, it cannot be overemphasized that the mainstay of management is the implementation of unhurried friendly discussions conducted in a spirit of open inquiry and genuine respect to encourage better communication between the principal parties.[16]

Advance Directives

General Background

There is now a strong societal and professional consensus in favor of patient self-determination in health care decision making, including decisions at the end of life. This consensus, which is reflected in legislation, judicial decisions, and official statements of professional societies and bioethics commissions, recognizes the right of competent adult patients to refuse or discontinue life-sustaining medical treatments.[17,18,19,20,21] Although little controversy remains regarding the rights of competent patients who can communicate their preferences directly, extending these rights to patients who have lost decision-making capacity, or who can no longer communicate, continues to present difficulties.

Traditionally, health care decisions for nonautonomous patients have been made by physicians according to their best medical judgment, with varying degrees of consultation with the patient's family. Particularly since the 1960s, there has been growing concern that decisions made on this basis were leading to overtreatment of critically ill patients, subjecting them to prolonged dying in inappropriate, acute-care, high-technology settings. These same concerns were instrumental in the growth of the modern hospice movement. The answer to this problem was to give a greater role to the patient in these decisions, and to extend that role to the nonautonomous patient in the form of a written document containing his or her treatment preferences in the case of terminal illness.

Terms such as "advance directive," "living will," "health care proxy," and "durable power of attorney for health care" often are used interchangeably to refer to any document that is designed to permit a nonautonomous patient to direct his or her medical care at the end of life. Such documents are of two broad types. The first records the patient's specific preferences for treatment or nontreatment in various clinical situations. Treatments addressed most frequently are cardiopulmonary resuscitation, antibiotics for infection, blood transfusions, kidney dialysis, and artificial nutrition and hydration. The second type authorizes another person to speak for the nonautonomous patient at the time decisions actually have to be made. This document may or may not include the patient's specific preferences. Its chief virtue is that it empowers someone to make decisions on the patient's behalf on the basis of the actual medical circumstances that have arisen, rather than relying on preferences that the patient expressed in the past, when all of the medical circumstances were hypothetical.

In the United States, the public's awareness of the potential importance of advance directives was dramatically heightened by the publicity surrounding the case of Nancy Cruzan, a young woman whose parents had been prohibited by the Missouri Supreme Court from discontinuing life supports for her, even though she had been in a persistent vegetative state for seven years. The court's reasoning, which was upheld in 1990 by the U.S. Supreme Court, was that there was insufficient evidence that the parents' desire to discontinue treatment was in accord with what Nancy herself would have wanted.[22]

Also in 1990, the U.S. Congress passed the Patient Self-Determination Act (PSDA). Effective since December 1, 1991, the PSDA requires health care institutions to inform all patients upon admission of their rights under state law to provide instructions regarding their medical treatment, their rights to refuse treatment, and their right to formulate advance directives.

Despite these influences, a growing body of empirical research has demonstrated that advance directives have had only a limited effect on health care decision making near the end of life. In part this is due to the small percentage of the population that has formulated an advance directive. Even among patients who have them, a significant number of advance directives either fail to come to the attention of health care providers at the time decisions have to be made, are too vague to give meaningful guidance, or are disregarded on the grounds that the actual medical circumstances make the patient's stated preferences appear contrary to the patient's best interests at the time.[23,24,25]

Research on the effectiveness of advance directives and attempts to improve their acceptability and influence on decision making will certainly continue in the future. What is important about advance directives, however, is not the form itself, but the process of discussion and clarification of values that patients, families, and health professionals go through when the subject of advance directives is raised. Indeed, a better way to think of these issues is in terms of *advance planning*, rather than advance directives. The goal is for patients, families, and professionals—conferring and working together—to arrive at medical care decision making at the end of life that reflects the values and priorities of the patient. The process of enhancing patients' self-determination begins well before end-of-life decisions actually have to be made; it should be built into patient-provider communication at the inception of the caring relationship.[26]

This requires physicians, for example, to communicate openly and honestly with patients regarding the patient's medical condition and the likely outcomes of various therapeutic options. It requires patients to examine their own goals and values in light of what they know or can reasonably anticipate about their medical condition, and to decide how they would want decisions to be made should they lose their own decision-making capacity. In short, advance planning requires of patients, families, and professionals the very candor and acknowledgement of the inevitability of physical decline and death that are hallmarks of hospice and palliative care.[27]

Advance Directives in Palliative Care

As Singer has pointed out, advance directives seem to be at once more and less relevant in the palliative care setting than elsewhere in health care.[28] They are more relevant because of the ubiquity of physical decline and death. They may be less relevant because patients who have elected to enter a hospice or palliative care setting are likely to have already decided to avoid many of the treatments that advance directives typically address.

As suggested earlier, however, there are still many decisions that have to be made within the hospice setting for which a clear sense of the patient's values and priorities is a critical ingredient in individualized decision making. Therefore, the broad guidelines for optimal advance planning and open communication mentioned in the previous section apply with equal force to hospice and palliative care, as well as in more active treatment settings. This reinforces the earlier discussion of the importance of open communication in clarifying goals and expectations for hospice and palliative care at the outset, thereby minimizing conflicts of expectations among the patient, family members, and hospice team.

Moreover, there are a number of issues not directly related to *medical* decision making about which patients may have strong preferences, and which the team will want to know about in advance. These might include which friends and family members should be called as the patient's condition worsens, or special requests for prayers or other rituals near or after the time of death. Eliciting preferences such as these is clearly part of comprehensive palliative care, and the skills necessary to bring these matters into the open with patients and families are part of the necessary education for the hospice and palliative care professional.

Physician-Assisted Suicide and Euthanasia

The subject of physician-assisted suicide and euthanasia has engaged philosophers, theologians, ethicists, health professionals, and policy makers for decades.[29,30,31,32,33] What follows is a necessarily brief summary of the key issues in the debate, with special reference to its implications for hospice and palliative care. The current debate is taking place in the context of referenda and legislative proposals in several states that would change current law to permit physician-assisted suicide and/or active voluntary euthanasia. On November 8, 1994, the citizens of Oregon approved the Death with Dignity Act, the only one of these proposals, so far, to be approved at the polls.[34] The Oregon experience with legalized physician-assisted suicide will provide a tentative conclusion to this chapter.

Definitions

Roy, Williams, and Dickens provide a clear and useful definition of euthanasia: "the deliberate, rapid, and painless termination of life of a person afflicted with incurable and progressive disease." What is usually referred to as "assisted suicide" they define as "assisted or self-administered euthanasia," that is, "when the sick person desiring to advance his or her death requires help from others, usually physicians or health care professionals, in obtaining lethal dosages of drugs and instructions on how to use these effectively."[35]

For the purposes of this discussion, euthanasia and assisted suicide are both to be distinguished from two other medical actions: withholding or discontinuing life-sustaining treatment, and the administration of drugs for the relief of intolerable symptoms with the foreseeable but unintended side effect of hastening the dying process. These distinctions are themselves controversial. Some have argued that there is no moral difference between allowing a patient to die by withdrawing necessary life supports, and acting with the deliberate intent to kill the patient. Both are deliberate actions that lead to the same result: The patient dies sooner than he or she otherwise would. To claim a moral difference between them, this argument runs, is to avoid facing up to the real issue: that health professionals sometimes do kill their patients, but that some acts of deliberate killing in medicine are justifiable.[29,36,37] In a similar vein, some would deny that a claimed difference in *intent* is sufficient to distinguish a lethal dose of pain medication, given for the relief of suffering, from an equivalent dose given to end the patient's life.[38]

The distinctions between withholding or withdrawing life-sustaining treatment, aggressive symptom control (to the point of terminal sedation), and active euthanasia can be subtle. Still, they remain useful and valid both clinically and socially. They have been widely endorsed by professional organizations, bioethicists, and the courts.[19,40,41,42,43,44,45,46] The issue of intent is crucial. In the case of withholding or withdrawing life-support, the primary intention is to refrain from useless or burdensome medical interventions that no longer benefit the patient. In the case of symptom control, the intent is to relieve suffering with the appropriate use of medications. In neither case is the death of the patient the primary goal, as it unquestionably is in the case of active euthanasia or assisted suicide.

The Paradigm Case and the Two Levels of Debate

The paradigm case for discussions of euthanasia and assisted suicide is that of a terminally ill patient who has concluded that his or her suffering—physical, psychological, or existential—is intolerable and beyond effective remedy, and who requests that he or she be helped to die, either by being given the knowledge and means to commit suicide, or by having his or her life ended quickly and painlessly through a lethal injection. The argument in favor of granting the patient's request rests on two main points: the patient's right to self-determination, and the obligation of health professionals to relieve suffering. An autonomous patient, who has concluded that his or her life is no longer of value to him or her because of extreme and irremediable suffering, ought to be able to choose the time and manner of his or her death. For a health professional to assist such a patient not only respects that patient's judgment regarding an acceptable quality of life and his or her autonomy, but also acts beneficently in providing the patient relief from otherwise continuous suffering.

How should the hospice and palliative care team respond to such a request? The answer to this question involves considerations at two levels, which are closely intertwined but logically distinct. At the level of *direct clinical care* the question is: *Is it ever appropriate and morally justifiable for a health professional to respond affirmatively to the patient's request?* At the level of *public policy* the question is: *Even assuming that it is morally justifiable for a health professional to grant the patient's request, should our laws be changed so that it would be legal to do so?*

Clinical Considerations   At the clinical level, the argument against granting the patient's request rests on the following main points. First, terminally ill patients who request help in hastening their deaths are frequently suffering from poorly controlled pain or other symptoms that are in fact amenable to effective palliative measures, or they are clinically depressed. Effective treatment of their symptoms or their depression usually results in the patient's repudiation of previously stated wishes to die.[47,48]

Second, the assumption that a patient who requests help in dying is truly autonomous is fallacious, not only because of the distorting effects of pain or depression, but also because dying patients are particularly vulnerable to feelings of worthlessness and of being a burden to others. These feelings make it likely that some patients' requests are not their own autonomous choices, but rather the choices they believe others want them to make.

Third, a patient's request for help in hastening death is often a way to express other things—loneliness, helplessness, fear—rather than a genuine wish for euthanasia. To take the request at face value without carefully probing its true significance for the patient would be a grievous error.

Thus, from the clinical standpoint, the appropriate and morally justifiable approach to a patient's request is to redouble efforts to identify the sources of the patient's suffering, and to apply palliative measures aggressively to alleviate them. This includes the full range of physical, psychological, and spiritual support.[49,50,51]

There are some who agree with the main thrust of these arguments and endorse aggressive palliative care as the appropriate clinical response to *most* patients' requests for assisted suicide or euthanasia, but nevertheless insist that there will always be two types of hard cases that urge us in the direction of complying with a patient's request. First, there are some patients whose pain or other symptoms are simply beyond effective palliative measures. Second, there are patients whose main source of suffering is not physical but existential: Life has simply become a torment and an intolerable burden to them for reasons that are rooted in their own deeply held, individual values. In this view, granting these patients' requests is morally and clinically justifiable, and public policy should be changed so that such acts on the part of physicians would be legal, or at least defensible in court in the case of attempted prosecution.[52,53]

There is, however, one more option that can be offered to these patients: continuous sedation.[54] The preference for continuous sedation over active euthanasia in these cases of extreme and otherwise irremediable suffering is based primarily on the broader public policy implications of professional or societal sanction of euthanasia.

Public Policy Considerations To those who believe that physician-assisted suicide and active voluntary euthanasia are sometimes morally valid and appropriate clinical responses, the distinction between continuous sedation and euthanasia seems vanishingly thin, if not hypocritical. And yet, in those rare cases where effective palliative measures are either lacking or are rejected by the patient, to offer sedation rather than to legalize euthanasia or physician-assisted suicide is the best social policy.

The overriding concern with the legalization of physician-assisted suicide or active euthanasia is the possibility of abuses. The major disagreement between advocates and opponents of changes in current law is over the nature and likelihood of potential abuses of a more permissive policy, and the reliability of various safeguards that have been proposed to prevent them.

Every plausible proposal for a change in the law restricts physician-assisted suicide and active euthanasia to the competent patient, suffering irremediably from a documented terminal illness, who makes repeated requests over time. Various safeguards, such as confirmation of diagnosis and prognosis, psychiatric examinations, and documented offers of "state-of-the art" palliative care, are proposed to prevent premature compliance with such a request, or the expansion of the policy to include patients for whom assisted suicide or euthanasia would be nonvoluntary or even involuntary. There are several reasons to worry, however, that the initial scope of the practice of assisted suicide and active euthanasia would in time expand beyond the original intent of the law. The current state of affairs in Oregon, where physician-assisted suicide has been legally practiced since 1998, provides an ongoing social experiment to test the validity of the concerns raised below.

First, recall that the foundations of the argument to adopt a more permissive policy are the values of *self-determination* and *relief of suffering*. The logic of the value of self-determination dictates that restricting the law to patients with a "terminal illness" is highly arbitrary. Who defines when a patient is "terminal," and therefore eligible for assisted suicide or euthanasia? Why shouldn't the patient—according to the value of self-determination—be able to preempt the suffering entailed in a long, progressive illness, and choose the time and manner of his or her death regardless of the timing of that decision? Similarly, if the motivation for the new law is the relief of suffering, why restrict its scope to the suffering that is due to a terminal illness? Why should it not be up to the individual to determine that his or her life is no longer of value, for reasons peculiar to him- or herself?

A second reason to anticipate the eventual expansion of the practices envisioned in a new law derives from the history of the movement to allow patients to refuse life support. Initially only a competent, terminally ill patient was allowed to do this. But it was soon convincingly argued that a person should not lose the right to decline burdensome life-supporting medical care simply because he or she had ceased to be competent or autonomous. Hence, as described above, advance directives and surrogate decision makers have been incorporated into policy and law to extend the right to refuse medical care to nonautonomous patients. There is no reason to suppose that a similar expansion of the "right" to assisted suicide and active euthanasia will not be similarly enacted, should an initially more restrictive policy be adopted.

Finally, the safeguards related to ruling out mental illness, and other attestations of the patient's genuine autonomy, may be illusory in practice. The aged and dying occupy vulnerable places in the social fabric as it is. Financial pressures, generational conflicts, the stigma attached to certain diseases such as AIDS, the enormous stresses associated with efforts to care for a dying family member at home, and the very uneven access to excellent palliative care, combine to create a societal context in which it is quite plausible to expect significant abuses of a more permissive policy for "voluntary" assisted suicide or euthanasia.

Statistics have been published for the first three years of the Oregon experience with legalized physician-assisted suicide (1998–2000).[55,56] In gross numbers, 95 patients received prescriptions for lethal doses of medication under the law. Sixty-nine of those patients died after ingesting the medication. Several other patients died of their underlying disease without using their prescription, and a few patients remained alive at the time of these reports. According to the reports published by the Oregon Center for Health Statistics, most of the patients who received prescriptions were receiving hospice care, and most had health insurance. Pain was *not* among the most frequently cited concerns among these patients according to their physicians. Rather, the most frequent concerns were becoming a burden, loss of autonomy or the ability to participate in enjoyable activities, and losing control of bodily functions.

These statistics have been cited by advocates of the Oregon law as reassuring indications that physician-assisted suicide has not been regarded as a shortcut to excellent palliative care, nor has it been motivated by financial pressures. Skeptics have questioned the completeness of this data, and point to the fact that we are still in the very early stages of the experiment. As has been the case with data regarding the Netherlands, where euthanasia is legal, the interpretations of the numbers commonly reflect the prior ideological commitments of the commentators.[57]

It is correct, as advocates of Oregon's approach argue, that maintaining other states' prohibitions against these practices is an abridgement of personal liberty. But such an abridgement still seems justified in light of the potential abuses and harms that could plausibly follow a new policy—and whose plausibility has not been eliminated by Oregon's early data. Moreover, the expansion of excellent palliative care services, which are severely underfunded and unevenly available to the population as a whole, and which can reduce even further the already small number of patients for whom assisted suicide or euthanasia are truly the only desirable options, is still an urgent societal need. Advocacy for these improvements, and not for more permissive policies for assisted suicide and euthanasia, is the proper ethical course for health professionals.

Summary

This chapter has discussed several ethical issues commonly encountered in hospice and palliative care: conflicting expectations of patients, families, and the hospice team; communication about diagnosis and prognosis; pain management; advance directives and decision making for the nonautonomous patient; and physician-assisted suicide and euthanasia. A common thread linking all of these issues is the importance of clear, sensitive communication with patients and families that respects the uniqueness of the individual. From its inception, the caring relationship should be characterized by open communication, the provision of accurate and realistic information, and clarification of values and preferences. This approach offers the best hope of avoiding serious ethical conflicts, and provides the foundation of trust and open communication necessary to resolve conflicts that do arise.

Clear, sensitive communication is especially important when patients' extreme suffering prompts requests for assisted suicide or euthanasia. The team must make every effort to understand the specific nature of the patient's suffering, and to provide the appropriate physical, psychological, or spiritual support, which may require attending to the needs of the patient's family as well. In the rare cases where palliative measures fail or are rejected by the patient, continuous sedation, and not compliance with the patient's request, is the morally preferable alternative.

References

1. Randall, F., and Downie, R. S. *Palliative Care Ethics: A Good Companion.* New York: Oxford University Press, 1996.
2. Christakis, N. *Death Foretold: Prophecy and Prognosis in Medical Care.* Chicago: University of Chicago Press, 1996.
3. Weisman, A. "The Patient with a Fatal Illness: To Tell or Not to Tell." *Journal of the American Medical Association,* 201:646–648, 1967.
4. Buckman, R. *How to Break Bad News: A Guide for Health Professionals.* Toronto: University of Toronto Press, 1992.
5. Fitch, M. I. "How Much Should I Say to Whom?" *Journal of Palliative Care,* 10(3):90–100, 1994.
6. Bowen, M. "Family Reaction to Death." In Phillip J. Guerin, Jr., ed. *Family Therapy: Theory and Practice.* New York: Gardner Press, 1976.
7. Northouse, P. G., and Northouse, L. L. "Communication and Cancer: Issues Confronting Patients, Health Professionals, and Family Members." *Journal of Psychosocial Oncology,* 5(3):17–46, 1987.
8. Vachon, M. L. S. "Emotional Problems in Palliative Care: Patients, Family, and Professional." In D. Doyle, G. W. C. Hanks, N. MacDonald, eds. *Oxford Textbook of Palliative Medicine.* Oxford: Oxford University Press, 1993.
9. Weisman, A. *On Dying and Denying: A Psychiatric Study of Terminality.* New York: Behavioral Publications, 1972.
10. Wool, M. S. "Understanding Denial in Cancer Patients." *Advances in Psychosomatic Medicine,* 18:35–53, 1988.
11. Psychological Work Group of the International Work Group on Death, Dying, and Bereavement. "A Statement of Assumptions and Principles Concerning Psychological Care of Dying Persons and Their Families." *Journal of Palliative Care,* 9(3):29–32, 1993.
12. Management of Cancer Pain: Clinical Practice Guideline Panel. Agency for Health Care Policy and Research. *Management of Cancer Pain: Clinical Practice Guideline No. 9.* AHCPR Publication No. 94-0592. Rockville, Md.: U.S. Dept. of Health Care Services, Public Health Service, 1994.
13. Burge, F. I. "I Would Never Do That!" *Journal of Palliative Care,* 10(3):73–75, 1994.
14. Henteleff, P. D. "We Don't Do That in Palliative Care." *Journal of Palliative Care,* 10(3):76–78, 1994.

15. Rait, D., and Lederberg, M. "The Family of the Cancer Patient." In J. C. Holland and J. H. Rowland, eds. *Handbook of Psychooncology*, New York: Oxford University Press, 1990.

16. Lederberg, M. "The Confluence of Psychiatry, the Law, and Ethics." In J. C. Holland and J. H. Rowland, eds. *Handbook of Psychooncology*, New York: Oxford University Press, 1990.

17. ACCP/SCCM Consensus Panel, "Ethical and Moral Guidelines for the Initiation, Continuation, and Withdrawal of Intensive Care," *Chest*, 97:949–958, 1990.

18. American Thoracic Society, "Withholding and Withdrawing Life-Sustaining Therapy." *Annals of Internal Medicine*, 115:478–485, 1991.

19. Council on Ethical and Judicial Affairs, American Medical Association. "Decisions Near the End of Life." *Journal of the American Medical Association*, 267:2229–2233, 1992.

20. Gostin, L. O., and Weir, R. "Life and Death Choices After Cruzan: Case Law and Standards of Professional Conduct." *Milbank Quarterly*, 69:143–173, 1991.

21. The Hastings Center. *Guidelines on the Termination of Life-Sustaining Treatment and the Care of the Dying.* Briarcliff Manor, N.Y.: The Hastings Center, 1987.

22. *Cruzan v Director.* Missouri Department of Health, 110 S.CT. 2841, 1990.

23. Teno, J. M., Lynn, J., Phillips, R. S., Murphy, D., Younger, S. J., Bellamy, P., Connors, A. F., Jr., Desbiens, N. A., Fulkerson, W., and Knaus, W. A. "Do Formal Advance Directives Affect Resuscitation Decisions and the Use of Resources for Seriously Ill Patients?" *Journal of Clinical Ethics*, 5(1):23–30, 1994.

24. Danis, M., Southerland, L. I., Garrett, J. M., Smith, J. L., Hielema, F., Pickard, C. G., Egner, D. M., and Patrick, D. L. "A Prospective Study of Advance Directives for Life-Sustaining Care." *New England Journal of Medicine*, 324:882–887, 1991.

25. SUPPORT Principal Investigators. "A Controlled Trial to Improve Care for Seriously Ill Hospitalized Patients." *JAMA*, 274:1591–1598, 1995.

26. Barnard, D. "Advance Directives." In R. C. Bone, et al., eds. *Pulmonary and Critical Care Medicine.* St. Louis: Mosby-Year Book, 1994.

27. Tulsky, J., Fischer, G. S., Rose, M. R., and Arnold, R. M. "Opening the Black Box: How Do Physicians Communicate About Advance Directives?" *Annals of Internal Medicine*, 129:441–449, 1998.

28. Singer, P. A. "Advance Directives in Palliative Care." *Journal of Palliative Care*, 10(3):111–116, 1994.

29. Brock, D. "Voluntary Active Euthanasia." *The Hastings Center Report*, 22(2):10–22, 1992.

30. Kamisar, Y. "Some Non-Religious Views Against Proposed 'Mercy-Killing' Legislation." *Minnesota Law Review*, 42(6):969–1042, 1958.

31. Quill, T. "Death and Dignity: A Case of Individualized Decision Making." *New England Journal of Medicine*, 327:691–694, 1991.

32. Singer, P. A., and Siegler, M. "Euthanasia—A Critique." *New England Journal of Medicine*, 322:1881–1883, 1990.

33. Weir, R. "The Morality of Physician-Assisted Suicide." *Law, Medicine, and Health Care*, 20(1–2):116–126, 1992.

34. Oregon State Legislature, Measure Number 16: Death with Dignity Act. November 8, 1994.

35. Roy, D. J., Williams, J. R., and Dickens, B. M. *Bioethics in Canada.* Ontario: Prentice Hall Canada, 1994, 411–412.

36. Rachels, J. "Active and Passive Euthanasia." *New England Journal of Medicine*, 292:78–80, 1975.

37. Brody, H. "Causing, Intending, and Assisting Death." *Journal of Clinical Ethics*, 4(2):112–117, 1993.

38. Quill, T. "The Ambiguity of Clinical Intentions." *New England Journal of Medicine*, 99:870–880, 1983.
39. Quill, T., Lo, B., and Brock, D. W. "Palliative Options of Last Resort: A Comparison of Voluntarily Stopping Eating and Drinking, Terminal Sedation, Physician-Assisted Suicide, and Voluntary Active Euthanasia." *JAMA*, 278:2099–2104, 1997.
40. American College of Physicians Health and Public Policy Committee. "Drug Therapy for Severe Chronic Cancer Pain in Terminal Illness." *Annals of Internal Medicine*, 99:870–880, 1983.
41. American Pain Society. *Principles of Analgesic Use in the Treatment of Acute Pain and Chronic Cancer Pain*, 4th ed. Skokie, Ill.: American Pain Society, 1992.
42. World Health Organization. *Cancer Pain Relief and Palliative Care.* Geneva, Switzerland: World Health Organization, 1990.
43. Spross, J. A., McGuire, D. B., and Schmitt, R. M. "Oncology Nursing Society Position Paper on Cancer Pain, Part I." *Oncology Nursing Forum*, 17(4):595–614, 1990.
44. Spross, J. A., McGuire, D. B., and Schmitt, R. M. "Oncology Nursing Society Position Paper on Cancer pain, Part II." *Oncology Nursing Forum*, 17(5):751–760, 1990.
45. Gostin, L. O. "Drawing a Line between Killing and Letting Die: The Law, the Law Reform, on Medically Assisted Dying." *The Journal of Law, Medicine, and Ethics*, 21(1):94–101, 1993.
46. Annas, G. "The Bell Tolls for a Constitutional Right to Physician-Assisted Suicide." *New England Journal of Medicine*, 337:1098–1103, 1997.
47. Foley, K. M. "The Relationship of Pain and Symptom Management to Patient Requests for Physician-Assisted Suicide." *Journal of Pain and Symptom Management*, 6(5):289–297, 1991.
48. Breitbart, W. "Suicide." In J. C. Holland and J. H. Rowland, eds. *Handbook of Psychooncology.* New York: Oxford University Press, 1990.
49. Byock, I. R. "Consciously Walking the Fine Line: Thoughts on a Hospice Response to Assisted Suicide and Euthanasia." *Journal of Palliative Care*, 9(3):25–28, 1993.
50. Moulin, D. E., Latimer, D. J., Macdonald, N., Scott, J. F., Scott, M. R., Deachman, M. J., and Mount, B. "Statement on Euthanasia and Physician-Assisted Suicide." *Journal of Palliative Care*, 10(2):80–81, 1994.
51. Saunders, C. "Voluntary Euthanasia." *Palliative Medicine*, 6(1):1–5, 1992.
52. Quill, T. *Death and Dignity: Making Choices and Taking Charge.* New York: Norton, 1993.
53. Brody, H. "Assisted Death: A Compassionate Response to a Medical Failure." *New England Journal of Medicine*, 3327:1384–1388, 1992.
54. Cherny, N. I., and Portenoy, R. K. "Sedation in the Management of Refractory Symptoms: Guidelines for Evaluation and Treatment." *Journal of Palliative Care*, 10(2):31–38, 1994.
55. Sullivan, A., Hedberg, K., and Fleming, D. W. "Legalized Physician-Assisted Suicide in Oregon—The Second Year." *New England Journal of Medicine*, 342:593–604, 2000.
56. Oregon Public Health Services Center for Health Statistics. "Oregon's Death with Dignity Act Annual Report 2000." www.ohd.hr.state.or.us/chs/pas/aresult.htm, accessed January 21, 2002.
57. Nuland, S. "Physician-Assisted Suicide and Euthanasia in Practice." *New England Journal of Medicine*, 342:583–584, 2000.

Legal Issues in Hospice and Palliative Care

8

Lynn McKeever, J.D.

Many of the legal issues in hospice and palliative care revolve around compliance with regulations, licensing requirements, and documentation for third-party payment from government agencies. These regulations vary from jurisdiction to jurisdiction, change frequently, and are well beyond the scope of this chapter. Because much of the interaction between team members and the legal system falls under the rubric of "so much paperwork," however, team members may be tempted to view the legal documents that patients sign as routine compliance measures. Merely obtaining patient or family signatures on documents without conversation about the contents of the papers deprives both patients and caregivers of an important opportunity to ritualize and communicate the shared values that make us a community. The deference that we render to our patients as persons is an expression of our cultural beliefs in human dignity and personal autonomy, and these are the beliefs enshrined in the law. They reflect the advance of our society in realizing itself as a unique civilization.

This chapter hopes to bring the law of patients' rights into the management of our service systems by presenting current legal thinking in plain language. Our focus is practical: to give professionals in the field access to the intellectual and applied discipline of the court-made law that dominates the areas of practice standards and consent to treatment. Although a lawyer generally does not work on the official hospice team, the concerns of the law are intrinsic to all team members' understanding of our roles as professionals. We look to the law for guidance, for wisdom, and for insight into how to think about our patients as people whose rights endure despite their physical and mental vulnerabilities. By incorporating the legal formalities of signing documents and obtaining consent into our practice routines, we grow in assurance that we are being attentive to the rule of law. Nothing can avoid lawsuits more certainly than conduct that consciously conforms to duty.

Introducing the Common Law

Most of the law regarding malpractice, patients' rights and privileges, and consent to treatment is not written in a statute or code book. This body of law comes from actions in tort, a creature of the common law. This law has grown and developed from very early English ideas of an implied social contract, the breach of which gave persons access to justice through the courts of the King. Rules of conduct shared by the community were applied to disputes between parties by traveling judges. The ruling of each case was announced to have the force of law in the land. Rulings of earlier cases became the expressions of the law that were applied to new cases and, over time, many legal precedents were established. By the apex of the British Empire, the common law was a sophisticated system of dispute resolution with many levels of courts, established procedures, well-kept records, and scholarly literature. British colonial courts throughout the world used common law. As colonies assumed their own sovereignty, separating from Britain, each jurisdiction developed its own lines of decision and precedents, adapting the common law precedents to diverse cultures in all kinds of urban and rural communities and post-colonial political systems. The common law tradition endures not only in the United States but also in Canada, Australia, New Zealand, India, and many countries of Africa.

The common law tradition has its own unique culture. Curious newcomers could approach it as a wise and eccentric senior citizen, whose methods of instruction are steeped in memories, lore, and circuitous method. Straightforward questions will not elicit crisp answers. In the next sections, I will attempt to describe a horizontal cross-section of important recent rulings and current thinking. But first, let us take a look at this thoughtful old codger, the common law, from the vantage of the more youthful sciences.

- *The common law is a normative system.* It creates categories that distinguish one person from another person and one situation from another situation. It solidifies the lines that draw these distinctions into fences, trying to assure that everyone understands the either/or nature of their choices about how to behave. In contrast, the sciences are systems of research and investigation. A scientist will look at data arranged along a continuum and see a continuum where the law has erected arbitrary fences. Scientists may find it difficult to interface their knowledge with legal thinking: Is this particular patient terminal or not, competent or not, eligible or not? The history of law and medicine is rich with instances of mutual bewilderment.

- *The common law waits for conflicts to ripen.* A court rules only upon issues that have ripened into full conflict and only when the parties whose actual interests are at stake stand before it. The sciences are grounded in underlying, discoverable realities from which facts can be established by experimentation, issues can be discussed and debated in abstract terms, problems can be anticipated, and disputes can be avoided.

- *The common law does not deduce from principle.* Legal thinking uses what Edward Levi terms *inductive reasoning*, a manner of sorting issues by similarities and differences to bring about a right result for the case at hand.[1] Science relies on logic. A law of physics moves from general principles to specific applications through a course of logical deduction. In contrast, the common law weaves and braids various strands into a tailored decision of the case.

- *The common law sets itself apart.* Courts employ customs and rituals to remove the judiciary from the messiness of life and project an elevated sense of stability, conformity, and order. Authorship of the law is attributed to the law itself; footnotes in legal opinions are to holdings and cases and only rarely to a work of scholarship. Workers in the realm of the sciences, on the other hand, claim personal ownership of their ideas, take pride in their personal reputations, advance their careers through invention and creativity, and aspire to be proactive colleagues. The extensive footnotes in scientific scholarship mention the work of mentors and friends, acknowledge the contributions of many individuals, and place the author in a milieu.

- *The common law is self-referential.* Its purpose is to reach the most appropriate legal decision, not necessarily to obtain the best practical result for the parties. A court listens to the cases before it to learn about the law. Much of what occurs before the case reaches a moment of decision is designed to create a written record that characterizes the facts of a case in light of existing precedents—the law as it is already known. The eventual decision must be supported by the record, and the record might not include what parties think of as their actual experiences. Rules of procedure, rules of evidence, and the unspoken economics of litigation all assure that the drama of the courtroom is quite different from the spontaneous life events that brought the parties into court. In contrast, when scientists work on their cases, they interact in real time with real facts, and often with real people whose very aliveness keeps data in a state of constant flux. The records they consult use statistical methods to stabilize their perceptions, provide bases for comparison, establish ranges for intervention, make reasonable projections of the future, and so on. As scientists work from case to case, they compile their records and employ empirical methods to achieve better results in the future. Science strives to break through strictures that doom future cases to past outcomes.

What Is a Right and Where Does It Come From?

Many of us were trained in childhood to recite Jefferson's famous declaration that people have "inalienable rights to life, liberty and the pursuit of happiness." Since the Enlightenment, we have carried forward an idea of a right as something "inalienable," an integral part of our being that cannot be separated. Through this lens of positive political thought and traditions, we see ourselves as cloaked with defined and certain freedoms as civilized people.

Unlike the Jeffersonian language in the Declaration of Independence, courts approach our rights not as affirmative expressions of power, but as boundaries that others are forbidden to cross. The original Bill of Rights to the U.S. Constitution conveys more of the actuality of how a right is made: "Congress shall make no law . . . ." The right is what is "carved out" by limiting the reach of those who may have power over us.

Long before the Enlightenment, the law began this process of delineating the boundaries between one person's liberty and the interests of his neighbor, landlord, employer, or agent. In the common law tradition of England, citizens began to bring actions before the King's judges in trespass: There were complaints allowed for trespass against property and trespass against the person. The current law that governs health care practice relies on precedents that date back to the late medieval concept of trespass against the person, a common law tort. The cultural norm that became a fundamental legal right was that a person should be free from trespass against their persons (i.e., free from being touched without consent). The law of negligence was born as a partner concept, implying a duty of care for those to whom consent to touch is given. These rights are not the same type of political rights as in Enlightenment, announced with rhetoric and flourish. They are older and perhaps more venerable because their contours have been hard-fought through eight hundred years of litigation. It is only through the trial of actual cases, decisions made after actual harm has been done, that the common law grows and changes.

In the spirit of the modern age, however, rights are expressed in the vernacular as powers, dignities, or privileges. We lay claim to a "right of choice," and a "right to live," and, more recently, a "right to die." Ethicists often approach the subject matter of health care with such positivist assertions on the part of patients and, when what ethicists say becomes an element of the local "standard of practice," their formulations find their way into cases.

Over the quilted fabric of the common law, legislatures from time to time do create positive law that reflects popular concepts, codifies the affirmative duties of health care providers, or limits the amount of damages a jury may award. This patchwork of legislation, jurisdiction by jurisdiction, adds texture to the law, but can never overtake the head start that the common law has in factually rich stories of where rights and duties meet.

The Common Law Rights of Patients, Plus One More

In this section we will discuss a patient's rights, stated in the affirmative, that derive from the common law:

- Right to receive care in keeping with current professional standards
- Right to confidentiality of medical records
- Right to make an informed consent regarding medical treatment
- Right to have a competent substitute decision maker in the event of mental incapacity
- Right to refuse medical treatment

In addition, we will discuss a right that can be created by statute:

- Choice of physician-assisted suicide

Right to Receive Care in Keeping with Current Professional Standards

This right is governed by the law of professional negligence, sometimes called malpractice. The law revolves around the right of a patient to receive care that meets objective standards established within the professional community. It is not the medical experts, however, but the judge and jury who apply the standards retrospectively to the facts of the case. Complaints of professional negligence, when presented to a jury to determine, are composed of four elements: What was the duty of care? Was the duty breached? Was the harm to the patient actually caused by the breach of duty? What is the loss or harm? The first two questions establish liability for negligence and the final two establish damages and the share attributable to the negligence of the tort-feasor, meaning one who commits a tort.

One of the results of the legal bifurcation between liability and damages is that similar breaches of duty to patients may result in quite disparate penalties, if the payment of compensatory damages were to be seen as a penalty. The common law does not see compensation of the victim as a punishment, however. The common law has another class of "punitive damage" awards that serve the purpose of deterrence. Under the tort law of all of the states of the United States, the measure of compensatory damages is victim-specific, meaning that monetary recovery depends on financial values associated with the loss to the actual victim and the victim's family, including loss of earnings. Thus, malpractice that causes death or disability to a young person with a promising future will result in a higher award of compensatory damages than a similar malpractice harming an old or poor person.

Despite the meaning of *negligent* in everyday speech as a kind of bad attitude, no evidence of the state of mind of the tort-feasor is necessary in the proof of failure to meet the duty of care. When evidence does show a willful breach or wanton disregard of the duty of care, courts may assess an extra measure of damages called *punitive damages.* These amounts are set by the jury (when a case is tried before a jury), and can range extravagantly depending on the facts of the case, the skill of the lawyers, and the influential voices on the jury. Trial judges and appeals courts have some authority to set aside punitive damage awards that are out of line.

Despite the disparity in damage awards, however, standards of care (the liability side of the decision) cannot and do not depend on the status or financial standing of the patient. Professional duties of care are established by the peer professional community in the locality and, as a matter of law, must rely on the testimony of at least one peer professional. In practice, both the plaintiff and the defense call peer professionals to give expert testimony regarding the practice standards in place at the time in the locality. Specialists are held to the standards of similar specialists. Here is an instruction to the jury in a physician's malpractice case:

> Duty of doctor. In treating a patient, the defendant is under the duty to possess and apply the knowledge and to use the skill and care ordinarily used by reasonably well-qualified doctors practicing under similar circumstances, giving due consideration to the locality involved. A doctor who fails to do so is negligent. The only way in which you may decide whether the defendant in this case possessed and applied the knowledge and used the skill and care which the law required of her is from evidence presented in this trial by doctors testifying as expert witnesses. In deciding this question, you must not use any personal knowledge of any of the jurors.[2]

Right to Confidentiality of Medical Records

Under the common law, a patient's communications with a physician was privileged, meaning that the physician could not disclose information learned in the course of treatment to anyone outside of the medical team without the consent of the patient. In most jurisdictions, this right has been abridged by statutes allowing the use of medical records for research and the disclosure of important information to agencies of government. Check on the law in your state!

The breach of the right to confidentiality by a patient's health care providers usually becomes an issue in court only when a patient has been harmed financially from the breach. Discussions with insurers, employers, or social workers should always be preceded by a written release or consent from the patient. Because the privilege is a common law right, and judges are the interpreters of the common law, judges can and do allow queries of the medical team when a medical fact is in controversy.

Outside of the courtroom, the issue of confidentiality is one of ethics. In the atmosphere of the hospice team, where information passes freely and often by spoken words in open rooms, it is important to recognize that only members of the team should have access to privileged information unless the patient has given permission for information to be shared with family and friends. The privilege, and therefore the right to release it, passes to an appointed surrogate in the event of a patient's incapacity.

Right of Informed Consent

The common law recognized a right to consent or to refuse consent to being touched. Touching someone without his or her consent still constitutes the tort of battery. Consent may be implied from circumstances, however, and most physical contact in social situations is both harmless and consensual. In a health care situation, where touching can be invasive and cause pain or harm, the issue of consent comes more clearly into play. Medical protocols usually involve obtaining express consent, either oral or written, for physical contact that may cause pain or discomfort. Emergency medical care relies on established legal doctrines of implied consent. Thus, the tort of battery arises most often in contemporary medical case law in instances of mistaken identity where a patient is subjected to surgery intended for another person.

The more common issue regarding consent in the context of hospice is the doctrine of *informed consent,* an expansion of consent that began in American law in the mid-1950s. This doctrine has found ground in malpractice actions throughout the country, where patients experienced unexpected outcomes that, in hindsight, they learned were foreseeable risks of treatment. Courts have ruled that patients must be afforded the choice of alternatives to recommended treatments and a prospective of the risks. Today, associations within the health care professions strive to meet the needs of their members by establishing standards for disclosure. Like the legal standard for professional negligence, the standard for informed consent is an objective one that is established by testimony of peer professionals. The jury is charged to determine whether the patient was informed of what a reasonably prudent patient would need to know in deciding whether to undergo the treatment.

Whether the law requires the disclosure of specific data about the track record and experience of the health care provider in comparison to other providers in the locality has come up as an issue in some state courts, and, if the standard takes hold, it will require health care providers to reveal statistical evidence that compares their past performance to their competitors. This comparative standard has been accepted in Wisconsin and is advocated by influential scholars in other jurisdictions throughout the country.[3]

The informed consent doctrine has special applicability to patients at the point of their admission to hospice care, when they adopt a treatment plan for palliative care rather than treatments aimed at prolonging life. But a blanket agreement opting for a treatment plan does not mean that consent cannot be later withdrawn.

Rights of Consent Exercised through Patient's Agent

Patients who are dying often lose the mental capacity to make rational choices. The patient's legal right of consent to treatment endures after the patient becomes incapacitated, even though the exercise of that right by the patient himself is no longer legally possible. The health care provider thus faces a dilemma of needing to obtain consent from a person who has legal authority to exercise the rights of the patient. This dilemma is usually anticipated by many patients while they still enjoy their rational faculties. With foresight of the vagaries of fate, many informed seniors sign a Durable Power of Attorney for Health Care, in which they appoint surrogate or proxy decision-makers. When a mentally competent patient enters hospice, an early inquiry about the existence of such a document may focus the family's concerns in time to discuss this issue.

When an incapacitated patient has not executed a written appointment of a substitute decision-maker, there are statutory legal procedures in every state that set out the manner of selection and appointment of a surrogate. Many states now have a statutory list of persons related to or knowledgeable of the patient with whom the health care provider may consult to obtain surrogate consent.

Although the Durable Power of Attorney for Health Care often contains a patient's expression of preferences in regard to drug therapies and end-of-life care, the legal document serves to delegate the right of consent to the surrogate or proxy. This is not the case with written advance directives that are executed under the several Right to Die statutes, where a patient anticipatorily exercises the right to withhold consent to treatments that are routinely used to prolong life. Troubling scenarios have emerged where such statements have prevented the use of a ventilator for a patient who suffers from pneumonia but is not in the terminal stages of her illness.

As with many of the other interfaces between law and medicine, the point at which loss of mental capacity is legally disabling is not an illuminated moment on medical charts or accessible to exact scientific determination. Furthermore, failure of the ability to communicate may not involve loss of cognitive faculties. Management of decisional conferences with patients through these marginal stages should include the participation of the surrogate as the patient's advocate, if not the patient's agent.

Pragmatism often rules in dealing with the ultimate decision to "let someone go." Whenever there is a strong objection by a person who claims to know what the patient would have wanted, the existence of written evidence to the contrary is merely that, *evidence.* The opinions of the caregivers are also merely *opinions.* The portent of being in a litigious situation where a deathbed drama over the evidence of consent is fought out among the survivors is a scenario that offends the spirit of hospice. Defer to the voices of the living unless their desires prolong the suffering of a patient in pain.

Right to Refuse Medical Treatment

Not only at the end of life, but also in regard to all proposed medical treatments, patients have the right to refuse or to withdraw their consent once given. This right is extended to their surrogate decision-makers and was the basis for allowing the discontinuance of artificial ventilation in the case of Nancy Cruzan.[4] Although sometimes popularly called the "right to die," the right to refuse medical treatment is not logically connected solely with treatments that prolong life. It surfaces in other contexts as well, especially in regard to patients with religious or philosophical beliefs that bring moral and ethical criteria to aspects of medical care.

The New Jersey case of Karen Ann Quinlan received widespread media attention. The story of Karen Ann's plight while her father fought an expensive and difficult legal battle to require the hospital to respect his decision to discontinue her life support systems fed the anxieties of an entire generation of baby-boom Americans who have taken up the subject of the right to choose death. They look for support to the law and customs of other countries and call into question the actual applicability of the common law precedents that pre-date the technology of the past 50 years. For now, however, their voice is a political one that has not found its way into the common law tradition, although it has spurred legislation, as we note in the next section.

Physician-Assisted Suicide

Despite increasingly popular philosophical beliefs, the common law recognizes no right to choose to die and no power to seek the assistance of a physician to carry out the suicide. On the contrary, suicide remains illegal in most jurisdictions of the United States.

The overview of current American legal precedents set out in the previous section describes a steady course of requiring medical service providers to supply more and better information about proposed treatments so that a patient can exercise judgment and choice. Medical professionals have gradually accommodated to a patient-centered decisional model, sometimes to the frustration of patients of the older generation who want and expect direction rather than guidance. Many patients' experience of choice in health care has been expanded by a consumer culture in which drugs and therapies are presented by advertisements and medical information is promulgated over public media like the Internet. Hospitals, clinics, HMOs, and pharmacies compete for local patronage through commercial media, emphasizing customer services. But none of these changes in the marketplace has provided a legal basis upon which an argument could arise that a person may choose to die as a matter of right. On the contrary, the current Supreme Court sees only a gradual enlargement through judicial precedents of the patient's right to consent or refuse medical treatment.

In 1997, the U.S. Supreme Court firmly denied appeals from physicians and their dying patients for authority to circumvent the existing state law criminalizing suicide.[5] Supported by an *amicus* brief signed by five noted philosophers, the plaintiff's argument that suicide was a political right founded on the concept of liberty was rejected. Several justices wrote separate opinions, but none could find a basis in law that would give an individual a right to commit suicide in a jurisdiction where state law forbade it.

In that same year, the State of Oregon passed a statute authorizing terminally ill patients to request and to receive lethal drugs administered by a physician. (At the time we go to press, the United States' Attorney General Ashcroft is battling to prevent the federal Medicare system from participation in payment for such procedures.) "Rights" created by statutes like the one in Oregon are different from both the common law rights discussed earlier and the constitutional rights set out in the founding philosophy of the nation. They are strictly delimited by the language of the legislation. The new laws will serve as exceptions to the general criminal prohibitions against murder and suicide in the jurisdictions in which they are enacted. And, in the absence of such an enactment, assisting a person in committing suicide may be a criminal violation.

Debate on the moral and ethical dimensions of the right to choose to die will remain with us regardless of statutory changes. Popular opinion in favor of a right to choose to die seems to be growing, increasing the probability that other states will follow Oregon's lead. Advocates for palliative care have visited the Netherlands, where physician-assisted suicide has been part of the medical culture for many years, in order to assess whether there is an inverse relationship between the availability of palliative care and the choice to die, but information gathering systems have not been in place to provide this data. Recent Dutch legislation has established reporting criteria that may help provide both qualitative and quantitative data about patients making the choice.

Documenting the Exercise of Patient Rights: A Guide to Forms

The five common law rights described in the previous section have given rise to standardized forms and procedures that educate patients and their families and offer them opportunities to exercise their rights in writing. Hospices may wish to have these forms available for their patients and they may improve their exercise of a duty of care by establishing a protocol for reviewing the law of consent with the family. The formality of writing becomes important in the face of likely incapacity and eventual death. As with all formally executed legal documents, people who are regularly represented by an attorney may feel more comfortable with an attorney present and they should not be discouraged from exercising their right to counsel.

Most lawyers who are engaged to write wills or other estate-planning documents will have prepared some of these documents for their clients' signatures. Patients or their families may bring them. As a matter of course, a more recently signed document supersedes all previous versions and there is nothing to fear in overriding a document that no longer expresses the wishes of the patient. Legal documents that may belong in a patient's file fall into three categories: (1) contracts and agreements, (2) advance directives, and (3) releases and consents.

Contracts

The agreement between the business entity that provides health care and the patient is a contract. Its terms are complex and often involve contingencies required because of the rules and regulations of third-party payers. It is wise to have a plain-language abstract of the contract that reviews business entities, contact names, and payment procedures. Void or voidable contracts for services are generally upheld as to the equitable value of the services that have been rendered.

Agreements for Future Performance

Agreements that are executed by a person who lacks legal capacity are not legally enforceable to require their performance. In most states, a spouse may enter into agreements to act for the benefit of a spouse. People are generally presumed to have legal capacity, but the circumstances of intimacy and specialized knowledge between a patient and her or his health care providers will require special caution in matters where the legal or financial interests of the patient may be involved. The legal standards of mental competence are prescribed by state law and do not require the support of a medical expert.

Advance Directives

An advance directive is a written statement, executed while a patient has legal capacity, containing directions to be followed after capacity is lost and/or after death. Some common advance directives include:

- *DNR/DNI orders.* These documents are part of the treatment plan and are placed prominently in the medical records. The patient's consent to these papers is a refusal of medical treatment in advance of its proposed intervention. Technically, the DNR order is not an "advance directive," but a medical order for which informed consent has been obtained.

- *"Right to die" statements.* By executing a written statement in anticipation of possible treatments for which patient consent is required, a patient may refuse to give consent to the treatment. This refusal of consent remains in effect even after the patient loses consciousness or capacity, and is self-executing (i.e., no surrogate's informed consent is required to give effect to the choice of the incapacitated patient). Many states enacted legislation after the case of Karen Ann Quinlan in New Jersey in the late 1970s that allowed patients to make a legally effective choice for the discontinuance of maintenance medical treatment. These statutes prescribe criminal penalties for persons who knew of the existence of such a "right to die" statement and failed to produce it or give it effect. The self-implementing provisions of these formal statements have proven troublesome in some palliative care situations, and the better format is to include authority for an agent appointed under a Durable Power of Attorney for Health Care to make further decisions consistent with the expressed wishes of the patient.

- *Instructions regarding cremation or embalming.* In many states, a person may execute written instructions regarding cremation or embalming in a form that the legislatures have promulgated. These statements have legal effect over the rights (and responsibilities) of survivors to dispose of a body. They are especially important when differing religious beliefs exist within a family. Other instructions in anticipation of death, including funeral arrangements, obituaries, and place of interment, are often signed with some formality but do not have the force of law.

- *Power of Attorney for Health Care.* Although sometimes combined into a single document with a General Durable Power of Attorney for financial matters when the appointees are the same people, this PoA document does not have the legal effect of creating an agency relationship over the patient's property or accounts. The Power of Attorney for Health Care is best not combined with a General Power of Attorney because copies of each will be made and distributed among an entirely different set of professionals and advisors. A Power of Attorney for Health Care appoints a surrogate or proxy to consent to treatment in the event of the lack of capacity of the principal. Language in this document may describe the patient's preferences in anticipated situations.

Consents and Releases

The consent to medical treatment does not need to be in writing. In fact, a written consent may always be orally rescinded. The primary purpose for obtaining written consent to palliative care treatment plans is to document the existence of "informed consent," by showing the subjects that have been discussed.

A valid release differs from a consent because it cannot be rescinded, either as a practical matter or under the law. Releases should always be in writing. Medical information, once released to third parties, cannot be returned. A Release of Legal Claims is a very serious contract matter for which patients are generally encouraged to obtain the advice of counsel. Because it is a contract, a patient who lacks legal capacity cannot execute a valid release, nor can a proxy decision-maker whose agency relationship is limited to health care decisions execute a release over money or property interests.

Dealing with Proxy Decision-Makers

The duty of care of health care providers is to the patient. When a family member steps into the role of proxy decision-maker, the consent to treatment or refusal of treatment is legally considered to be the action of the patient. However, it may be difficult for the substitute decision-maker to imagine the state of mind the patient would have in the drama of the moment. Whether the proxy actually carries out the wishes of an incompetent person is not a cause that a court will entertain, however, as long as a decision is made by the person wtih the legal authority to make it. In most instances, the person with that authority is clearly designated by a signed Health Care Power of Attorney or state statues. Courts will hear and decide cases when the authority of the proxy is challenged (rather than the proxy's decision).

The legal literature is beginning to take note of a duty of care to persons serving as substitute decision-makers. The persons who are so appointed are close to the patients in whose stead they are acting and are involved emotionally. In their grief after the death of the patient, they may dwell upon their decisions, thinking they should have or could have acted differently. Medical records should contain contemporaneous reports of the condition of both the patient and the decision-maker at the time any consent is obtained.

Managing the Flow of Legally Significant Documents and Conversations

Timing is perhaps the most sensitive parameter that affects the quality of agreements, releases, and consents. Of course, very few cases come through the door that present the ideal for easy flow from setup to performance. Many patients are enrolled in hospice long after they have lost the capacity for making choices, and some will not have communicated their intentions to their families. An important focus at the intake sessions must be to ascertain whether there are any written or oral instructions from the patient. If the patient has the legal capacity to sign advance directives, the hospice team may assist by providing forms. Most localities have agencies that distribute legally sufficient standardized forms of advance directives, or the hospice attorney may draw up generic documents.

The member of the hospice team who presents legally significant documents to a patient for signature should be in a position to provide the information necessary for "informed consent." Sometimes, however, it is advisable to include more than one team member in these sessions, so that the medical advice can be distinguished from the counseling regarding the patient's rights. Management can assist this process by establishing protocols for the timing and sequence of legally significant conversations and document signing sessions.

Questions of legal capacity arise in response to conflicts among family members. Because it is extremely rare for a court to issue a declaratory judgment regarding a patient's legal capacity while the patient is living, contemporaneous medical records that would have the qualities of legal evidence are the next best thing. A written certification by a professional (usually the primary care nurse or treating physician) that the patient meets the legal criteria established by statute can be inserted into the medical record on the date that sensitive decisions are made.

Members of the hospice team are cautioned to avoid taking positions of advocacy or giving advice in any conflict situation. Merely repeating that the rights of the patient belong to the patient, even when the patient is unable to exercise them, may at first frustrate the family members, but is more likely to result in acquiescence in a decision than more complicated explanations of surrogate decision making and agency relationships.

Table 8-1 may be helpful as a checklist in planning.

TABLE 8-1   A Document Presentation Checklist

Document	Who Present	Who Signs	When
Contract for Services	Patient, spouse, member of management, member of service team	Patient, spouse, or surrogate	On admission
Release of Medical Information to Third Parties	Patient, member of management	Patient or agent	On admission
Consent to Treatment Plan, DNR/DNI Order	Patient, spouse, family members, medical director, or primary care nurse	Patient or surrogate	After initial assessment
Advance Directives and Power of Attorney for Health Care	Patient, social worker or chaplain, significant family members, witnesses as required by statute	Patient, witnesses	Soon after admission if not recently signed
Durable Power of Attorney	Patient, patient's attorney, notary public	Patient, notary	Soon after admission if not recently signed
Consent to Change in Treatment Plan	Patient, primary caregiver	Patient or surrogate	At time of significant change
Certification of Capacity	Primary care team member	Caregiver	At time of patient's execution of legal document
Certification of Incapacity	Primary care team member	Caregiver	At time of execution of legal document by surrogate or attorney in fact

References

1. Levi, Edward H. *An Introduction to Legal Reasoning*, Chicago: University of Chicago Press, 1962.
2. New Mexico Uniform Jury Instructions, 13–1101.
3. Twerski, Aaron, and Cohen, Neil. *The Second Revolution in Informed Consent: Comparing Physicians to Each Other*, 94 NW U.L. REV. 1 (1999).
4. *Cruzan v. Director MDH*, 497 US 261, 1998.
5. *Washington v. Glucksberg*, 521 US 702, 1997; *Vacco v. Quill*, 521 US 793, 1997.

Resources

Rudd, Merri. *Life Planning in New Mexico*, Albuquerque, N.M., Abogada Press, 2003 Update, abogada@aol.com.

Leitzer, Stelzner, Rudd et al., *Elder Law Manual*, Senior Citizens Law Office, Albuquerque, N.M., 2003.

Sabatini et al., *The American Bar Association Guide for Older Americans*, Times Books, NY, NY, 1998.

Loverde, Joy. *The Complete Eldercare Planner*, Times Books, NY, NY, 2000.

The American Association of Retired Persons engages in education and political awareness on issues of medical care and provides countless resources. Consult your local chapter or visit www.aarp.org.

Lynn McKeever, J.D., is Founder of Lynn McKeever & Associates, LLC, a training and coaching company based in Grinnell, Iowa.

Spiritual Care of the Dying Person

9

Constance B. McPeak

Dying is a spiritual event. For the purposes of this chapter, I will use the term spirituality to describe one's relationship with one's deeper self, one's relationship with other persons, and one's relationship with the ineffable. In traditional parlance spirituality is normally associated with organized religious movements. The fact is that it is more widespread and ubiquitous than institutional forms. It is the role of those who provide hospice care to recognize and care for the spiritual needs of the dying person and those who are significant in their lives. We cannot wait for the minister, rabbi, chaplain, or other designated "spiritual caregiver" to arrive to address the patient's spiritual issues because these concerns cause suffering just as profound and immediate as physical pain. The difference between pain and suffering is in the patient's sense of meaning. Palliative care of physical pain does not necessarily mean the patient is no longer suffering. The diminution of meaning to life often brings suffering even without any physical cause. It is essential that all hospice caregivers have some understanding of the basis of this suffering so that they are able to provide appropriate interventions.

As a person approaches death, his or her whole life is reordered. Much of what has been important in the past may either grow significantly or diminish in importance. How people identify themselves in relation to the world changes. The sphere of the dying person's influence and interaction narrows. His or her relationships with others are examined and ultimately must be relinquished. At the end, dying people return to a state of absolute vulnerability, requiring assistance with all of their very basic needs, letting go of all that keeps them connected to the outer world and to life itself.

Religious beliefs and practices may be of great comfort during a terminal illness. These beliefs and practices can help to continue to give meaning to what is happening. Facilitating and participating in these practices may be the most therapeutic thing the hospice caregiver can do. It should be part of the development of the plan of care to explore what religious practices have been and are meaningful to the patient, and to include support of these practices by the hospice caregivers. These practices might include the reading of sacred texts, prayer, listening to religious music, and exploring with the dying person their and their family's religious beliefs about life and death, and what happens after death.

More universal than specific religious practice and expression is the spiritual work of examining purpose and meaning, relationship work, and the return to essential self.[1] We will look at each of these in turn. By our openness and authenticity as caregivers we may support the dying person in this work. The degree to which we are able to be open and authentic will largely determine the degree to which we are able to give genuine support.

Exploration of Purpose and Meaning

When a person is faced with impending death, many questions about purpose and meaning may arise. Dying persons may question why this is happening to them, and ask what is going to happen to them. Did they do something to bring on this situation? Are they being punished? Is there life after death? Do heaven and hell exist? Have they been a good person? How would they hope to be remembered? What was the purpose of their life? Were they successful? What is the point of being ill and having diminishing functioning? The dying person may or may not articulate these questions.

As caregivers, it is our responsibility to recognize that this work is probably going on whether spoken or not and to be the listeners to the dying person's story. When caregivers take the time and sit down to listen we may help this process of exploration of meaning. Open-ended statements or questions such as "Tell me your story," "How are you doing with this?", or "What are you thinking about all of this?" can be very helpful. Ira Byock, MD, a palliative care physician and author of *Dying Well* would ask "How is your heart?"[2] Byock is asking the patient to speak about his or her internal emotional and spiritual journey. He is inviting the person to speak of yearnings and apprehensions. He is indicating to the person that not only is her physical condition of concern but also her emotional and spiritual conditions. When the dying person feels that the questioner is genuinely interested in her life and has the time to listen, she may tell stories never told, integrate difficult times into a cogent whole, and leave her loved ones a legacy of story. The following stories illustrate this profound work.

The hospice team had been seeing Whitey, an elderly gentleman with congestive heart failure, for a year. A new nurse came to see the patient. The patient was severely debilitated, meeting all of the noncancer diagnosis criteria for congestive heart failure.[3] He was on maximum medication therapy. His ejection fraction was less then 20%. He had been bed-bound for more than six months with dyspnea at rest and cyanosis from his fingertips to his elbows. He was unable to perform any activities of daily living without extreme fatigue. The newly assigned nurse coming to see Whitey assumed that the patient had shared his life story and was simply waiting to die. At the end of her first visit the nurse asked the patient what he might like to be doing if he were well and not bed-bound. He replied that he thought he might be fishing. The nurse asked him to tell her his best fish story during her next visit.

The following week the nurse asked the patient about his fish story and he told her he had been fishing off the coast of Florida in about 1930. The nurse, acting from the premise that everything the dying person says is significant until proven otherwise, did some quick thinking about who might have been in the population in Florida in the 1930s. The patient had a sixth-grade education, had worked for the railroad, and as far as the nurse had known, had never been any-where outside of the small Midwestern town where he now lived. As the nurse thought about this man she had a hunch and asked him a question: "Were you a hobo?" The patient responded in surprise that indeed he had been. His wife of fifty years was equally surprised and apparently had not known this about her husband. The patient, supported by the nurse's questions, started to tell his story. It seemed clear to the nurse that this was one of the most important and formative experiences of this man's life and had been unspoken for more than sixty years. The nurse suggested that this story was precious and constituted a significant part of the patient's legacy and should be preserved for future gener-ations. The nurse suggested that the patient wait until they met again and have as many of his family as could come be there for the telling of his story. The nurse said she would bring a recorder so that the story could be taped.

For the following three weeks the patient told this life story. He would talk nonstop for an hour, filled with an astounding energy despite his dyspnea and fatigue. Finally he spoke about how he had come to be a hobo from the age of 14 to the age of 24. He spoke of the Depression, when his father was out of work. The patient had four younger siblings. In the desperate situation of the family, his father asked him to pay for his room and board. He told of hopping a train to try to reach an uncle in a faraway city, and being picked up by the railroad police and put in jail. He spoke of the horror of that experience. He sobbed as he spoke and said he would kill the jailer if he ever saw him again. He reflected a minute, and then said that he believed that his father was a good man who loved him and had done the best he could. After this last sen-tence there were no more words. There was a profound silence, a time of hon-oring the intense pain of this life experience and perhaps a time of integrating it finally into the dying man's full life. After the silence the patient said "I'm done now, you can turn that thing off." The nurse turned off the recorder, thanking the patient as she had each week for the gift of his story. The patient died peacefully before the nurse's next scheduled visit. At the very end of his life this gentleman was able to tell his story, feel his pain, and find validation, honor, and closure. He left a legacy to his children.

One of the very significant ways that the dying person and their family may continue to find meaning and purpose is in the recognition of a person's legacy of life story. Byock believes that it is through the telling of this story that a person may "find a sense of an emerging soul that can survive beyond."[4] Sometimes the meaning is supplied by looking at the present situation in a new way, so that the legacy is not so much an "old" story but the creation of a "new" ongoing story.

Millie was a seventy-five-year-old Italian woman who went from being a healthy older person to a dying person in a matter of days. Millie had stomach cancer, too extensive for surgery, and had developed a gastric outlet obstruction. Millie had been hospitalized for about two weeks in a palliative care unit when she was transferred to a nursing facility with a hospice unit. Millie was on several medications in an attempt to control her vomiting and nausea, including intravenous odansetron. The report the hospice nurse was given stated that this medical regime was the only way that Millie's nausea had been able to be controlled. Millie continued to vomit regularly and was fearful of aspirating her emesis. She was suffering terribly from the vomiting even though she reported not feeling nausea. After establishing a trusting relationship with the patient and her family, the hospice nurse and social worker suggested that there might be another way to manage or treat Millie's symptoms. The nurse explained the disease process to Millie and her daughter. The nurse told them, in simple terms, that Millie had a blockage and so when she ate there was no place for the food to go. Millie asked the nurse what was causing the blockage. The nurse responded that it was the tumor causing the blockage. Millie asked if it could be removed and the nurse responded that it could not. Millie asked why not and the nurse told her that there was too much tumor to remove. Millie nodded her head in understanding. It seemed that even if Millie had been given this information earlier, she had not been able to process it or take it in, but now she was able to understand her situation.

At this point the spiritual work or focus consisted in trying to discover a higher purpose or meaning for this dire situation. Millie was a devout, practicing Roman Catholic. Within the practice of Catholicism, as with most religions, is the making of a pilgrimage to a shrine or holy place. In Christianity the journey may be to Jerusalem, or perhaps to the site of a reported miracle such as Lourdes, or to Rome, the home of the Catholic Church. In Judaism the journey may be to Jerusalem; in Islam, to Mecca; and in Hinduism to the Ganges River. There are often ways to make the pilgrimage without taking the outward journey. During the Crusades, Christian pilgrims could go to Chartres and walk the Labyrinth in place of going to Jerusalem. Retreats with fasting and time for prayer are one form of making the spiritual pilgrimage. Recognizing the possible need for a sense of meaning and comfort in her last days, and the physiologic dilemma, the team suggested that the patient could make such a pilgrimage. The nurse suggested that if the patient stopped eating, she would stop vomiting and feel better. If there was no food going into her stomach, then her stomach would not have anything to reject, peristaltic action would slow down, and the vomiting would stop. It was suggested that this secession of eating could be seen as a fast, a spiritual exercise often practiced over the ages by the saints and other holy people. The promise was made that the team would see to it that Millie was kept comfortable with medications if there was any pain or other discomfort. It was also explained that most people find that due to the metabolic changes that occur during a fast they actually feel better. The nurse offered that the hospice team and Millie's family would provide sacred music and help the patient to pray and read sacred writings during her pilgrimage. Millie would be able to continue to have Holy Communion.

With tears in her eyes and a smile on her face the patient agreed to this plan of care by nodding yes. Millie spent her last few days surrounded by the love of her family in a prayerful environment with religious music playing at her bedside. Her parish priest visited, as did the spiritual care coordinator from the hospice team. The team freely entered into prayer with the patient and her family on each visit. Millie was no longer suffering from vomiting. The central line was removed. There was no further need for intravenous medications. Millie died very peacefully several days later, holding her rosary with her daughter at her bedside. Her daughter reported that Millie's death was "so gentle that she didn't even know that her mother was gone for several minutes." After her mother's death, Millie's daughter said that the last few days had indeed felt like a sacred pilgrimage to her. Her mother had seemed very serene, "almost as if she was surrounded by angels" and that she would cherish the memory of this time with her mother forever.

These two stories illustrate the importance of continuing to find meaning in one's life, and the ongoing necessity to find this meaning even at the end of life. They also point to the crucial importance of the hospice caregivers as catalysts in facilitating the process of finding meaning.

Relationship Work: Saying Goodbye

Another area of deeply spiritual work done by the dying person is in the realm of relationships. As one is dying it is possible to address unresolved issues with loved ones, to reconcile, and to let go. Byock describes five tasks of the dying and their loved ones.[5] These tasks constitute recognizing the need for and asking for forgiveness, forgiving, expressing love, saying thank you, and saying goodbye. Shaver says that as the dying say goodbye to their loved ones, they fear being left alone, abandoned in the face of death.[1] As hospice caregivers we can be present to them in their letting go. It is not uncommon for the dying person to withdraw emotionally from their loved ones but to continue to speak with the hospice team. There is no emotional investment in staying connected to the hospice team. There is no need to let go of the team in the same way that it is necessary to let go of loved ones. So the team may provide the security of ongoing human contact needed as a person is facing death, without the emotional entanglement that can make peaceful dying difficult. In order to die peacefully a person must let go of those dear ones they are about to leave behind. They may also need to know that these loved ones are ready to let them go. Byock's five tasks are part of the spiritual process in which dying persons and their families may be intentionally assisted. Simply naming the process, the five tasks, can give a structure to the work being done. They serve as a road map along the way for both the dying person and their loved ones.

During our dying we may be able to become the person we had hoped to be. As we reflect on our relationships with others we may see times when we have been unloving, or perhaps unkind. It is possible as a part of our preparation for death to alter the results of our previous actions. We may have the opportunity to ask for forgiveness and to forgive both ourselves and others. Our caregivers may provide the safe spiritual space in which to do this work.

William's story illustrates this well. When William came to hospice care he was arrogant, controlling, and had an unkind remark for everyone. He had been a nursing home administrator and ironically found himself dying in a nursing home. The hospice team believed that underneath his behavior was deep-seated fear and shame. The caregivers set gentle limits on his behavior, asking him not to say unkind things about the staff. The team continued to show up cheerfully even when he was overly demanding or critical and they actually increased their time with him even as they encouraged the use of proper channels of communication for his complaints. The team encouraged him to tell us his story. He first told of all his successes, and the power he had had in his work. But after a time, as he developed a trusting relationship with his hospice caregivers, he spoke of the mistakes he had made in his life, his regrets about his failed marriage, another failed relationship, and then finally his feelings of failure in relation to his grown children. William was uncomfortable with expressions of strong emotion. He had been told as a child that it was weakness to cry, so that now he could speak about the places of the most emotional pain for only very short periods of time. But William kept coming back to his unfinished business.

The hospice team explored ways that he might make contact with his estranged children. The team encouraged him to tell his children of his feelings for them, his regrets about the past, and his love for them. William did so. His children became more present in his life. They forgave him and in turn asked his forgiveness for their anger. As William grew closer to death a gentleness overcame him. He became appreciative of his care, quick to praise his caregivers and openly concerned about the lives of all who came to see him. There were no more bigoted remarks. Tears came more easily as William remembered the sweet times of his childhood and the love of his family. William seemed to become the person he had always hoped to be, allowing love in and in turn reflecting it back to his family and all who came in contact with him. He had come to hospice care alone, isolated, and afraid. At the end of his life he was surrounded by people who accepted him as he was, vulnerable and imperfect. He was able with this acceptance to face his fears, resentments, disappointments, and feelings of failure. He was then able to forgive, feel forgiveness, and die peacefully with loving family at his bedside.

The Return to Essence 125

It is a privilege for hospice caregivers to participate in such sacred work of forgiveness and reconciliation. In order to facil tate this work, caregivers must be alert to possibilities, and put the spiritual we fare of the patient above their own irritation and frustration.

The Return to Essence

In the final days and hours of a person's life the hospice team may be able to help create an atmosphere of deep healing, meaning, and sacred space. As the dying person returns to the helpless state of the infant, requiring assistance with all basic needs, there is the opportunity for actions of profound unconditional love and healing. These actions may be seen as spiritual practices. When the caregivers of the dying person have a clear understanding of the dying process, when the dying person is peaceful and symptom free, and when the hospice team can model and support caring for the physical needs of the dying person with reverence for that person's life there can be a sense of deep peace. Encouraging ongoing life review, storytelling, spiritual practice, and final goodbyes to the dying person, even when the person can no longer respond, can be final acts of love, forgiveness, meaning, and faith. In reflecting back after the person's death, loved ones will often speak of this time as one of the most meaningful of their lives.

Peter's story is about faith, religious expression, and the constant dynamic experience of the dying person and their loved ones. Peter lay dying, comatose, stripped of all external controls, in a state of total dependence. Peter was still present in the state of essential self, as unencumbered as an infant. During these last days, Peter required acts of unconditional love, without the expectation of any response from him. During this time of dependence his family expressed a profound experience of community with one another and of transcendent love.

Peter was a 40-year-old artist who had been struggling with a low-grade glioblastoma for eleven years. He spent his last two months in a hospice care facility. Peter and his wife, Claire, had been raised Roman Catholic but in their young adult years had chosen a different expression of their spirituality. Peter was a successful artist and had one of his large vibrant oil portraits hanging on the wall in his room at the hospice care facility. He had said, "I felt most connected to God as I was painting." His wife found deep personal satisfaction and a sense of unity with all things as she worked in her flower garden. They both expressed belief in God and prayed together daily. The final weekend of Peter's life, as he lay in a coma, friends came and said their goodbyes. They reminisced and laughed and cried with Claire and the rest of Peter's family. The family said that they had a clear sense that Peter was listening, as well, and enjoying the party. They said it felt like a celebratory time. The love was palpable in his room. There was a feeling of peace and deep caring and support for each other. During the final hour Claire became restless and requested a priest. The priest came and administered the sacrament of the sick. Claire had also hoped to have the sacrament of communion but the priest had not brought the Host with him. The nurse suggested to Claire that perhaps they had been experiencing the true spirit of Holy Communion in this time of being together in the presence of unconditional love. The hospice nurse suggested that it was this unconditional love that was God's presence manifest. Claire looked up with shining eyes and responded "Oh! You are right!" Within minutes Peter died with his family and close friends forming a circle of love around his bed. In the months to come Claire spoke often of the deeply spiritual nature of the last hours of Peter's life.

The spiritual work of the family is of equal importance in the hospice experience. Claire found deep meaning in the experience of her husband's death and was able to share eloquently with others what she had learned.

The hospice worker has the opportunity to participate in the profound work of helping the patient and family discover the spiritual meaning at the time of a person's death by being present and authentic. To be authentic is to not be afraid to be truthful about what one does and doesn't know and understand about the dying process. Authenticity requires being in touch with one's own feelings and the impact these have on one's work. In order to be truly open to seeing and addressing the individual needs of the dying person and their family the hospice workers need to be doing their own internal work about what they believe, fear, and understand. Ongoing learning is essential. When the hospice workers are anxious, due to insecurity in relation to their clinical expertise, fear of death and dying, personal grieving, or unresolved questions about their own beliefs, they are likely to find it difficult to be genuinely open and attentive to the needs of the patients and their loved ones. All who work with the dying will have their own questions about life and death. This questioning can be very valuable in helping one be attentive to the dying. When the hospice workers can assess and recognize their own feelings, and validate them in themselves, they may then set these aside so as to be more able to empathize with and be genuinely open to the needs of the patients and their families.

Summary

In conclusion, hospice care should be viewed as spiritual as well as physical and psychosocial. The alleviation of pain and suffering often, if not always, requires deep internal work by the dying person and their loved ones in the realm of purpose and meaning, relationships, and return to essential self. This work should be understood by all hospice practitioners because the patient's work will be facilitated and supported by this understanding. Hospice caregivers should be prepared to respond in the moment, with authenticity and sensitivity, to the spiritual needs of the dying person. Each of us as caregivers may need to do our own exploration of our personal sense of purpose and meaning, relationships and values, in order to be prepared to be present for the dying as they explore these essential questions.

References

1. Shaver, William, MD, "Suffering on the Way to Transcendence," address to the NHPCO Conference, April 2000.
2. Byock, Ira, MD. *Dying Well.* New York: Riverhead Books, 1997, p. 140.
3. Medical Guidelines for Determining Prognosis in Selected Non-Cancer Patients. National Hospice and Palliative Care Organization, Oliver Printing, Washington, D.C., 1996. Available at the NHPCO website: http://www.nhpco.org.
4. Webb, Marilyn. *The Good Death, the New American Search to Reshape the End of Life.* New York: Bantam Books, 1997, pp. 234–236.

For Further Reading

Broyard, Anatole. *Intoxicated By My Illness.* New York: Clarkson Potter Publishers, 1992.

Callanan, Margaret, and Kelley, Patricia. *Final Gifts.* New York: Bantam Books, 1992.

Cassell, Eric. *The Nature of Suffering and the Goals of Medicine.* New York: Oxford University Press, 1991.

Dowrick, Stephanie. *Forgiveness and Other Acts of Love.* New York: W. W. Norton and Co., 1997.

Frankl, Viktor E. *Man's Search for Meaning.* New York: Washington Square Press, Pocket Books, 1984.

Hargrove, Terry D. *Families and Forgiveness: Healing Wounds in the Intergenerational Family.* Levittown, Pa.: Brunner/Mazel, Inc., 1994.

Rinpoche, Sogyal. *The Tibetan Book of Living and Dying.* San Francisco: HarperSanFrancisco, 1994.

Storch, Susan C., RN, MA. *Dying into Freedom: A Nurse's Handbook to Conscious Dying.* self-published, email address: **storch@silcom.com**.

General Issues: Fatigue, Dyspnea, and Constipation

10

Diletta M. Renier-Berg

The patient with a terminal illness presents a challenge for the treatment of symptoms such as fatigue (also known as asthenia), dyspnea, and constipation. In many instances these symptoms prompt the patient to seek medical attention long before the diagnosis of the disease is made. The prevalence and pattern of asthenia, dyspnea, and constipation vary greatly according to different studies. Most patients with terminal illnesses report at least one symptom, and a small number of patients report more than five symptoms.

Regardless of gender, asthenia, dyspnea, and constipation are the most frequent complaints for patients with terminal illnesses; this seems to be true for cancer and noncancer patients. These symptoms may be caused directly by the primary disease or they may appear as side effects of the treatment course. They occasionally are very severe and may lead patients to refuse potentially helpful therapy.

The best way to approach patients with a complex symptomatology always begins in the same way by taking a careful history. Particular attention should be given to the level of activity performed by the patient prior to and after the diagnosis of the terminal illness. All medications must be reviewed, including the use of over-the-counter preparations, which the patient may not consider necessary to report to the health care professional. A careful history is then followed by a review of symptoms and a thorough physical examination. It is always very important to ask the patient what his or her goal for the treatment plan is. In palliative care, helping the patient set realistic goals and expectations may ultimately help him or her to better control the symptoms without any added frustration. We must always remember that explaining the disease process allows the patient and the family to understand why certain symptoms are present and why they change during the course of the disease.

Asthenia (Fatigue)

Asthenia, from the Greek word *asthenos*, means the absence or loss of energy and strength. Asthenia, which we will refer to as fatigue, has a significant impact on quality of life for the patient and his or her family, and can be a very frustrating aspect of symptom management. Fatigue is the most common complaint given to health care providers in the setting of terminal illness and, by definition, is a very broad, ill-defined symptom. Patients may complain of tiring easily and of having a decreased ability to maintain previous performance. They may also complain of difficulty in initiating certain activities, impaired mental ability, and/or impaired concentration.

Fatigue is always present in patients with advanced and terminal disease and unfortunately its basic pathophysiology is poorly understood. Usually in cancer patients the reasons for the generalized sense of fatigue are multiple and frequently coexist. The general causes of fatigue are malnutrition, infection, anemia, chronic hypoxia, metabolic and electrolyte disorders, psychogenic, and pharmacological. It is known that many types of cancers release a number of substances considered to be important factors in the pathogenesis of fatigue. These include tumor degradation products, cachexin, PEG-2, IL-2, IL-6, TNF, and other substances still being investigated. This systematic approach will help provide the patient with the most realistic goals.

The most widely used tools in clinical practice for the assessment of fatigue are the Fatigue Self Report Scale and the Edmonton Functional Assessment Tool (see Table 10-1). Occasionally the use of a numerical scale or a visual analogue scale, such as those used in the assessment of pain, can guide the health care professional in evaluating changes in fatigue and the effectiveness of therapy.

Pathophysiology of Fatigue

Cachexia (Malnutritionment) and Failure to Thrive   The patient with an advanced disease usually has a poor appetite and shows the physical signs of weight loss and wasting. The association between cachexia and fatigue is very frequent in cancer patients, and the anorexia associated with cachexia is one of the major contributors to fatigue. The loss of muscle mass can only partially explain the symptoms of weakness. The concomitant presence of pain, nausea, emesis, and constipation can make anorexia very difficult to treat. Further, the patient may become cachectic despite a normal, or even above normal, caloric intake as the result of tumor or disease-related processes.

Anemia   Although the role of anemia in the terminally ill patient is still somewhat controversial, it is well known that a sudden change in the patient's hemoglobin value can make fatigue much worse. In such cases, blood transfusions can help the patient feel better. On the other hand, treating chronic

TABLE 10-1 **Edmonton Functional Assessment Tool (EFTA).**

	0 *Functional*	1 *Minimal Dysfunction*	2 *Moderate Dysfunction*	3 *Maximum Dysfunction*
Communication	Independent	Effective >50% but <100% of time	Effective <50% of time	Unable to communicate
Mental Status—six tasks on memory and orientation	Oriented with intact memory	2–6 tasks impaired but follows simple commands	3–4 tasks impaired or responds inconsistently	5–6 tasks impaired or unresponsive to verbal commands
Pain	No impact on function	Inhibits function minimally	Inhibits function moderately	Unable to perform any activity
Dyspnea	No SOB (Shortness of Breath)	Urgency with counting of SOB on exertion or intermittent O_2 use	One extra breath with counting or O_2 at 1–3 liters	>2 breaths with counting or O_2 at >4 liters
Balance (sitting or standing)	Independent	Requires equipment or 1 person; minimal safety risk	Requires moderate assistance ($\geq$1 persons); unsafe on own	Requires maximum assistance or unable to evaluate
Mobility (bed mobility and transfer)	Independent and safe	Requires 1 assistant to move safely	Requires 2 assistants to transfer safely	Unable to assist with positioning; requires lift
Locomotion (walking or wheelchair)	Independent	Requires walking aid or 1 person to walk or wheelchair supervision	Requires 2 persons to walk or assistance with wheelchair	Unable to walk; dependent wheelchair management
Fatigue	Rarely needs to rest	Rests <50% of the day	Rests >50% of the day	Bedridden due to fatigue
Motivation	Participates in all activities	Participates >50% of the time	Participates <50% of the time	No desire to participate
ADL (Activities of Daily Living)	Independent	Independent using equipment	Requires some assistance	Totally dependent
Performance Status	Independent	Independent with minimal assistance	Requires moderate assistance	Requires maximal assistance

anemia with continuous and systematic transfusions may improve the patient's symptoms only minimally or not at all.

Infection   Protracted and recurrent infection may be the sole cause of the patient's feelings of fatigue and weakness. A terminal illness always compromises the immune system, increasing the incidence of infection. This is a very difficult problem for the patient who is immunosuppressed by palliative chemotherapy and should be addressed by experienced clinicians.

Pharmacological Therapy

In many instances, therapy for the primary disease, or for symptoms associated with the disease, causes fatigue for patients. Examples include surgical procedures, chemotherapy, radiation therapy, opioid agonists, antiemetics, and other medications. Further, symptoms of the disease or side effects of the therapy used to treat it, such as nausea, emesis, pain, and infection, may increase the feeling of fatigue or weakness.

Psychological Distress

Many terminally ill patients present with depressive symptoms, especially when the disease is initially diagnosed. Although depression is rather common, it is rare to see patients with adjustment disorder and/or with major depressive episodes. There is a clear association between fatigue and mood changes where, again, the influence on mood can result from the disease or from the therapeutic measures taken to treat the disease.

Treatment

The terminally ill patient with fatigue must be evaluated carefully. During the initial evaluation all concomitant symptoms that may cause a more generalized malaise need to be addressed promptly; that is, pain, nausea, emesis, dyspnea, and flu-like symptoms need to be treated appropriately. The simple treatment of these problems may be all that is needed to improve the patient's sense of well-being. After these problems are resolved, more specific measures can be taken to address the patient's fatigue.

General Measures

It is of paramount importance to discuss with the patient and his or her family the disease progression. The patient will then be more likely to understand suggestions such as decreasing their workload, taking more frequent periods of rest, and improving their nutritional status. Goal setting is, once again, very important. Many terminally ill patients can see an improvement in their fatigue, although few of them can ever eliminate this problem completely. Emotional support of the primary caregiver can also indirectly affect the patient's sense of improvement and well-being.

Corticosteroids   In several studies, corticosteroids were found to produce a feeling of well-being and increased energy in patients with terminal cancer. Their mechanism of action is not well understood. The agents most often used are dexamethasone (0.75–4.0 mg in the morning) and prednisone (10–30 mg in the morning). Prednisone causes fewer problems with myopathy than dexamethasone. The improvement seen with steroids is usually appreciable after 10–14 days of therapy; however, it may diminish after four weeks.

Psychostimulants Fatigue associated with depression or opioid-induced sedation may respond to psychostimulants. Methylphenidate may be initiated at 5 mg in the morning and at noon, avoiding doses later in the day to prevent interference with sleep, and titrated to effect up to doses of 40 mg per day. The antidepressant effect is rapid, usually within a few days, and the antisedative effect may be seen with the first dose. Dextroamphetamine and pemoline may also be used in this setting, although there is considerably less medical literature discussing their use.

Erythropoietin The growth factor erythropoietin (EPO) may be of value in increasing hemoglobin and hopefully reverse the fatigue associated with anemia. EPO should be dosed at 40,000 units subcutaneously once weekly for four weeks. Hemoglobin should then be assessed and if it has risen by 1 gm/dl or more, therapy should be continued. If it has not, the EPO dose should be increased to 60,000 units weekly. If after four weeks, hemoglobin has risen by 1 gm/dl or more, continue therapy; if it has not, the patient is a nonresponder and EPO should be discontinued. Adequate iron stores are required for EPO to function properly.

Antibiotics All episodes of infection, especially those in the immunocompromised and the very elderly, should be immediately addressed by the health care professional. In addition to contributing to fatigue, infections are often life threatening.

Dyspnea

The role of the airways is very important in palliative care. Any decrease in airflow caused by any type of obstruction and/or narrowing can cause physical and psychological distress to the patient and psychological stress for the family. Dyspnea is defined as the subjective symptom of difficulty in breathing and it may or may not be related to exertion. The word dyspnea comes from the Greek *dyspneoa* meaning "bad breathing." The fear and anxiety associated with dyspnea are directly related to the sensation of suffocating experienced by the patient.

The prevalence of dyspnea in terminally ill patients varies greatly according to the main pathology affecting the patient and the different studies examined. In the National Hospice Study (USA), which collected data from hundreds of patients in different programs, dyspnea was seen in 70% of patients during the last six weeks of life. Preexisting lung disease may influence greatly the sensation of dyspnea. Unfortunately, good symptom control for respiratory distress is achieved less frequently than for other symptoms such as pain and nausea.

Pathophysiology of Dyspnea

Dyspnea is associated with clinical conditions where 1) the respiratory system is subject to an increased mechanical workload, 2) ventilation needs to be increased, and 3) there is respiratory muscle weakness due to fatigue, paralysis, or lung volume increase. The causes of respiratory distress are linked not only to the respiratory system's inadequate function, but also to the psychological condition of the patient. Various etiologies of dyspnea are shown in Table 10-2.

TABLE 10-2 Causes of Dyspnea	
Pulmonary	Airway malignancy
	Airway collapse
	Tracheo-esophageal fistula
	Inhalation
	Consolidation
	Infection
	Fibrosis
	Vasculitis
	Radiation exposure
	Embolism
	Lymphangitis carcinomatosa
Pleural	Effusion
	Malignancy
	Pneumothorax
	Embolism
Cardiac	Ischemic heart disease
	Cardiac failure
	Pericardial disease
	Superior vena cava obstruction
Other	Chest wall malignancies (primary or metastatic)
	Diaphragmatic malignancy
	Respiratory muscle fatigue (primary or secondary)
	Severe anemia
	Chemotherapy
	Surgical procedures
	Psychological factors

TABLE 10-3	The Borg Scale
	BORG SCALE
10	Maximal
9	Very, very strong
8	
7	Very strong
6	Strong
5	Somewhat strong
4	
3	Moderate
2	Weak
1	Very weak
	Very, very weak
0	None

The quantification of symptoms is always difficult, particularly after such symptoms have become chronic. Several tools for measuring dyspnea are available. For bedside clinical purposes, the Borg Scale (Table 10-3) seems to be the simplest and most effective method available. It combines a numeric scale with a descriptive one, making it very easy for the patient to quantify his or her breathlessness. This tool is also used for follow-up evaluation, allowing the clinician to assess the efficacy of the treatment for dyspnea. The Borg scale is similar to scales used for measuring other symptoms, such as those used for pain evaluation. The regular evaluation of dyspnea in patients with severe respiratory disease is absolutely necessary because it cannot be extrapolated from objective parameters such as pulse oxymetry, respiratory rate, or arterial blood gases.

Anxiety is strongly correlated with dyspnea. This correlation is difficult to interpret because anxiety may contribute to dyspnea and may also be caused by dyspnea. Hence, quantifying anxiety is also very important.

Treatment

Multiple different mechanisms of dyspnea may coexist in a given patient, so a comprehensive approach to treatment is of paramount importance. The clinician should try to treat the underlying causes of breathlessness. The risk benefit of all treatment should always be considered and explained to the patient and his or her family. Thus, when treating shortness of breath, many approaches are available.

In patients with congestive heart failure, the simple use of appropriate doses of diurectics may be all that is needed to relieve the respiratory discomfort. The drainage of a large pleural effusion, even if partial, may dramatically improve the patient's dyspnea. The risk versus benefit of all such treatments must be evaluated carefully. For patients with cancer, palliative chemotherapy and radiotherapy, when feasible, are often included as part of the therapeutic regimen. Both are used to improve the quality of life of the terminally ill patient rather than to achieve cure. Radiotherapy and endobronchial laser treatment may help to shrink the tumor to the point where it no longer causes obstruction. Stent placement is also used to alleviate obstruction. The role of chemotherapy in palliative care is more controversial than other treatments, and is generally reserved for tumors highly sensitive to chemotherapy, such as small cell lung cancer.

Long-term oxygen therapy has been shown to have a beneficial effect on patients with chronic obstructive pulmonary disease (COPD). However, some hospice studies suggest that chronic oxygen administration has no symptomatic effect on dyspnea caused by malignancy or end stage congestive heart failure. The decision of when to use chronic oxygen therapy lies in determining when the patient is hypoxemic. Usually this is easily accomplished with the use of a pulse oximeter. In general, there is compelling evidence that the use of oxygen may produce symptomatic relief of cancer-related dyspnea for patients who are hypoxemic at room air. A mixture of helium and oxygen is occasionally used to relieve the respiratory distress of patients with severe stridor caused by tracheal obstruction. This treatment modality is effective because the gas mixture is much lighter than air and can be inspired effortlessly. The patient should be advised that this therapy is known to change the pitch of the voice.

A number of drugs have been used to treat the dyspnea of cancer and other chronic disease conditions. In the case of cancer-related dyspnea, many published studies have demonstrated the efficacy of opioid analgesics; however, the optimal medication, schedule, and route of administration have not been determined because therapy is highly individualized and may be dependent on other treatment modalities. The general consensus at this time is that the opioids should be used on an "as needed" schedule and taken orally, parenterally, or, more controversially, via nebulization.

Benzodiazepines are commonly used for the treatment of dyspnea in dying patients; however, most of the studies have found no significant difference between the use of placebo and benzodiazepines. There is a definite role for such medications when the shortness of breath is a manifestation of anxiety or causes panic or anxiety disorder.

Corticosteroids are used in the management of bronchospasm of asthma and COPD. They are also used in the management of superior vena cava syndrome and for the treatment of dyspnea associated with carcinomatous lymphangitis. Their use should be carefully monitored in terminally ill patients because of their effect on several muscle groups. For example, it has been suggested that the effects of corticosteroids may be more pronounced on the diaphragm, which can lead to bouts of intractable hiccough.

Many patients with terminal cancer and dyspnea have a prior history of COPD and it is known that there is a strong association between air flow obstruction and the sensation of shortness of breath. Patients with this kind of pathology may benefit from the use of simple bronchodilator treatment. Those terminally ill cancer patients with asthenia and muscle weakness may benefit from treatment with xanthines that act to enhance respiratory muscle contractility.

Many nonpharmacological interventions are routinely employed in the treatment of dyspnea. Positioning the patient with the head elevated, teaching pursed-lip breathing, and keeping a window open or a fan nearby to provide cool air to the patient are all techniques found to decrease the dyspnea of the terminally ill patient. Relaxation therapy, biofeedback, and the presence of a caregiver with a calming effect have all been shown to be effective in improving the symptoms of respiratory distress.

Constipation

Constipation is an extremely common problem in the hospice patient. The word derives from the Latin *stipare* which means *to cram*. The most general and widely accepted definition of constipation involves the infrequent, difficult passage of small, hard stool. The term often has different meanings for different people. Many patients will include with it the sense of abdominal discomfort, bloating, flatulence, and low stool weight. Stool frequency is typically the most common parameter considered, with a frequency of at least three bowel movements per week considered normal. However, frequency alone cannot define constipation. Although the frequency and consistency of bowel movements are obviously dependent on oral intake, it should be recognized that stool continues to be produced with very low oral intake. Ultimately, the presence of constipation should be determined from frequent evaluation of the patient. In the general population, the prevalence of constipation ranges from 5% to 20%; however, it appears to be more prevalent in patients dying of cancer than of other terminal illnesses. Two British studies found that at least 50% of patients admitted to hospice care complained of constipation, despite the fact that many of them were already using laxative preparations regularly. The goal of symptom control therapy in the terminally ill is not just relief, but prevention. For constipation, as with most other symptoms, this requires anticipation and frequent review of the underlying pathophysiology.

Pathophysiology and Etiology

Effective control of constipation requires a basic understanding of normal bowel function. An average person ingests two liters of fluid per day; an additional seven liters of fluid is secreted into the gut system by the salivary glands, the stomach, the biliary system, the pancreas, and the small intestine. The total volume is reduced to 1.5 liters by the time it reaches the colon, where further absorption reduces the total volume of stool to 150–200 cc. This movement of the food bolus is accomplished through peristalsis, which consists of coordinated circular constrictions and longitudinal shortening of the gut musculature. Peristalsis is stimulated by the ingestion of food, psychogenic factors, and somatic activity. The residual bolus distends the rectum, initiating defecation. In patients with cancer, constipation may be secondary to systemic disease or to disease afflicting the gastrointestinal tract. It is usually multifactorial, most of the time caused by poor oral intake of food and fluids, impaired mobility, and the use of opioid analgesics and other medications for symptom control. Some causative factors involved with the development of constipation are shown in Table 10-4.

Treatment

Following the quantification of constipation, a complete history of the patient's bowel habits before and after the diagnosis of terminal illness must be obtained. The first principle of bowel control is to anticipate and prevent constipation. The second principle is to reverse specific causes with specific therapy. Although the patient should be encouraged to increase his or her oral intake, with an emphasis on dietary fiber, and to increase appropriate physical activity, these measures are generally not successful and can be poorly tolerated in unselected patients. Furthermore, the lack of available facilities and the lack of privacy can exacerbate constipation. The use of bedpans for the bedrid-

TABLE 10-4   Causes of Constipation

Causes	Examples
Cancer	Primary bowel cancer, secondary bowel cancer, pelvic cancer, pheochromocytoma, glucagonoma, malignant paraneoplastic autonomic neuropathy, dermatomyositis, peritoneal mesothelioma
Cancer-related	Inanition, dehydration, weakness, pain, dyspnea, paralysis, disturbance of prior bowel function, bed rest, confusion, inadequate food and fluid intake, low fiber diet, depression
Coincidental	Prior laxative habituation, hemorrhoids/anal fissures, diabetes, hypothyroidism, scleroderma, chronic neurological disease, hypokalemia, hernia, diverticular disease, rectocele, colitis
Cancer therapy	Bowel surgery, vincristine, vinblastine, vinorelbine, diagnostic barium
Symptom control therapy	Opioid analgesics, anticholinergic drugs, antihistamines, tricyclic antidepressants, antispasmodics, neuroleptics, anticonvulsants, muscle relaxants, aluminum antacids, iron, anti-Parkinson's agents, diuretics

den terminally ill patient not only causes an uncomfortable circumstance for defecation but the posture necessary to use this technique increases the pressure needed to expel stool. An individual laxative regimen generally leads to the best results. The selection of the laxative is made by considering its mechanism of action and the characteristics of the patient's constipation. Laxatives are grouped according to their primary action on the bowel tract. In general, oral laxatives should be used for around-the-clock administration and rectal laxatives should be reserved for "as needed" use.

There is no optimal way to normalize bowel function and no optimal choice of laxative. Therapy should be individualized based on the cause of the constipation, patient history of and preference for specific laxative regimens, and the patient's clinical history. The following principles should be kept in mind when considering laxative therapy: 1) it is better to prevent constipation than wait to treat it, 2) if there is a fecal impaction, evacuation will not occur until manual rectal disimpaction is performed, 3) intestinal obstruction must be ruled out, and 4) combining agents with different mechanisms of action often will improve results.

Bulk-Forming Laxatives   These agents contain polysaccharides or cellulose derivatives resistant to bacterial breakdown. They may take more than 24 hours to have an effect, and they are often ineffective in the terminally ill patient. They are inappropriate for use in opioid-induced constipation.

Emollient Laxatives   The well-known agent in this class is mineral oil. These agents lubricate the stool surface and penetrate the feces to soften and promote easier passage. They also act to decrease the colonic absorption of water. Mineral oil may be administered at a starting dose of 15–30 cc daily, and it will produce an effect in 8–48 hours. Although usual directions are to give the dose at bedtime, caution is advised in the elderly or debilitated patient, who is at greatest risk for aspiration. Aspiration of mineral oil can cause acute or chronic lipid pneumonitis.

Fecal Softeners   This class is composed of the surfactant agents not absorbed by the gut. They act as detergents to increase water penetration in the stool bolus, making it softer and easier to expel. They also promote water and electrolyte secretion. Agents in this class include the sodium, calcium, and potassium salts of docusate, and poloxamer 188. Docusate may be used alone or in formulations combined with the stimulant laxatives danthron, senna, or casanthranol. The initial dose of docusate is usually 200 mg daily, and it usually produces an effect in 24–72 hours.

Stimulant or Irritant Laxatives   These agents directly stimulate the myenteric plexus to induce peristalsis. They are the most commonly used preparations to stimulate bowel movement. They include senna, cascara sagrada, danthron, bisacodyl, and casanthranol. A reddish discoloration of alkaline urine or a yellow-brown discoloration of acidic urine may occur with senna or cascara sagrada. All of these drugs may cause severe cramping and abdominal discomfort. This side effect may be avoided by careful dosage titration and by using them in combination with a stool softening agent.

Osmotic Laxatives   These agents exert an osmotic effect, increasing the intraluminal volume by retaining water. They also appear to directly stimulate peristalsis and to increase water secretion. They are not broken down nor absorbed in the small gut. Their latency of action is very short, usually producing a response within a few hours. Lactulose and sorbitol are oral agents initiated at 15–30 cc one to two times daily. Flatulence is one of the most reported undesirable side effects of lactulose, and its taste is often unpalatable. Sorbitol is the most economical agent and reportedly has a better taste. Glycerin is a rectal preparation formulated as a liquid or suppository.

Saline Laxatives   These agents include the sulfate and citrate salts of magnesium, the oral sodium phosphates solutions, and milk of magnesia. Refrigeration of the magnesium citrate solution will help retain potency and enhance palatability. Doses vary with preparations. Continuous use of these agents may lead to electrolyte imbalances, such as an undesirable sodium or magnesium load, which may present problems for patients with hypertension, congestive heart failure, or significant renal dysfunction.

Enemas   Rectal enemas are available formulated with sodium phosphate, bisacodyl, or mineral oil. The oil retention enemas are especially useful in the setting of constipation with very hard, impacted stool. Generally, rectal preparations should be used as an adjunct to a prophylactic oral regimen.

Summary

The terminally ill patient has a multitude of symptoms that cause distress and compromise quality of life. Although it is impossible to relieve all symptoms completely, it is of paramount importance that each one be addressed individually and as frequently as is appropriate. It is also very important for the patient and family to be proactive and involved in the choice of treatment. The role of the health care provider in the palliative care setting is to give their expert knowledge and provide the available tools to alleviate symptoms so that each patient's quality of life may be the best possible until death.

Further Reading

Back, I. N. "Terminal restlessness in patients with advanced malignant disease." *Palliat Med*, 6:293–298, 1992.

Bruera, E. "Current pharmacological management of anorexia in cancer patients." *Oncology*, 16:125–130, 1992.

Bruera, E. "Clinical management of cachexia and anorexia in patients with advanced cancer." *Oncology*, 49(suppl 2):35–42, 1992.

Bruera, E., Brenneis, C., Michaud, M., Jackson F., MacDonald, R. N. "Association between asthenia, nutritional status, lean body mass, anemia, psychometrical status and tumor mass in patients with advanced breast cancer." *J Pain Sympt Manage*, 4:59–63, 1989.

Bruera, E., and MacDonald, R. N. "Asthenia in patients with advanced cancer." *J Pain Sympt Manage*, 3:9–14, 1988.

Bruera, E., MacEachern, T., Ripamonti, C., and Hanson, J. "Subcutaneous morphine for dyspnea in cancer patients." *Ann Int Med*, 119:106–107, 1993.

Bruera, E., Macmillian, K., Pitche, J., and MacDonald, R. N. "Effect of morphine on dyspnea of terminal cancer patients." *J Pain Sympt Manage*, 5:341–344, 1990.

Bruera, E., Ripamonti, C. "Dyspnea in patients with advanced cancer." In *Principle and Practice of Supportive Oncology*. A. Berger, R. Portenoy, and D. E. Weissman (eds.). Philadelphia: Lippincott-Raven, 1998.

Bruera, E., Schmitz, B., Pither, J., Neuman, C. M., and Hanson J. "The frequency and correlates of dyspnea in patients with advanced cancer." *J Pain Sympt Manage*, 19:357–362, 2000.

Casarrett, D. J., Hirschman, K. B., and Henry, M. R. "Does hospice have a role in nursing home care at the end of life?" *J Am Ger Soc*, 49:1493–1498, 2001.

Cherney, N. I., and Portenoy, S. K. "Sedation in the management of refractory symptoms: Guidelines for evaluation and treatment." *J Palliat Care*, 10:31–38, 1994.

Della Cuna, G. R., Pellegrini, A., and Piazzi, M. "Effect of methylprednisolone sodium succinate on quality of life in preterminal cancer patients: A placebo-controlled, multicenter study." *Eur J Cancer Clin Oncol*, 25:1817–1821, 1989.

Farncombe, M., and Chater, S. "Case studies outlining use of nebulized morphine for patients with end-stage chronic lung and cardiac disease." *J Pain Sympt Manage*, 8:221–225, 1993.

Gift, A. "Therapies for dyspnea relief." *Holistic Nurse Pract*, 2:57–63, 1993.

Gift, A., Moore, T., and Soeken, K. "Relaxation to reduce dyspnea and anxiety in COPD patients." *Nursing Res*, 4:242–246, 1992.

Grond, S., Zech, D., Diefenbach, C., and Bishcoff, A. "Prevalence and pattern of symptoms in patients with cancer pain: A prospective evaluation of 1635 cancer patients referred to a pain clinic." *J Pain Sympt Manage*, 9(6):372–382, 1994.

Heyes, J. R. "Depression and chronic fatigue in cancer patients." *Primary Care*, 18:327–339, 1991.

Janssens, J. P., Muralt, B., and Titelion, V. "Management of dyspnea in severe chronic obstructive pulmonary disease." *J Pain Sympt Manage*, 19:378–392, 2000.

Johanson, G. *Physician's Handbook of Symptom Relief in Terminal Care*, 4th edition. Santa Rosa, Calif.: Sonoma County Academic Foundation for Excellence in Medicine, 1993.

Kaasa, T., Gillis, K., Middleton, E., and Bruera, E. *The Edmonton Functional Assessment Tool (EFAT) for Terminal Cancer Patients*. Presented at the 9th International Congress on Care of the Terminally Ill. Montreal, Nov. 1–2, 1992.

Kaye, P. *Notes on Symptoms Control in Hospice and Palliative Care.* Essex: Hospice Education Institute, 1989.

Levy, M. H. "Constipation and diarrhea in cancer patients: Part I." *Primary Care Cancer,* 12(4):11–18, 1992.

Levy, M. H. "Constipation and diarrhea in cancer patients: Part II." *Primary Care Cancer,* 12(5):53–57, 1992.

Love, R., Leventhal, H., Easterlin, M., and Nerenz, D. "Side effects and emotional distress during cancer chemotherapy." *Cancer,* 63:604–612, 1989.

McNamara, P., Minton, M., and Twycross, R. G. "Use of midazolam in palliative care." *Palliat Med,* 5:244–249, 1991.

Mercadante, C. "Diarrhea, malabsorption and constipation." In *Principles and Practice of Supportive Oncology.* A. Berger, R. Portenoy, and D. E. Weissman (eds.). Philadelphia: Lippincott-Raven, 1998, pp. 191–205.

Neuenschwander, H., and Bruera, E. "Asthenia." In D. Doyle, G. W. C. Hanks, and N. MacDonald (eds.) *Oxford Textbook of Palliative Medicine,* 2nd edition. Oxford University Press, New York: 1998, pp. 573–581.

Plum, F. "Asthenia, weakness and fatigue." In *Cecil Textbook of Medicine.* Philadelphia: W. B. Saunders Company, 1985, p. 2044.

Rousseau, P. "Existential suffering and palliative sedation: A brief commentary with a proposal for clinical guidelines." *Am J Hospice Palliat Care,* 3:151–153, 2001.

Saunders, C. *The Management of Terminal Malignant Disease.* London: Edward Arnold, 1989.

Sheehan, D. C., and Forman, W. B. *Hospice and Palliative Care.* Sudbury, Mass.: Jones and Bartlett, 1996.

Sykes N. P. "Constipation and diarrhea." In D. Doyle, G. W. C. Hanks, and N. MacDonald (eds.) *Oxford Textbook of Palliative Medicine,* 2nd edition. Oxford University Press, New York: 1998, pp. 513–526.

Twycross, R. G., and Lack, S. A. *Therepeutics in Terminal Cancer,* 2nd edition. London: Churchill Livingstone, 1990.

Zerwelkh, J. V. "Comforting the dying dyspneic patient." *Nursing,* 87:66–69, 1987.

Principles of Pain Management

11

Marijo Letizia, R.N.C., Ph.D.

The undertreatment of pain is a widely recognized, well-documented health care problem. In light of this fact, management of pain has become a priority in recent years. For example, the World Health Organization (WHO) has urged all nations to establish pain relief policies. In the United States, the National Cancer Institutes (NCI) have placed a great emphasis on pain education and research, and other professional regulatory agencies and health care professionals have responded to this problem as well. For example, the Agency for Health Care Policy and Research (AHCPR), now known as the Agency for Healthcare Research and Quality (AHRQ), published a Clinical Practice Guideline on the Management of Cancer Pain, emphasizing the numerous and complex barriers to pain management that must be addressed in order to improve this very significant problem. The Joint Commission on Accreditation of Healthcare Organizations (JCAHO) instituted policies in 2000–2001 accreditation manuals addressing the need for more effective ways to manage pain. Health care providers are now required to recognize patients' rights to pain assessment and management; assess the nature and intensity of pain; record results of assessment to aid in follow-up; ensure staff competency in pain assessment and management; support appropriate prescribing of pain medications; and address the need for pain management in discharge planning.

Unrelieved pain is associated with considerable detrimental physiologic and psychosocial consequences. Pain can affect every aspect of a person's quality of life; unremitting pain can consume every aspect of that life. Changes in sleep patterns and concentration can cause interference with work and relationships and create a burden for loved ones. Those in pain may find themselves unable to participate in family and leisure activities, leading to feelings of isolation. Emotionally, there can be expressions of hopelessness, helplessness, anger, anxiety, depression, and frustration. Physical symptoms of pain that are detrimental to health include anorexia, tachycardia, increased blood pressure, increased oxygen demand, and hypercoagulation. Decreased mobility that can occur with pain may lead to cough suppression and shallow breathing, resulting in retained secretions and pneumonia. The effect this type of chronic pain can have on quality of life is shown in Table 11-1.

The health care community has embraced McCaffery's (1968) classic definition of pain: "Pain is whatever the person says it is, and existing whenever the person says it does." This definition designates the patient as the authority about pain. It also points to the self-report as the most reliable indicator of pain. Pain is an inherently subjective phenomenon. It is a sensation that is influenced by physical, psychosocial, and spiritual circumstances. For example, the experience of pain can be impacted by knowledge and beliefs about pain; previous pain experiences; particular styles of coping; educational level; age; gender; availability and type of social support systems; role models and family members; and cultural, religious, and social influences. These variables must be considered in the pain management plan of care.

Etiology of Pain

The dying patient can experience pain from tumor progression, toxicities of chemotherapy and radiation, nerve injury, infection, inflammation, and ischemic changes in the tissues. Pain can be acute or chronic in nature; this distinction is made according to the duration of the discomfort. Acute pain typically has a well-defined onset, lasts a relatively short period of time, and responds well to treatment. Acute pain often signals an injury and when the injury heals, the pain disappears. In contrast, chronic or persistent pain may

TABLE 11-1   Activities Impaired by Increasing Pain

Pain Level	3	4	5	6	7	8
	enjoy	enjoy	enjoy	enjoy	enjoy	enjoy
		work	work	work	work	work
			mood	mood	mood	mood
			activity	activity	activity	activity
			sleep	sleep	sleep	sleep
					walk	walk
					eat	eat
						talk
						relate

not have a defined onset, can be mild or severe, and is present for an extended period of time. Chronic pain often responds unpredictably to treatment. In the dying, this pain can be unrelenting and is often progressive.

When a person experiences pain, the body attempts to respond as the brain produces protective natural opioids (endorphins and enkephalins) to lessen the perception of painful nerve signals. These chemicals are produced in the pituitary gland. They attach to the outer surfaces of the brain cells like chemical keys fitting into locks to help stop neurons from sending a pain message. Communication about pain originates in distinct ways in the body; two physiologic classifications of the messages are "nociceptive" and "neuropathic." Nociceptive pain results when tissue is damaged by electrical, thermal (hot or cold), mechanical (stretching of organs or pressure), or chemical (ischemic) stimuli. The stimulus causes a chemical change in the tissues, activating sensory neurons called "nociceptors" that transmit information about the damage to the central nervous system. This electrical activity becomes the experience of pain when it reaches the brain. Nociceptive pain originates in either the soma (skin, muscle, fascia, deep tissues, and joints) or viscera (hollow organs). This pain is described as aching, throbbing, burning, or cramping and may be well localized. In contrast to nociceptive pain, neuropathic pain is more complex because it involves injury to the structures of the peripheral or central nervous system itself. This pain is described as a sharp, tingling, burning, or shooting sensation. Neuropathic pain can occur with mild stimuli such as clothing touching the skin. This phenomenon is called allodynia.

It is important to recognize the differences between the types of pain, because the treatment approach is based in part on the etiology of the pain. For example, consideration must be given to the site and mechanism of action of different types of medications. Nonopioid medications act to alter the breakdown of cell membranes in an area of inflammation, reducing the stimulation of the sensory neurons. In contrast, opioid medications bind to the end of the primary neuron, stopping the release of neurotransmitters. Other medications are called "adjuvants" because they have been found to be effective in analgesia but are primarily prescribed for other clinical conditions. Drugs used as adjuvants for pain control include antidepressants, anticonvulsants, and corticosteroids. Specific information about all of these medications is covered in the next chapter.

The WHO has conceptualized a ladder approach to the management of pain, with adjustment of the class and dose of medications as the patient's pain increases (see Figure 11-1). At the first rung of the ladder, patients who are in mild pain are treated with around-the-clock doses of nonopioids; adjuvant medications may also be used at this level. As pain increases, the second step of the ladder incorporates the use of an opioid for mild to moderate pain. Nonopioid and adjuvant medications can also be used. As pain continues to increase, on the third rung of the ladder, a strong opioid is provided for moderate to severe pain. Again, a nonopioid and adjuvant may also be used. It is important to recognize that the pain treatment plan can be initiated at any of

FIGURE 11-1 **WHO 3-Step Analgesic Ladder**

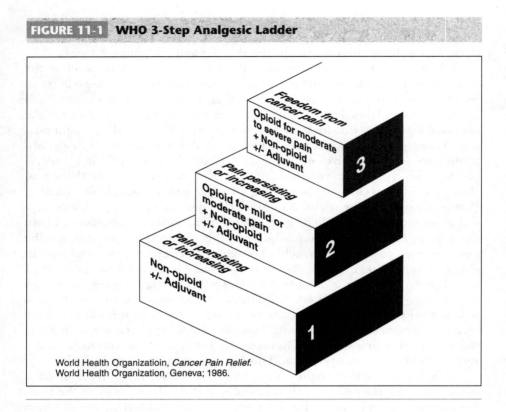

World Health Organizatioin, *Cancer Pain Relief.*
World Health Organization, Geneva; 1986.

the three levels. Because the dying may experience pain from both a nociceptive and neuropathic etiology, and in both an acute and chronic nature, healthcare providers must first base the pain management plan on a thorough pain assessment.

Assessment of Pain

Pain is now designated as the "fifth vital sign," demonstrating that pain assessment is an essential responsibility of the health care team. Total pain assessment includes consideration of the physical, psychosocial, spiritual, and financial components associated with pain. To begin, assessment includes noting the intensity, location, and quality of pain as well as the level of distress that it causes; Table 11-2 outlines components of a comprehensive pain assessment. Brief and easy-to-use assessment tools such as the numeric rating, visual analog, and categorical scales allow patients to quantify pain (see Figure 11-2). Appendix 1 contains other useful pain assessment tools. Ongoing assessment must be made and documented at regular intervals and with each new report of pain. Even those who do not freely report pain must be asked about the presence of pain. Each report of pain must be accepted, documented, and acted on.

TABLE 11-2 Components of an Initial Pain Assessment

I. Assessment of pain intensity and character
    a. Onset and temporal pattern
    b. Location
    c. Description
    d. Intensity
    e. Aggravating and relieving factors
    f. Previous treatment
    g. Effect of pain on physical and social function

II. Psychosocial assessment
    a. The effect and understanding of the diagnosis and treatment on the patient and caregiver
    b. The meaning of the pain to the patient and family
    c. Significant past instances of pain and their effect on the patient
    d. The patient's typical coping responses to stress or pain
    e. The patient's knowledge of, curiosity about, preferences for, and expectations about pain management methods
    f. The patient's concerns about using controlled substances such as opioids, anxiolytics, or stimulants
    g. The economic effect of the pain and its treatment
    h. Changes in mood that have occurred as a result of the pain

A number of behaviors can be observed that are related to the experience of pain. Patients may grimace, cry, moan, seem restless, and/or guard or rub a painful area. Objective indicators of pain are related to stimulation of the sympathetic nervous system. These include diaphoresis, tachycardia, and blood pressure changes. However, it is important to recognize that not all patients in pain will display these signs. For instance, the body's autonomic nervous system adapts to pain that is experienced over time, returning the patient to normal vital signs and other physiologic indicators. Likewise, the individual experiencing chronic pain may develop adaptive coping mechanisms that mask the characteristic findings seen in people with acute pain. Coping behaviors include humor and distraction through conversation or music. Some patients may report pain only if they are asked directly. They may exhibit sleepiness that can also occur secondary to the pain. It is essential to understand that the lack of pain expression does not necessarily mean lack of discomfort. Likewise, the inability of a health care provider to identify a specific cause of the pain does not negate that the pain exists.

A number of individuals are at risk for undertreatment of pain, primarily because of inherent difficulties in communicating information about their

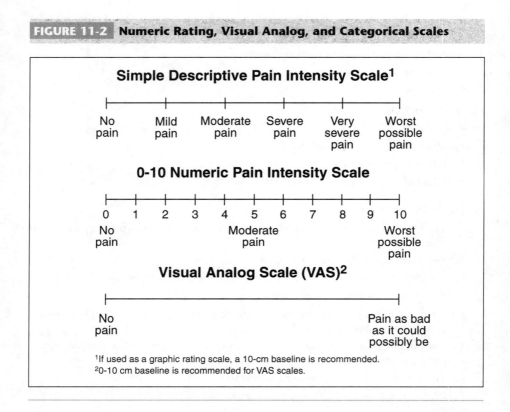

FIGURE 11-2 Numeric Rating, Visual Analog, and Categorical Scales

Simple Descriptive Pain Intensity Scale[1]

No	Mild	Moderate	Severe	Very	Worst
pain	pain	pain	pain	severe	possible
				pain	pain

0-10 Numeric Pain Intensity Scale

0   1   2   3   4   5   6   7   8   9   10

No   Moderate   Worst
pain   pain   possible
                                   pain

Visual Analog Scale (VAS)[2]

No pain   Pain as bad
                                            as it could
                                            possibly be

[1]If used as a graphic rating scale, a 10-cm baseline is recommended.
[2]0-10 cm baseline is recommended for VAS scales.

pain. These include patients who are infants, young children, women, elderly, cognitively impaired, ethnic minorities, and those with a language barrier. Patients also at risk for undertreatment of pain are those with a history of substance abuse and the poor and uninsured.

In the pediatric population, care providers rely on behavioral observation when verbal communication about pain is not possible. Typical behaviors include crying, grimacing, grunting, guarding, withdrawing, and clinging to loved ones. Regression of motor, verbal, and social skills may also be present. When asked, the older infant may be able to point to the location of the pain. Of those children who are able to participate in a self-report of pain, the "Pain Faces Scale" has been used effectively to provide quantitative information for documentation and intervention (see Figure 11-3).

On the other end of the age spectrum, physiologic changes in the older adult also impact pain assessment and treatment. For example, hearing, visual, cognitive, and motor impairments may impede the self-report of pain. In addition to providing an elderly patient with more time to process information, approaches such as the use of good lighting, hearing devices, and large-print written material may be helpful in assessing for pain. It is important to face the patient directly, speak slowly and clearly, present information in short seg-

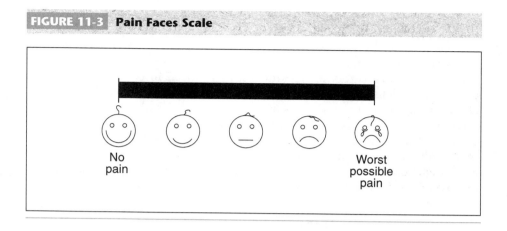

FIGURE 11-3 **Pain Faces Scale**

ments, and repeat or reword information. When there are difficulties in communication, or when the patient is unable to communicate, facial expressions, body position, the appearance of fatigue, and depression may be valuable nonverbal indicators of pain.

Barriers to Pain Management

Although great emphasis is currently placed on pain assessment and management, the literature suggests that patients who are dying continue to experience pain that is not well controlled. Efforts have been focused on identifying those impediments that prevent adequate management of pain at the end of life. The AHCPR has devised an organizing framework of the barriers involved in the suboptimal treatment of pain (Jacox, Carr, Payne et. al, 1994). Three problem areas are identified in this framework: problems related to the health care system, problems related to health care professionals, and problems related to patients and families.

Problems related to the health care system include low priority placed on pain treatment, inadequate reimbursement, restrictive regulation of controlled substances, and problems of availability/access to treatment. Problems related to health care professionals include inadequate pain management knowledge, poor pain assessment, concern about regulation of controlled substances, fear of addiction, concern about side effects, and concern about the development of tolerance to analgesics. Problems related to patients and families involve beliefs and attitudes about pain and pain medications that result in reluctance to report pain and reluctance to take pain medications. Reluctance to report pain may involve concern about distracting physicians from treatment of the underlying disease, fear that pain means the disease is getting worse, and concern about not being a good patient. Reluctance to take pain medications may involve fear of addiction, worries about unmanageable side effects, and concern about becoming tolerant to pain medications.

In caring for the dying, control of pain is a major concern, and possibly the greatest area of burden for family caregivers. As the dying process and change in level of functioning progresses, hospice patients become quite dependent on the family caregiver for administration of pain medication. When this occurs, caregivers are inherently involved in communicating with the hospice/palliative care staff about the patient's pain and making decisions about the administration of medications. These individuals are responsible for increasingly complex protocols that often include the use of multiple medications, adjuvant drugs, and complicated delivery systems. It is therefore crucial that health care providers consider the impact of the caregivers' concerns about reporting information regarding their loved one's pain and administering analgesics, as well as their skill level in administering the medications.

Misconceptions about Pain

Health care providers can begin to address the barriers to pain management by discussing myths surrounding the use of analgesics with the patient and caregiver. For example, it is crucial that staff members understand and clarify the differences between tolerance, dependence, and addiction, as illustrated in Table 11-3 (American Pain Society, 1999). Tolerance is a physiological state characterized by a decrease in the effects of a drug over time. Because of this phenomenon, patients may require a higher or more frequent dose of pain medication to achieve continued relief of discomfort. Over time, tolerance to the nonanalgesic effects of opioids such as sedation, nausea, and vomiting is also expected. In this way, undesirable side effects often dissipate after two to three days of opioid use. However, tolerance to the constipating effect of opioids does not develop. This can also be expected following repeated administration of an opioid over two to three days. The body becomes dependent on the opioid and an abrupt cessation or reduction in the dose may result in withdrawal symptoms. Exhibited symptoms are opposite to the initial effects of an opioid, and include diaphoresis, diarrhea, tachycardia, and anxiety.

One of the most misunderstood terms related to pain management is that of addiction. Concern about addiction impacts health care provider, patient, and caregiver approaches to treatment of pain. Whereas tolerance and physical dependence are purely physical phenomena, addiction is characterized by a psychological dependence on a drug. Addiction is defined as a pattern of compulsive drug use characterized by a continual craving for an opioid and the need to use the opioid for effects other than pain relief (McCaffery & Pasero, 1999). Addiction to opioid medications taken by patients in pain is extremely rare.

Overview of Approaches to Pain Management

In the care of the dying, general principles of pain management include using the simplest dosing schedules and least invasive route of administration; using

TABLE 11-3	Definitions Related to the Use of Opioids for the Treatment of Pain
Addiction	Addiction is a primary, chronic, neurobiologic disease, with genetic, psychosocial, and environmental factors influencing its development and manifestations. It is characterized by behaviors that include one or more of the following: impaired control over drug use, compulsive use, continued use despite harm, and craving.
Physical Dependence	Physical dependence is a state of adaptation that is manifested by a drug class-specific withdrawal syndrome that can be produced by abrupt cessation, rapid dose reduction, decreasing blood level of the drug, and/or administration of an antagonist.
Tolerance	Tolerance is a state of adaptation in which exposure to a drug induces changes that result in a diminution of one or more of the drug's effects over time.

the right drug for the right pain; anticipating, preventing, and treating medication side effects; giving medications for persistent pain around the clock; respecting individual differences, and including nonpharmacologic treatment approaches in the plan of care. The overall pain management goal is to achieve that level of pain management identified by the patient that allows for maintaining or improving quality of life. The mnemonic "ABCDE" is a helpful guide for pain management (see Table 11-4).

In most instances, medications should be given on an around-the-clock schedule. Attention also must be given to breakthrough pain that occurs on the background of otherwise controlled pain and in spite of taking pain medication around the clock. Breakthrough pain is typically of rapid onset, moderate to severe intensity, and relatively short duration. It can be triggered by various activities or be entirely unpredictable. In managing breakthrough pain, the goal is to treat the pain without overmedicating the patient. It may be helpful to visualize the management of breakthrough pain as similar to the use of rapid-onset insulin when a diabetic patient has varying blood glucose levels.

At the end of life, patients can experience various types and intensities of pain. It is essential to recognize pain crises that demand immediate intervention. These crises can result from a number of factors, including bone fracture, bowel perforation, brain and/or spinal cord metastasis, and septicemia.

Nonpharmacologic Approaches to Pain Management

Most often, health care providers approach pain management by first carefully considering available and appropriate pharmacologic agents, which will be covered extensively in the next chapter. However, nonpharmacologic therapies are also important to consider in the patient's plan of care (Decker,

TABLE 11-4	ABCDE Approach to Pain Assessment and Management
A	Ask about the pain regularly. Assess pain systematically.
B	Believe the patient and family in their reports of pain and what relieves it.
C	Choose pain control options appropriate for the patient, family, and setting.
D	Deliver interventions in a timely, logical, and coordinated fashion.
E	Empower patients and their families. Enable them to control the course to the greatest extent possible.

2000). Alternative and complementary therapies are nontraditional practices that can be used instead of or in conjunction with more conventional means of pain management. Whereas drug therapy tends to focus on isolated symptoms, alternative therapies involve a more holistic approach. Each requires the team to have a clear understanding of the therapy's purpose and a means of evaluating the patient's response to the treatment.

The National Institutes of Health (NIH) established an Office of Alternative Medicine (OAM) in 1992. The purpose of this division is to identify, evaluate, and provide information about alternative treatments for health problems. The OAM designated seven categories or specialty practice areas of alternative treatments. Three areas that have been particularly useful in the care of the dying are behavioral interventions, manual healing methods, and bioelectromagnetic therapies. The other categories that are also available are alternative systems of medical practice, herbal medicine, diet and nutrition therapies, and pharmacologic/biologic treatments.

Behavioral interventions are mind/body approaches based on the mind's important connection to and relationship with the function of body systems. With the belief that thoughts and emotions can exert great influence on health, behavioral interventions include relaxation, imagery, and hypnosis. In these therapies, breath, body relaxation, and imagination are used to promote relaxation. Meditation is a related behavioral technique that induces relaxation by focusing attention on the present moment using an image, sound, thought, or breathing. Music, dance, and art therapy promote relaxation and feelings of well-being by allowing the release of energy through expression as the patient draws, paints, sculpts, sings, dances, or simply views art or listens to music. Prayer, psychotherapy, and support groups are seen as offering more conventional complementary interventions that are also useful in the management of pain. Another mind/body intervention, aromatherapy, uses oils obtained from the root, flower, bark, leaves, or rind of a plant or fruit for therapeutic purposes. These oils are inhaled, massaged into the skin, or placed in bath water. Because the sense of smell is so acute, benefits from this therapy are thought to occur by evoking pleasant memories and emotions to enhance well-being.

Manual healing therapies include techniques such as physical therapy, massage, and therapeutic touch in which the health care provider uses his or her hands to enhance health. In physical therapy multiple modalities can be used to decrease muscle spasm and soft tissue discomfort. These include range of motion and muscle conditioning exercises as well as hydrotherapy or heat/cold applications. In therapeutic massage, manipulation of the soft tissues of the body enhances blood and lymph flow to the tissues and facilitates waste product removal from the muscles. Therapeutic touch is performed as a trained practitioner places his or her hands on or near the patient's body. The practitioner acts as a transmitter of energy within and around the patient while attempting to restore energy equilibrium.

Bioelectromagnetic therapies are intended to produce changes in the body's electromagnetic field to promote healing. These energy-based changes are thought to occur primarily at the level of the cell membrane. For management of pain, bioelectromagnetic therapies have the same intent as conventional approaches such as nerve blocking, in which local anesthetic agents are injected into an area of the body to prohibit the transmission of pain signals. In contrast, the aim of acupuncture is to control the sensation of pain by the insertion of special thin needles under the skin at designated points on the body. This technique is intended to correct the flow of painful stimuli away from its source. A transcutaneous electric nerve stimulation (TENS) therapy differs in that a battery-operated device applies a mild electric current to the surface of the skin to interrupt pain messages. As with other nonpharmacologic approaches, each of these therapies can be used in conjunction with medication to alleviate discomfort.

Alternative and complementary pain management therapies involve a holistic approach to care; this approach addresses physical, psychosocial, and spiritual components involved in the experience of pain. Today's health care team must be knowledgeable and prepared to provide comprehensive pain management that incorporates both alternative and conventional treatment strategies. In considering alternative approaches, the provider must have a clear understanding of what the therapy entails, including its benefits, therapeutic uses, practical applications, and risks. In all cases, it is crucial to both consider and respect the patient's values and belief systems, cultural customs and habits, and expectations in outlining the plan of care.

Summary

Unrelieved pain leads to unnecessary suffering and has a profound impact on quality of life. This problem is one of the most common and most feared of all symptoms encountered at the end of life, yet it is one that can be controlled. Every hospice and palliative care professional must act to treat pain by having a basic understanding of the physiology of pain and an awareness of the tools available for pain assessment and documentation. Team members must become comfortable and skilled in using the multiple pharmacologic and nonpharmacologic interventions and specific treatment guidelines for the management of pain. Professional resources are abundant, including clinical programs and specialists dedicated to pain management. Health care providers must be dedicated to improving the care of patients in pain in their practice.

Further Reading

1. American Nurses Association. *Position Paper on the Promotion of Comfort and Relief of Pain in Dying Patients.* Washington, D.C.: American Nurses Association, 1990.
2. American Pain Society. *Principles of Analgesic Use in the Treatment of Acute Pain and Cancer Pain.* 4th Edition. Glenview, Ill., American Pain Society, 1999.
3. Decker, G. "An overview of complementary and alternative therapies." *Clinical Journal of Oncology Nursing,* 4(1):49–52, 2000.
4. Management of Cancer Pain Guideline Panel. Agency for Health Care Policy and Research. *Management of Cancer Pain: Clinical Practice Guideline No. 9.* AHCPR Publication No. 94-0592. Rockville, Md.: U.S. Dept. of Health and Human Services, Public Health Service, 1994.
5. McCaffery, M. *Nursing Practice Theories Related to Cognition, Bodily Pain, and Man-Environment Interactions.* Los Angeles: UCLA Press, 1968, 95.
6. McCaffery, M., and Pasero, C. *Pain: Clinical Manual.* 2nd Edition. St. Louis: Mosby, 1999.
7. World Health Organization. *Cancer Pain Relief.* Geneva: World Health Organization, 1986.

Resources

Agency for Healthcare Research and Quality: **http://www.ahrq.gov**
American Academy of Pain Management: **http://www.aapainmanage.org**
American Pain Society: **http://www.ampainsoc.org**
American Society of Pain Management Nurses: **http://www.aspmn.org**
City of Hope Pain Resource Center: **http://prc.coh.org**
Joint Commission on Accreditation of Healthcare Organizations:
    http://www.jcaho.org/standards/
Mayday Pain link: **http://edc.org/painlink/**
Office of Alternative Medicine: **www.altmed.od.nih.gov**
Pain Link: **http://www.edc.org/PainLink/**
Roxanne Pain Institute: **http://www.roxane.com/pain/**
Wisconsin Cancer Pain Initiative Cancer Society: **http://cis.nci.nih.gov**

Pain Guidelines from the Agency of Health Research and Quality

Management of Cancer Pain, Clinical Practice Guideline Number 9, AHCPR Pub. No. 94-0592, March 1994.
Management of Cancer Pain: Adults, Quick Reference Guide for Clinicians, Number 9, AHCPR Pub. No. 94-0593.
Managing Cancer Pain, Consumer Guide Number 9, AHCPR Pub. No. 94-0595, March 1994.

Initial Pain Assessment Tool

Date _____

Patient's Name _____ Age _____ Room _____

Diagnosis _____ Physician _____

Nurse _____

I. LOCATION: Patient or nurse mark drawing

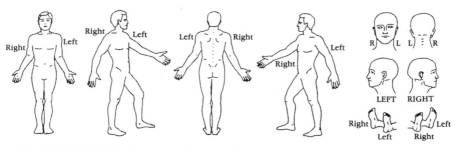

II. INTENSITY: Patient rates the pain. Scale used _____

Present: _____
Worst pain gets: _____
Best pain gets: _____
Acceptable level of pain: _____

III. QUALITY: (Use patient's own words, e.g. prick, ache, burn, throb, pull, sharp)
_____
_____

IV. ONSET, DURATION, VARIATIONS, RHYTHMS: _____
_____

V. MANNER OF EXPRESSING PAIN: _____
_____
_____

VI. WHAT RELIEVES THE PAIN? _____
_____

VII. WHAT CAUSES OR INCREASES THE PAIN? _____
_____

VIII. EFFECTS OF PAIN: (Note decreased function, decreased quality of life.)

Accompanying symptoms (e.g. nausea) _____
Sleep _____
Appetite _____
Physical activity _____

Relationships with others (e.g. irritability) _____
Emotions (e.g. anger, suicidal, crying) _____
Concentration _____
Other _____

IX. OTHER COMMENTS: _____
_____

X. PLAN: _____
_____

Brief Pain Inventory (Short Form)

Study ID # _____   Hospital # _____

Do not write above this line

Date: _____/_____/_____

Time: _____

Name: _____   _____   _____
             Last   First   Middle Initial

1) Throughout our lives, most of us have had pain from time to time (such as minor headaches, sprains, and toothaches). Have you had pain other than these everyday kinds of pain today?   1. Yes   2. No

2) On the diagram, shade in the areas where you feel pain. Put an X on the area that hurts the most.

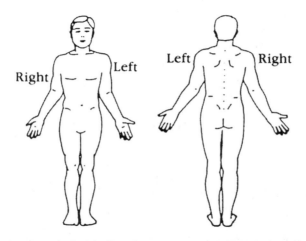

3) Please rate your pain by circling the one number that best describes your pain at its worst in the past 24 hours.

0   1   2   3   4   5   6   7   8   9   10
No   Pain as bad as
pain   you can imagine

4) Please rate your pain by circling the one number that best describes your pain at its least in the past 24 hours.

0   1   2   3   4   5   6   7   8   9   10
No   Pain as bad as
pain   you can imagine

5) Please rate your pain by circling the one number that best describes your pain on the average.

0   1   2   3   4   5   6   7   8   9   10
No   Pain as bad as
pain   you can imagine

6) Please rate your pain by circling the one number that tells how much pain you have right now.

0	1	2	3	4	5	6	7	8	9	10

No
pain

Pain as bad as
you can imagine

7) What treatments or medications are you receiving for your pain?

_____

8) In the past 24 hours, how much relief have pain treatments or medications provided? Please circle the one percentage that most shows how much relief you have received.

0%	10%	20%	30%	40%	50%	60%	70%	80%	90%	100%

No
relief

Complete
relief

9) Circle the one number that describes how, during the past 24 hours, pain has interfered with your:

A.   General activity

0	1	2	3	4	5	6	7	8	9	10

Does not
interfere

Completely
interferes

B.   Mood

0	1	2	3	4	5	6	7	8	9	10

Does not
interfere

Completely
interferes

C.   Walking ability

0	1	2	3	4	5	6	7	8	9	10

Does not
interfere

Completely
interferes

D.   Normal work (includes both work outside the home and housework)

0	1	2	3	4	5	6	7	8	9	10

Does not
interfere

Completely
interferes

E.   Relations with other people

0	1	2	3	4	5	6	7	8	9	10

Does not
interfere

Completely
interferes

F.   Sleep

0	1	2	3	4	5	6	7	8	9	10

Does not
interfere

Completely
interferes

G.   Enjoyment of life

0	1	2	3	4	5	6	7	8	9	10

Does not
interfere

Completely
interferes

Source: Pain Research Group. Department of Neurology, University of Wisconsin-Madison. Used with permission. May be duplicated and used in clinical practice.

Memorial Pain Assessment Card

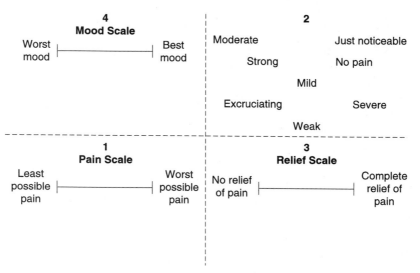

Note: Card is folded along broken line so that each measure is presented to the patient separately in the numbered order.

Source: Fishman, B., Pasternak, S., Wallenstein, S.L., et al. The Memorial Pain Assessment Card: A Valid Instrument for the Evaluation of Cancer Pain. *Cancer*, 60(5):1151–1158. 1987. Used with permission.

Pharmacotherapy for Chronic Pain

12

Robert P. Anderson, RPh

pharmacological approach, using opioid and adjuvant medications, remains the cornerstone of therapy for cancer-related pain and an appropriate therapy for many pain syndromes not related to cancer. Thus, a thorough understanding of the actions of these medications, both pharmacokinetic and pharmacodynamic, is essential to optimize pain control and minimize adverse events. Cancer pain may be continuous, intermittent, or, most frequently, a combination of the two. Continuous pain requires around-the-clock (ATC) analgesia, preferably with a long-acting or sustained release preparation. Intermittent pain requires the as-needed (PRN) dosing of immediate release medication. The patient suffering both continuous and intermittent pain is then best treated with an ATC and PRN medication regimen. With respect to the particular agent and specific dose, the key principle to keep in mind is the *individualization of therapy* to each patient.

Nonopioid Analgesics

The nonsteroidal anti-inflammatory drugs (NSAIDs) possess analgesic, anti-inflammatory, and antipyretic properties. The mechanism of action of this heterogeneous group of agents involves the inhibition of cyclooxygenase, the enzyme responsible for the biosynthesis of the prostaglandins. The NSAIDs may be used initially for mild cancer pain or as an adjuvant to the opioids for bone pain or soft tissue damage, where pain is generally well localized and constant and where inflammatory processes are present. The major side effects associated with the NSAIDs include gastrointestinal bleeding (ulceration), renal dysfunction, and blockade of platelet aggregation. Before initiation, the patient's history should be reviewed for allergies, renal or hepatic dysfunction, and gastrointestinal bleeding or ulceration. If long-term NSAID use is anticipated, ulcer prophylaxis should be initiated. Other potential side effects to be aware of include hepatic dysfunction, hypersensitivity reactions, and gastrointestinal intolerance manifested by nausea and/or vomiting, dyspepsia, bloating, heartburn, and/or constipation.

Unlike the opioid analgesics, the NSAIDs are characterized by a maximum tolerable dose (Table 12-1). Exceeding this dose provides only a minimal increase in analgesia while significantly increasing the side effect profile. Dosages should be individualized, starting low, and therapy should take into account any significant gastrointestinal or renal history. There has been no conclusive evidence that demonstrates the superiority of one agent over any other. If a trial with one specific NSAID, titrated to maximum dose, does not result in optimal pain control, rotation to another NSAID before discontinuing therapy with this class of drugs is a rational approach.

Celecoxib and rofecoxib are two new agents that selectively inhibit COX-2, one isoenzyme of cyclooxygenase. Although the exact mechanism of action has not been clearly defined, it is thought that the analgesic, anti-inflammatory, and antipyretic effect of the NSAIDs is mediated via inhibition of COX-2 and that the adverse effects on the gastrointestinal mucosa and on platelet aggregation is mediated via inhibition of COX-1. Thus, the selective inhibition of COX-2 is thought to result in equivalent benefits with fewer side effects when compared to the nonselective NSAIDs. Given their high cost and the relatively short experience with evaluating fully their side effect profiles, these agents should be reserved for those patients who have failed therapy with other nonopioid analgesics. Celecoxib is dosed at 100–200 mg once daily or twice daily in equally divided doses. Doses greater than 400 mg/day do not appear to provide added benefit. Rofecoxib is initiated at 12.5 mg once daily with a maximum dose of 50 mg/day. As with the other agents, dosing should be individualized and titrated to pain control.

The nonacetylated salicylates include choline salicylate, magnesium salicylate, salsalate, diflunisal, sodium salicylate, and sodium thiosalicylate. These agents have fewer adverse gastrointestinal effects and less adverse effects on platelet aggregation than the NSAIDs, so they may be beneficial in the patient with existing risk factors. Acetaminophen is a para-aminophenol derivative, with good analgesic and antipyretic activity; however, it does not provide clinical anti-inflammatory activity. The major side effect with chronic use is hepatic dysfunction; however, renal dysfunction may also present following long-term use of doses greater than 2000 mg/day. Initial dosing starts with 325–650 mg every four hours; maximum daily doses, when used chronically, should not exceed 4000 mg/day. Often patients with cancer present with liver disease; in this case, or for patients with active liver disease or a tendency toward alcohol abuse, acetaminophen should be used with caution, in lower doses, or simply not used as a chronic adjuvant. Both acetaminophen and aspirin are formu-

TABLE 12-1 Nonsteroidal Anti-Inflammatory Drugs

Agent	Peak Onset (h)	Initial Dosing	Maximum Dose	Serum Half-Life (h)	Duration of Analgesia (h)	Duration of Antiplatelet Effect
Aspirin	0.5–2.0	325–650 mg q4h	3900 mg	6–12	2–4	14 days
Diclofenac	2–3	75 mg bid 25–50 mg tid-qid	200 mg	1–2	?	5–10 hours
Etodolac	0.5–2.0	200 mg tid-qid 300 mg bid, tid, qid 400 mg bid-tid	1200 mg	3.3–11.3	4–12	36 hours
Fenoprofen	1–2	200–600 mg tid-qid	3200 mg	2–3	?	15–24 hours
Flurbiprofen	1.5	50–100 mg bid-tid	300 mg	5.7	?	24–48 hours
Ibuprofen	0.5–2.0	300–600 mg tid-qid	2400 mg	1.8–2.5	4–6	5–10 hours
Indomethacin	0.5–2.0 (SR 2–4)	25 mg bid-tid 75–150 mg bid or hs	200 mg	4.5 (SR 4.5–6.0)	4–6	24–48 hours
Ketoprofen	0.5–2.0	75 mg tid 50 mg qid	300 mg	2–4	?	5–10 hours
Ketorolac	0.5–1.0	30–60 mg IM load 15–30 mg qid	120 mg	2.4–8.6	IM: 6	24–48 hours
Nambumetone	2.5–4.0	1000 mg qid-bid	2000 mg	22.5–30.0	?	4–7 days
Naproxen	1–4	500 mg then 250 mg tid-qid	1500 mg	12–15	7	4 days
Naproxen Na	1–2	550–825 mg then 275–550 mg bid	1375 mg	12–13	7	4 days
Oxaprozin	3–5	600–1200 mg qid	1800 mg	42–50	?	8–10 days
Piroxicam	1–5	20 mg qid	20 mg	30–86	48–72	7–20 days
Sulindac	2–4	150–200 mg bid	400 mg	16.4	?	4 days
Tolmetin	0.5–1.0	400 mg tid	1800 mg	1–1.5	?	8–16 hours

? = unknown/unclear.

lated in combination with opioids. It is important to remember that although there is no ceiling dose associated with the opioid, there is a maximum daily dose for each of the nonopioid analgesics.

When significant pain relief cannot be achieved with the foregoing agents, a trial of corticosteroids may be initiated. Tapering doses of prednisone, starting at 20 mg twice daily, or dexamethasone, starting at 16 mg once daily, often provide relief for a wide variety of pain syndromes such as metastatic bone pain, visceral pain, neuropathic pain, pain due to spinal cord compression or from inflammatory lesions (soft tissue or musculoskeletal), or nerve compression from a tumor mass. Advantages of corticosteroid therapy include an increased appetite, antiemetic effects, and a sense of well-being. Gastrointestinal bleeding, infections, and blood sugar fluctuations are potential serious adverse events. When using corticosteroids long term, prophylactic H_2 blockers are recommended.

Opioid Analgesics

Opioid pharmacotherapy is well established as the cornerstone of treatment for moderate to severe cancer-related pain. As a class, the opioid analgesics have many advantages when used for the treatment of pain. There is no maximum dose associated with the pure opioid agonist, a characteristic that allows for the titration to pain control in most clinical situations. The medical literature has reported up to 50-fold differences in interpatient doses required for pain relief. Unlike the renal or gastrointestinal insult seen with the nonsteroidal anti-inflammatory drugs, opioids are not associated with any end-organ damage. These agents provide an excellent risk:benefit ratio for the majority of patients, that is, efficacy is obtainable without significant side effects. All types of pain respond to opioids; however, the degree of response is variable. Somatic and visceral pain respond well, whereas neuropathic pain is often poorly responsive and will require adjuvant therapies. Finally, the opioid analgesics represent a very cost-effective therapy for pain when the loss of productivity, hospitalization, and consequences to quality of life are considered. The opioids used for moderate to severe pain are shown in Table 12-2.

Morphine is considered the gold standard for the treatment of moderate to severe cancer-related pain. This superiority resides in the comprehensive clinical experience with dosing, side effect profiles, changes in route of administration, and rotation to other opioids. Further, morphine is available in several formulations that allow for a wide variety of routes of administration. These include long-acting, immediate release, solution, suppository, and parenteral formulations for oral, sublingual, rectal, subcutaneous, intravenous, and intraspinal delivery. There is no evidence that morphine provides superior efficacy or a more benign side effect profile when compared to the other pure opioid agonists. It is generally considered that when dosed in appropriate equianalgesic doses, no one opioid analgesic is superior to another.

Codeine, hydrocodone, and oxycodone are formulated in combination with acetaminophen, aspirin, and, in the case of hydrocodone, ibuprofen. The

TABLE 12-2 Opioid Analgesics for Moderate to Severe Pain

Classification	Agent	Parenteral Equivalency Dose (mg)	Conversion Parenteral to Oral	Oral Equivalency Dose (mg)	Half-Life (hr)	Duration of Analgesia
Phenanthrene Derivatives	Codeine	120	1.67	200	3	3–6 hr
	Hydrocodone	—	—	60	4	3–6 hr
	Oxycodone[1]	—	—	15–30	3	3–6 hr
	Morphine[2]	10	2–3	30	3	3–6 hr
	Hydromorphone[3]	1.5	5	7.5	2–3	3–4 hr
	Levorphanol	2	2	4	12–16	6–8 hr
	Oxymorphone	1–1.5	—	—	3	3–6 hr
Phenylpiperidine Derivatives	Fentanyl[4]	300 mcg	—	—	3–4	1–2 hr
	Sufentanil	30 mcg	—	—	2	1–2 hr
Diphenylheptane	Methadone[5]	3	3	10	15–40	4–8 hr

1. Oxycodone may be up to twice as potent orally as morphine. Studies with the parenteral formulations determined the morphine to oxycodone ratio to be 0.7:1.

2. In opioid-naïve patients the morphine parenteral to oral ratio is 1:6. With chronic dosing this ratio becomes 1:2–3.

3. Hydromorphone appears to demonstrate a directional difference in equianalgesic dose. When rotating from morphine to hydromorphone the ratio is 5:1 (M:H); however, when rotating in the other direction, the ratio is 3.5:1 (M:H).

4. 25 mcg/hr transdermal patch (600 mcg/day) is equivalent to 60 mg of oral morphine daily.

5. Equianalgesic dosing of methadone is based on total daily morphine equivalents. Use (morphine to methadone) 3:1 for doses <100 mg, 6:1 for doses 100–400 mg, and 10:1 for doses >400 mg. Some clinicians recommend 15–20:1 for patients receiving daily morphine equivalents >1000 mg. With chronic dosing, the half-life of methadone may increase in some individuals to 150 hours.

clinical importance of these combination products is that they are characterized with a maximum dose, defined by the nonopioid agent. Codeine is the
weakest of the opioid analgesics and may result in greater constipation and
thus may be better reserved for those patients where diarrhea presents a problem. Codeine is available in combination as oral tablets, capsules, or solution
and as a single entity formulated for oral (tablets and solution) or parenteral
use. Hydrocodone is formulated only in combination as tablets, capsules, or
solution. The combination products of oxycodone are available as tablets, capsules, and in solution. Oxycodone as a single entity is a potent analgesic and
appropriate for use in the setting of severe pain. The drug is available in a
long-acting tablet as well as immediate release tablets, capsules, and solution.

Hydromorphone has a more rapid onset and shorter duration of action
than morphine. These characteristics provide advantages for this agent when
used in the setting of breakthrough pain, which is generally characterized by a
relatively rapid onset and short duration. Thus, pain relief is swifter and, as the
breakthrough pain episode concludes, the time the patient may experience
toxicity from overmedication will be shorter. Hydromorphone is available as
immediate release tablets and solution for oral use, rectal suppositories, and
parenteral injection including a high potency 10 mg/ml formulation. An
extended release formulation is available in Canada and is currently being
studied for release in the United States.

The characteristics of fentanyl have been exploited to formulate a very
attractive breakthrough pain medication. Fentanyl is a very lipophilic agent,
lending itself to reliable and fast sublingual or buccal absorption. The formulation of an oral transmucosal lozenge resulted in an oral analgesic with a very
sudden onset of action (~5 minutes). Fentanyl's short duration of action (1–2
hours) further reduces exposure to overmedication following termination of
the breakthrough pain episode. In addition to the lozenge, fentanyl is available as a topical transdermal system and a parenteral solution for injection.
Sufentanil is an analogue of fentanyl that is approximately ten times more
potent than fentanyl. Sufentanil is available only in a parenteral solution for
injection; however, this solution has been used sublingually for pain control.

Levorphanol and oxymorphone are relatively infrequently used opioid
analgesics. Both are potent analgesics capable of providing relief for moderate
to severe pain. The disadvantage of levorphanol resides in its long half-life relative to its duration of action. Caution must be used to prevent toxicity from
an accumulation of parent drug or metabolites. Levorphanol is available only
as a 2 mg tablet and a parenteral solution for injection. Oxymorphone is available only as a 5 mg rectal suppository and a parenteral solution for injection.

Methadone is a structurally unique pure opioid agonist that presents several advantages and disadvantages for use in the cancer pain setting.
Methadone is an immediate release product with a duration of action ranging
from 4 to 8 hours following a single dose; however, due to a high volume of
distribution, there can be a substantial increase in the duration of action following chronic dosing. This allows for 2–3 times daily dosing while providing

the relatively rapid pain relief of an immediate release product. There are no known active metabolites associated with methadone, circumventing the toxicity seen following accumulation of metabolites from morphine and probably other opioids. The lipophilic nature of the drug allows for increased sublingual and buccal absorption. Methadone is also very inexpensive when compared to the other commercially available extended release preparations. The major disadvantage is a very long half-life—15–40 hours, with outliers to 150 hours. Caution and vigilance must be exercised, especially with initiation of therapy, to prevent accumulation of the drug and serious, even life-threatening, toxicity. This, coupled with the limited knowledge concerning titration, dose schedule, and equianalgesic conversion, demand highly individualized, time-intensive therapy be directed to the patient initiated on or converted to methadone. The drug is available as an oral tablet or solution and a parenteral solution for injection.

Methadone has been termed a "broad spectrum" analgesic because of its multiple mechanisms of action. In addition to its activity at the opioid receptor, methadone is also postulated to act antagonistically at the N-methyl-D-aspartate (NMDA) receptor and to inhibit the reuptake of norepinephrine and serotonin. The NMDA receptor has been implicated in the amplification of pain impulses to higher cortical centers. Further, metabolites of morphine, and possibly hydromorphone, may act at the NMDA receptor to facilitate hyperalgesia in a manner similar to that seen with chronic C-fiber input. The inhibition of bio-amine reuptake would enhance activity at inhibitory pathways, further reducing pain. Thus, rotation from morphine to methadone could result in pain relief from action at the opioid receptor, desensitization of the NMDA receptor as metabolites of morphine are eliminated, blockade of the NMDA receptor, and increased activity at descending inhibitory pathways.

In the chronic pain setting, one could speculate that the ability to interact with both opioid and nonopioid receptors could result in decreased analgesic requirements that would translate to an increased relative potency for methadone when compared to other opioids. Thus, when rotating from methadone to morphine or another opioid, caution must be exercised to prevent serious overmedication. Although many equianalgesic charts show a relative equivalence between methadone and morphine, methadone may be as much as 10–20 times more potent than morphine in the patient tolerant to opioids, especially high doses of opioids. Clinicians must be wary of assuming that the level of tolerance for patients receiving relatively high doses of opioids will protect them from serious toxicity during conversion to methadone. On the contrary, increased vigilance during the conversion is essential for a positive outcome. For these reasons, conversion to methadone for patients receiving >400 mg morphine equivalents should be undertaken in the hospital following a strategy that provides for patient safety. One such approach involves reducing the opioid by one-third each day over three days. Methadone is initiated at 10% of the morphine equivalent dose eliminated each day. The immediate release characteristics of methadone allow it to be used as a PRN supplement for breakthrough pain during this rotation of opioids.

Several opioids are generally not recommended for routine clinical use. The partial agonist buprenorphine and the agonist-antagonists pentazocine, nalbuphine, and butorphanol are characterized with maximum tolerated doses and psychomimetic side effects, and have the potential to precipitate withdrawal in the patient tolerant to a pure opioid agonist. Meperidine is metabolized to normeperidine, which due to its half-life of 15–18 hours may accumulate, especially in the setting of renal dysfunction, and cause myoclonus and seizure. Propoxyphene, an agent whose efficacy has been questioned in several clinical trials, is also associated with a potentially toxic metabolite, norpropoxyphene. Given the variety of available pure opioid agonists, these agents are generally best avoided for the control of chronic pain.

Adverse Effects

The adverse effects associated with opioid analgesics should be anticipated and rigorously attended to. The primary side effects include constipation, nausea and/or vomiting, and sedation. Less common side effects include dysphoria, mental confusion, delirium, pruritis, urinary retention, mood disturbances, sexual dysfunction, and myoclonus. There appears to be no evidence of major organ dysfunction associated with the opioids, and there is minimal risk of respiratory depression, which will not occur until both analgesia and sedation present, with chronic opioid use. Tolerance will generally develop to the side effects of opioids relatively quickly with the exception of constipation, which should be anticipated by initiating prophylaxis with the start of the opioid analgesic regimen. Factors that influence the incidence of side effects should be considered in all patients initiated on opioid analgesics. The elderly are more sensitive to both the beneficial and adverse effects of opioids. Hepatic and/or renal dysfunction may result in less predictable opioid effects due to changes in metabolite concentrations. Concurrent medications should be reviewed for potential additive toxicity.

Management strategies to reduce side effects begin with careful monitoring of the patient until tolerance develops. The patient should be informed about the potential side effects and what measures will be taken to alleviate the problem. This is important in view of the potential for the interference of the side effect profile with maintaining pain control. If a given side effect persists (i.e., tolerance develops partially or not at all) symptomatic management of the side effect may be considered. Another approach is to reduce the dosage of the opioid with the addition of another analgesic (e.g., the use of NSAIDs or pamidronate for bone pain) or nonpharmacologic treatment. In either of these approaches, the risk:benefit ratio of the added medications must be taken into account. A further approach involves switching the route of administration. Very limited evidence suggests that switching to rectal, subcutaneous, or transdermal delivery may reduce some side effects of oral opioids. Finally, because no opioid (except meperidine) is universally better or worse than any other with respect to its side effect profile (or analgesia) and each varies with respect to the side effect profile (or analgesia) manifest in an individual patient, opioid rotation is a reasonable approach. Careful monitoring of the patient is essential to recognize an unfavorable outcome should the approach fail. Minimizing polypharmacy is an obvious advantage of this approach.

Opioid analgesics act on receptors in the gastrointestinal tract to slow motility, thus, constipation will manifest itself in the majority of patients receiving opioid medications. Exceptions will include patients with cancers that cause diarrhea (e.g., carcinoid tumors) or those receiving chemotherapy that may cause diarrhea (e.g., cisplatin). In the former, opioids may counter the diarrhea either partially, in which case additional antidiarrheal agents may still be required, or completely. It is rare that these patients will require laxative therapy; however, patients receiving chemotherapy may require titration of laxative therapy; downward for the day of and a few days following chemotherapy, with a return to increased laxatives until the next chemotherapy cycle. Care should be taken to recognize the addition of medications that may exacerbate constipation, such as vinca alkaloids and iron therapy.

Laxative therapy should be initiated with the start of opioid pain management. Exercise and fluids should be encouraged; however, they are rarely adequate for the treatment of opioid-induced constipation. Bulk-forming laxatives also do not generally provide adequate therapy. A history of the patient's bowel habits and laxative use should be obtained. In the patient with minimal prior laxative use, stimulant laxatives in combination with stool softeners (e.g., Pericolace® or Senekot-S®) often provide a good starting point, initiated at 1 tablet every 12 hours and titrated to 3 tablets every 8 hours. If, during titration, the patient experiences cramping, the dose should be reduced to the prior tolerated dose and a laxative from a different class (e.g., osmotic) added to the regimen. In general, oral laxatives are preferred for ATC use, with rectal enemas reserved for PRN use. The goal of therapy should be a comfortable bowel movement every two to three days.

Nausea/vomiting are seen in approximately 50% of patients following initiation of opioid therapy or when there is a large dosage increase. Tolerance often develops within three to five days and these symptoms often decline. Because up to 50% of patients will not suffer from nausea/vomiting, prophylactic antiemetics are not indicated, unless the specific clinical situation requires their use. For the patient who develops nausea/vomiting, several agents may be used. Antivertigenous drugs (e.g., scopolamine, meclizine) may be used for the patient with a history of vertigo. More frequently, prochlorperazine (5–10 mg every six hours), metoclopramide (10 mg every six hours), or haloperidol (2–5 mg two to three times daily) functions well to control nausea/vomiting. If the nausea/vomiting persists, antiemetics can be continued or rotation to another opioid may be tried in an attempt to alter the side effect profile.

Sedation is another side effect for which tolerance often develops quickly with chronic opioid use. Again, patient education is important to prevent the early discontinuation of pain therapy. Initial sedation is often the result of poor sleep hygiene that has resulted from significant pain. Chronic pain will interfere with sleep patterns and following good pain control the patient may doze frequently as the body attempts to "catch up" on its sleep. The principle of "easy arousal" is important. If the patient is easily aroused and cognizant of his surroundings when aroused, he or she is not overly sedated. If, however, he or she cannot be easily aroused, dosage adjustments should be made. If sedation persists in the presence of good pain control, several approaches should be considered. The patient's medication profile should be examined for any central nervous system depressants and those that can should be discontinued. Other causes, such as metabolic abnormalities (e.g., hypercalcemia, uremia) and CNS tumor involvement (e.g., carcinomatous meningitis, brain metastases) should be ruled out. Psychostimulants may overcome sedation in the setting of good pain control and may provide adjuvant analgesia when analgesia has not been maximized. These agents include methylphenidate (5–20 mg in the morning and at noon), dextroamphetamine (5–20 mg in the morning and at noon), and pemoline (18.75–75 mg every morning). Care should be taken not to dose these agents late in the day because they can interfere with normal sleep. Haloperidol should be used only when cognitive function is affected resulting in mental confusion or delirium. Again, opioid rotation is also an option.

Mental confusion, dysphoria, mood disturbances, and myoclonus are thought to result from the accumulation of morphine, and possibly other opioid, metabolites. Rotation to an alternate agent is generally the best approach.

Routes of Administration

The preferred route for the administration of opioid analgesia is by mouth. This route is, when it can be used effectively, the most convenient for the patient, the least invasive, and the most cost effective. It is the simplest method, which in turn minimizes the burden on the family and caregivers. In the main, oral opioids can often be used until death is imminent; however, this route becomes unreliable in the clinical setting of persistent nausea and vomiting, dysphagia, significant somnolence or drowsiness, malabsorption, and bowel obstruction. Further, this route is unsuitable for patients who require rapid titration for the relief of severe pain. Current sustained release formulations for morphine and oxycodone allow for one to three times daily around-the-clock dosing and immediate release preparations of these agents formulated as tablets or solutions allow for breakthrough pain management. Methadone, although an immediate release preparation, may also be used for ATC dosing because of its long half-life, generally administered every eight hours, although occasionally every six hours or every twelve hours may be required.

If oral dosing is not feasible, the relatively noninvasive rectal route or transdermal route should be considered next. Rectal suppositories are available for morphine, hydromorphone, and oxymorphone as immediate release preparations. Sustained release suppositories are available in Canada and may be compounded in the United States by specialized pharmacies. Conversion from the oral dose should start at a 1:1 ratio. This route is most useful in temporary or terminal care situations. Disadvantages include rectal irritation and mechanical or spontaneous expulsion of the suppository. This route should be used with caution or avoided in the neutropenic patient.

MS Contin® (an oral sustained release formulation of morphine) has been shown to be effective when used rectally. Dosing is based on a 1:1 ratio with oral dose. The tablet(s) may be placed in an empty gelatin capsule for easier insertion. For the dehydrated patient, 5 cc of water should be placed in the rectum to facilitate dissolution. Oral solutions of morphine have also been used successfully as a micro-enema.

Often the use of rectal preparations is distasteful to the patient or the caregiver. In this setting, transdermal preparations provide another noninvasive, convenient alternative for the patient unable to tolerate oral medication. Currently the only opioid available in this formulation is fentanyl. The transdermal patch should be applied to clean dry skin and held in place for a minimum of 30 seconds, and preferably for up to 2 minutes, to prevent detachment of the patch. This formulation is designed to improve compliance by supplying a given amount of drug hourly for 72 hours; however, a small number of patients may experience significant breakthrough pain during the last 24 hours; in these patients the patch may have to be changed every 48 hours. Once applied, it may take from 8 to 18 hours before blood levels produce analgesia. Release rates may be affected by fever and by the cachectic condition of the patient. Therefore, it is crucial to maintain pain control with immediate release analgesics until the patient has stabilized. Further, dosage adjustments based on breakthrough medication usage should not be made until analgesia from the transdermal patch has stabilized. It is also important to recognize that when the patch is removed, the drug depot in the skin will confer analgesia for the same 8 to 18 hours. Titration should not be attempted with this formulation; it is best adapted to the patient with relatively stable pain.

Oral transmucosal delivery of pain medication has several advantages. The oral mucosa is highly permeable and highly vascularized. Lipophilic drugs are able to cross the oral mucosa, enter the systemic circulation without hepatic first-pass metabolism, and produce a rapid onset of action. This rapid action allows for dosing to effect, a crucial component for the optimal management of breakthrough pain. Currently fentanyl is the only opioid available in a transmucosal formulation. This lozenge formulation has an onset of action of 5–8 minutes, a peak effect at 15–30 minutes, and a 60–120 minute duration of action, again, characteristics that help provide for the optimal management of breakthrough pain. It is more comfortable for the patient than parenteral administration and often less expensive.

The parenteral route affords the quickest way to achieve pain control. Delivery may be intravenous or subcutaneous. Intramuscular injections should be avoided because they are painful to the patient and absorption is erratic. For the patient with severe out-of-control pain, titration with parenteral opioids can provide fast, effective relief; however, this approach requires infusion pumps and invasive techniques. Subcutaneous and intravenous delivery shows comparable kinetics and dosing; however, subcutaneous administration is less invasive to the patient and more readily taught to the family or caregiver. Both approaches allow for the continuous delivery of drug, bolus delivery of patient-controlled dosing for breakthrough pain, or a combination of the two when appropriate infusion devices are used. Subcutaneous access may be kept in place for up to seven days if the pump and tubing remain uncompromised, whereas intravenous access sites often require change every two to three days. Continuous subcutaneous infusion, with or without bolus capability, is a safe and effective method of outpatient management of chronic pain when the oral, rectal, and transdermal routes are not feasible. Although this method of administration requires diligence and commitment from all health care personnel involved, it can shift the burden of care from the hospital to the home, thereby decreasing health care costs and maximizing quality of life for the patient.

Adjuvant Medications

Adjuvant medications may be used to enhance analgesia or to provide relief from the side effects of the primary analgesic. Often, adjuvant analgesics are necessary to optimize pain control. As with opioid analgesics, underdosing or use of an incorrect adjuvant may result in suboptimal pain control. Several factors should be considered when choosing a specific adjuvant medication, including the pathophysiology of the pain, medical and analgesic history of the patient, opioid poorly-responsive pain, and the adverse events being experienced by the patient.

Antidepressants have been used as adjuncts to the opiate analgesics to enhance pain control, especially in the setting of neuropathic pain. Although their exact mechanism of action is unknown, they are thought to exert an analgesic effect via their ability to prevent the synaptic reuptake of the neurotransmitters dopamine, serotonin, and norepinephrine. There are several agents in this class, each with unique characteristics. Thus, the clinician should become familiar with a given agent before prescribing it.

The tricyclic antidepressants (TCAs) have been studied most extensively, and their efficacy has been defined. They are composed of the tertiary amines (e.g., amitriptyline, doxepin, and imipramine) and the newer secondary amines (e.g., desipramine and nortriptyline). Lower doses suffice for analgesia when compared to those used for depression. Initial doses for those agents mentioned are 10–25 mg with maximum doses in the 100–150 mg range. Each dose should be taken once daily at bedtime. The secondary amines have fewer, less intense anticholinergic effects and would be appropriate in the patient where sedation, constipation, dry mouth, or urinary retention are present or could become a problem. On the other hand, if insomnia were a problem, amitriptyline may be more suitable. The onset of analgesia for the TCAs often occurs within a few days to a week, much shorter than that required for their antidepressant effect. Caution must be exercised if they are to be used in any patient with a significant cardiac history.

The selective serotonin reuptake inhibitors (SSRIs) have been studied in a relatively small number of controlled trials. These agents (e.g. fluoxetine and paroxetine) have, in general, demonstrated little advantage over placebo, with lesser efficacy when compared to the less selective TCAs. Other antidepressants that have been reported to provide pain relief include the serotonin/norepinephrine reuptake inhibitor venlafaxine and the tetracyclic antidepressant mirtazipine. Venlafaxine provides a second line option for patients with problematic sedation or those suffering hot flashes. Mirtazipine, with its rapid antidepressant effect (usually within five to seven days), potential antiemetic effects, appetite stimulatory effects, and sedative properties, might be useful in the patient who would benefit from any or all of these other properties.

The antiepileptic agents have activity in a variety of neuropathic pain syndromes. They appear to be particularly effective in patients complaining of "lancinating" or "burning" pain. Carbamazepine has a relatively rapid onset of analgesic action and has been commonly used for diabetic neuropathy and trigeminal neuralgia. Common side effects associated with carbamazepine include nystagmus, dizziness, diplopia, lightheadedness, and lethargy. Baseline liver function tests should be obtained as well as complete blood counts in order to monitor for the rare toxicity to these organ systems. Initial dosing of 50–100 mg twice daily may be increased to a maximum of 1200 mg per day, although reports of up to 1600 mg per day have appeared in the medical literature. Gabapentin is another antiepileptic with significant activity against neuropathic pain. The medical literature supports its use in a wide range of neuropathic syndromes including reflex sympathetic dystrophy, diabetic neuropathy, trigeminal neuralgia, postherpetic neuralgia, radiation myelopathy, central poststroke pain, and neuropathic cancer pain. Despite its higher cost, it is often used first line because it is better tolerated and has fewer drug interactions than carbamazepine. Common side effects include somnolence, dizziness, ataxia, and fatigue. A dose of 900 mg per day is generally considered the minimum effective dose; however, an initial dose of 100 mg every eight hours titrated to 300 mg every eight hours over a few days may prevent the onset or minimize the severity of the more common side effects. A dose of 3600 mg per day is generally considered the maximum, although the use of 4500 mg per day has been reported. Gabapentin is eliminated almost entirely unchanged by the kidney; therefore, caution should be used when dosing the drug in the presence of renal dysfunction.

Bone pain related to metastatic cancer may respond to calcitonin, pamidronate, or radiopharmaceuticals such as strontium chloride SR-89. Practitioners should consider these alternatives, especially when NSAIDs are contraindicated. Corticosteroids are also useful in this setting because of their anti-inflammatory activity. Additionally, they may be of value for treating pain caused by soft-tissue infiltration, visceral distention, or increased intracranial pressure. The added benefit of mood elevation, appetite stimulation, and antiemetic activity may be particularly useful in the terminal patient. Adverse events associated with long-term use are generally not of consequence in the terminal patient. Those seen with short-term use include hypertension, hyperglycemia, immunosuppression, psychotic reactions, and cognitive impairment.

Further Reading

American Pain Society Quality Care Committee (consensus statement). "Quality improvement guidelines for the treatment of acute and cancer pain." *JAMA*, 274(23):1874–1880, 1995.

Bruera, E., and Neumann, C. M. "Role of methadone in the management of pain in cancer patients." *Oncology*, 13:1275–1282, 1999.

Cherny, N. "Opioid analgesics. Comparative features and prescribing guidelines." *Drugs*, 51(5):713–737, 1996.

Cherny, N., Ripamonti, C., Pereira, J., Davis, C., Fallon, M., McQuay, H., Mercadante, S., Pasternak, G., and Ventafridda, V. "Strategies to manage the adverse effects of oral morphine: An evidence-based report." *J Clin Oncol*, 19(9):2542–2554, 2001.

Coluzzi, P. H., and Fairbairn, B. S. "The management of pain in terminally ill cancer patients with difficulty swallowing." *Amer J Hospice Palliat Care*, 16(6):731–737, 1999.

Davis, M. P., and Walsh, D. "Methadone for relief of cancer pain: A review of pharmacokinetics, pharmacodynamics, drug interactions and protocols for administration." *Support Care Cancer*, 9(2):73–83, 2001.

Ferrante, F. M. "Principles of opioid pharmacotherapy: Practical implications of basic mechanisms." *J Pain Sympt Manage*, 11(5):265–273, 1996.

Foley, K. M. "Controlling cancer pain." *Hosp Pract*, 35:101–112, 2000.

Foley, K. M. "The treatment of cancer pain." *N Engl J Med*, 313:84–95, 1985

Jacox, A., Carr, D. B., Payne, R. *Management of Cancer Pain: Clinical Practice Guidelines No. 9* AHCPR publication No. 94-0592. Rockville, Md.: Agency for Health Care Policy and Research, U.S. Department of Health and Human Services. Public Health Services, March 1994.

Joint Commission on Accreditation of Healthcare Organization. *Comprehensive Accreditation Manual for Ambulatory Care* (section R1.27 to P1.3.1) (1999). Available at: **www.jcaho.org/standard/pmac.htlm**.

Mays, T. A., "Antidepressants in the management of cancer pain." *Curr Pain Headache Rep*, 5(3):227–236, 2001.

Mercadante, S. "Opioid rotation for cancer pain: Rationale and clinical aspects." *Cancer*, 86(9):1856–1866, 1999.

Mercadante, S., Casuccio, A., Fulfaro, F., Groff, L., Boffi, R., Villari, P., Gebbia, V., and Ripamanti, C. "Switching from morphine to methadone to improve analgesia and tolerability in cancer patients: A prospective study." *J Clin Oncol*, 19(11):2898–2904, 2001.

Mercadante, S., and Fulfaro, F. "Alternatives to oral opioids for cancer pain." *Oncology*, 13(2):215–225, 1999.

Mercadante, S., and Portenoy, R. K. "Opioid poorly-responsive cancer pain. Clinical strategies to improve opioid responsiveness." *J Pain Sympt Manage*, 21(4):338–354, 2001.

Milch, R. A. "The dying patient: Pain management at the hospice level." *Curr Rev Pain*, 4(3):215–218, 2000.

Pappagallo, M., Dickerson, E. D., and Hulka, S. "Palliative care and hospice opioid dosing guidelines with breakthrough pain (BP) doses." *Amer J Hospice Palliat Care*, 17(6):407–413, 2000.

Payne, R., Coluzzi, P., Hart, L., Simmonds, M., Lyss, A., Rauck, R., Berris, R., Busch, M. A., Nordbrook, E., Loseth, D. B., and Portenoy, R. K. "Long-term safety of oral transmucosal fentanyl citrate for breakthrough cancer pain." *J Pain Sympt Manage*, 22(1):575–583, 2001.

Pereira, J., Lawlor P., Vigano, A., Dorgan, M., and Bruera, E. "Equianalgesic dose ratios for opioids: A critical review and proposals for long term dosing." *J Pain Sympt Manage*, 22(2):672–687, 2001.

Portenoy, R. K. "Cancer pain management." *Sem Oncol*, 20(2)(suppl 1):19–35, 1993.

Portenoy, R. K, and Lesage, P. "Management of cancer pain." *Lancet*, 353:1695–1700, 1999.

Sarhill, N., Walsh, D., and Nelson, K. A. "Hydromorphone: pharmacology and clinical applications in cancer patients." *Support Care Cancer*, 9(2):84–96, 2001.

Seaman-Wrede, L. D. "Treatment options to manage pain at the end of life." *Amer J Hospice Palliat Care*, 18(2):89–101, 2001.

Twycross, R. G., and Lack, S. A. *Symptom control in far advanced cancer: Pain relief.* London: Pitman, 1983, pp. 43–55.

Vigano, A., Bruera, E., Suarez-Almazor, M. E. "Age, pain intensity and opioid dose in patients with advanced cancer." *Cancer*, 83:1244–1250, 1998.

Walsh, D. "Pharmacological management of cancer pain." *Sem Oncol*, 27(1):45–63, 2000.

Cultural Competence in Hospice and Palliative Care

13

Polly Mazanac, MSN, APRN, BC
Judith Kitzes, MD, MPH

Culture is a patterned behavioral response that develops over time and is shaped by the values, beliefs, norms, and practices that are shared by members of the same cultural group.[1] Culture is broader than ethnicity and race, and encompasses many dimensions including gender, age, differing abilities, sexual orientation, religion, financial status, residency, employment, and educational level. See Table 13-1.[2]

Every person has a cultural heritage.[3] The values, beliefs, norms, and practices of this heritage guide thinking, decisions, and actions in a patterned way.[4] In a pluralistic society, health care professionals need to provide culturally appropriate care.[5] This care must be individualized for each person and family. Nowhere in the health care continuum is this more significant than in the provision of hospice/palliative care.

The population statistics of the United States demonstrate that cultural diversity is increasing among the five panethnic groups identified as White, Black, Hispanic, Asian/Pacific Islander, and American Indian/Alaskan native (Table 13-1). The population of the United States derived from the 2000 Census report is 281,421,906.[6] By 2030, the population of Hispanics and Asian/Pacific Islanders will nearly double that of 1998.[3] Immigrants and their children will account for nearly one-half of the growth of the U.S. population. By 2050, 50% of Americans will claim a relationship to an ethnic minority group.[7] The increasing diversity of treasured beliefs, shared teachings, norms, customs, language, and meaning challenges the ability of hospice and palliative care team members to provide holistic care that is culturally competent.[8, 9]

TABLE 13-1 U.S. Racial and Ethnic Population Projections for the 21st Century	White	Hispanic	Black	Asian/ Pacific Islander	American Indian/ Alaskan Native
2000	75.1%	12.5%	12.3%	3.7%	0.9%
2005	69.9%	12.6%	12.4%	4.4%	0.8%
2010	68.0%	13.8%	12.6%	4.8%	0.8%
2015	66.1%	15.1%	12.7%	5.3%	0.8%
2020	64.3%	16.3%	12.9%	5.7%	0.8%
2030	60.5%	18.9%	13.1%	6.6%	0.8%

Adapted from Andrews, M. "Theoretical foundations of transcultural nursing." In *Transcultural Concepts of Nursing Care*, 3rd ed. M. Andrews and J. Boyle, eds., New York: Lippincott, 1999, p.13, and the U.S. Bureau of the Census (2000).

Cultural Competence

Cultural competence refers to a dynamic, fluid, continuous process of awareness, knowledge, skill, interaction, and sensitivity.[4, 8, 9-13] It is more comprehensive than cultural sensitivity, implying not only awareness of cultural differences, but also the ability to intervene appropriately and effectively.[2, 5, 9-13] Seeking to become more culturally competent requires learning in the affective (attitudes, values, feelings, and beliefs), cognitive or intellectual, and psychomotor or behavioral domains, and assumes skill in critical thinking.[3, 5] Cultural competence is an ongoing process, not an end point. Campinha-Bacote has identified four components necessary in pursuing cultural competence: cultural awareness, cultural knowledge, cultural skill, and cultural encounter.[14]

Cultural Awareness

Cultural awareness begins with an examination of one's own heritage, family's practices, experiences, and religious or spiritual beliefs. It is essential to identify and acknowledge the role that one's own belief system plays in interactions with others.[12] Each member of the hospice and palliative care team brings his or her own cultural and philosophical views, education, religion, spirituality, and life experiences to the care of the patient and family.[13, 15, 16] Cultural awareness encourages each of us to examine the influence cultural stereotypes have on our beliefs, values, and clinical practices. These stereotypes can foster prejudice and discrimination and could interfere with holistic care.[15]

We are challenged to look beyond our ethnocentric view of the world.[16] Each one of us is called to identify how I am different from the individual and family being cared for, rather than how the individual and family are different from me.[17] In that examination, it is likely that we will find many similarities rather than differences. In hospice/palliative care, the universal aspects of life, family, trust, love, hope, understanding, and caring unite us in our efforts to care for those at the end of life.[8] Assessing one's own attitudes, beliefs, and practices surrounding the end of life provides an important cultural awareness (Table 13-2).[15]

TABLE 13-2 Know Your Own Attitudes, Beliefs, and Practices

- To what extent do you believe in a life after death?
- How appropriate is it for children to attend funerals?
- How was death talked about in your family?
- How significant is religion in your death attitudes?
- To what extent do you believe in reincarnation?
- How often do you think about your own death?
- If you could choose, when would you die?
- What do you believe causes most deaths?
- What kind of death would you prefer?
- How do you feel about having an autopsy done on your body?
- To what extent should suicide be prevented?
- If you were diagnosed with a terminal disease, would you want to be told?
- What efforts should be made to keep a seriously ill person alive?
- What circumstances would prompt you to refuse medical treatment for a dying family member?
- Are you willing to be an organ donor?
- If a close friend were dying and wanted to talk, how would you feel?
- How helpful to a survivor's grief is viewing the body?
- What is your experience of participating in rituals to remember the dead?

DeSpelder, L. "Developing cultural competence." In *Living with Grief,* K. Doka and J. Davidson, eds., Philadelphia: Hospice Foundation of America, 1998, pp. 97–106.

Cultural Knowledge

Improving cultural knowledge about different cultural groups is essential to gaining cultural competence. However, knowledge alone is insufficient in providing quality care. Knowledge serves as a guide to assist the hospice/palliative care team members in gaining a better understanding of the individual and family. Numerous resources are available to assist the team members in acquiring knowledge about specific groups. Table 13-4 defines end-of-life care practices and beliefs of a variety of religious groups.

It *is* within the framework of this chapter, however, to caution readers in the use of these resources. Acting on assumptions without validating their significance to the individual and family may lead to harmful stereotyping.[7, 8] Stereotyping occurs when one makes an assumption about an individual based solely on the individual's group membership.[15] It does not recognize the uniqueness of the individual or that differences exist even within groups.[15] Of particular significance is the variation in values, beliefs, and practices among generations of a particular group. The first-generation immigrant may retain cultural norms of their country of origin, whereas the second- or third-generation caregiver may have beliefs more consistent with present-day American culture. These differences must be identified to provide culturally appropriate care to the patient and to the family.

Cultural Skill

Cultural skill in hospice and palliative care is required for competency. Cultural assessment, cross-cultural communication, cultural interpretation, and appropriate intervention are skills that can be acquired. Multiple tools are available to assess cultural behavior and beliefs. These tools focus on cultural affiliation, values orientation, cultural sanctions and restrictions, communication, health-related beliefs and practices, nutrition, socioeconomic considerations, organization, education, religion, cultural aspects of disease, incidence, biocultural variations, and developmental considerations across the life span.[16] However, a thorough cultural assessment tool is time-consuming and may be too fatiguing for hospice/palliative care patients. Lipson and Meleis have identified the essential cultural assessment questions that should be asked about or observed when developing the plan of care. These questions are applicable to the hospice/palliative care setting (Table 13-3).[18]

TABLE 13-3   Key Cultural Assessment Questions

- Where was the patient born? If an immigrant, how long has the patient lived in this country?
- What is the patient's ethnic affiliation and how strong is the patient's ethnic identity?
- Who are the patient's major support people: family members, friends? Does the patient live in an ethnic community?
- What are the primary and secondary languages, speaking and reading ability?
- How would you characterize the nonverbal communication style?
- What is the patient's religion, its importance in daily life, and current practices?
- What are the patient's food preferences and prohibitions?
- What is the patient's economic situation, and is the income adequate to meet the needs of the patient and family?
- What are the health and illness beliefs and practices?
- What are customs and beliefs around such transitions as birth, illness, and death?

Lipson, J., and Meleis, A. "Culturally appropriate care: The case of immigrants." *Topics in Clinical Nursing,* 7(3):48–56, 1985.

Cultural Phenomenon

The Giger-Davidhizar Transcultural Assessment model is an excellent theoretical framework for culturally competent care.[1] This model has been applied to various settings, across various disciplines. It focuses on six phenomena: communication, space, social organization, time, environmental control, and biologic variations. In becoming more knowledgeable about different cultures, one can learn the cultural norms surrounding these phenomena. However, it must be stressed that each individual should be assessed to identify the relevance of specific cultural values, beliefs, and practices to the individual.

Communication

Becoming competent in cross-cultural communication involves recognizing the ways in which people of different backgrounds communicate with each other. An assessment of verbal communication includes identifying the language spoken in the home, how the patient prefers to communicate, and the patient's speaking and reading ability. Keep in mind that the stress of illness and the progression of disease in hospice/palliative care patients may cause a person to return to his or her most familiar language.

When language is a barrier, an interpreter may be necessary. Asking if the patient needs an interpreter, or if there is someone whom the patient would not prefer as an interpreter, such as a member of the opposite sex, is important. The implications of using a family member as an interpreter should be considered. Family members who are pressed into service as interpreters, may have difficulty with this responsibility because of role conflicts or lack of ability to freely translate medical terminology to the patient. In addition, family members may choose to withhold critical information to spare the patient from bad news or sensitive issues.[13]

It is important to recognize the overall characteristics of language and the communication process. Respect the way a person wishes to be addressed. Be aware of the rules of communication within the culture. Listen to the tone and quality of voice to help understand the message. A loud voice may mean anger or simply emphasis.[13] (Remember that amplifying the volume of the voice does not equate with improving understanding.) The meaning of silence in conversation varies among cultural groups. It may indicate apprehension or discomfort, or it may be a sign of thoughtful reflection or respect.[13] Verifying the meaning is important to the communication.

It is necessary to vary techniques of communication depending on the individual. Respect cultural differences regarding the appropriate tempo of the conversation, use of nonverbal behaviors, sensitive topics such as prognosis, and with whom one should be communicating. It is critical to communicate in a nonhurried manner, to listen carefully, to allow time, and to speak slowly and distinctly. Repeat the message in different ways and do not assume the meaning is interpreted as it was sent. Nonverbal behaviors are important in every culture.

Every culture also has acceptable practices concerning the use of touch.[1, 13, 16] In some cultures touch is a powerful tool. It can connect the patient and hospice/palliative care team member. It can decrease loneliness, reassure others, provide stimulation, and improve self-concept. In other cultures, however, touch is seen as a negative experience. It may appear as an invasion of personal space and privacy, and can convey a subservient relationship. Cultural rules for touch can also vary by gender.[16] Cultural prohibitions on touching certain parts of the body also exist.[13]

The use of eye contact is an important consideration when communicating with persons of different backgrounds. This nonverbal technique implies different meanings to different cultures. In some cultures, eye contact communicates warmth, and lack of eye contact communicates rudeness, low self-esteem, and dishonesty. In other cultures, eye contact is regarded as a sign of disrespect or an inappropriate behavior between different genders.[13, 16]

Space

Cultural conceptions of personal space vary. These conceptions may lead to misinterpretation of nonverbal communication depending on the individual's need for personal space. The dimensions of one's comfort zone vary from culture to culture. In the Euro-American culture, there are three primary dimensions of space: the intimate zone (0–18"), the personal zone (18–36"), and the social/public zone (3'–6').[20] Consequently, where one sits or stands may communicate different messages. In the Euro-American culture, standing or sitting within the personal zone may communicate caring and respect. However, in some cultures, this action may be considered aggressive and disrespectful.[13, 16]

Social Organization

Social organizations are structured in various groups, such as family, religious, ethnic, and racial. These groups define acceptable behavior and responses to significant life experiences such as disease/illness, dying, death, and grief. The role of the family is particularly important in hospice and palliative care. The definition of family has changed to encompass anyone whom the patient considers as family.[21, 22] Identification of family members and recognition of acceptable caregiving practices within this social structure are essential.

The religious practices of the patient and family should be assessed to identify their importance in daily life. Religious and spiritual beliefs may influence a patient's explanation of the cause of illness, pain, and suffering. Important religious traditions, such as the use of prayer, religious objects, and spiritual healers, should be incorporated into the plan of care. Restrictions associated with religious practices must be honored. Religious customs for the care of the body after death should be known and respected. Knowledge of acceptable grief and mourning behaviors and practices are significant when continuing to care for the family after the patient has died.[23]

Time

Implications of how a cultural group views the concept of time is especially important in understanding the patient's response to prognosis and duration of illness, and anticipated death. Campinha-Bacote compared time orientation among certain groups in the United States.[24] Future-oriented groups may defer gratification of personal pleasure until future obligations have been met. As a result, an early death may rob a patient and family from this group of future goals and dreams. Present-oriented groups focus on living in the present and are not overly concerned with the future. Time is flexible; what happens now is far more important than what happens later on. Individuals who are present-oriented may have difficulty discussing advance care planning.

Environmental Control

Complex systems of health beliefs and practices exist within cultural groups. Environmental control is the ability of individuals to plan activities that control nature. Recognizing cultural factors that affect illness behaviors related to environmental control is important in hospice/palliative care. Health is a balance between the individual and the environment. According to Western medical standards, effective health practices are those that are viewed as improving health status. However, an effective plan of care must be consistent with individuals' beliefs and practices, and not just consistent with Western medical practice.[7] For example, integrating folk healers into the plan of care may improve symptoms and quality of life for individuals of some cultural groups. Recognizing theories, such as the use of "hot/cold" compresses, and incorporating them into medical management may improve compliance with, and responses to, evidence-based medical practice.[16, 25]

Symptoms are believed to have cultural meanings.[16] It should not be assumed that symptoms are equivalent to syndromes commonly associated with Western medicine. As individuals experience symptoms, they may interpret them in ways consistent with their cultural norms. For example, in some cultures, hallucinations may be thought to be caused by ghosts, and gastrointestinal symptoms may be the result of a hex or witchcraft. Implications for management of these symptoms emphasize an understanding of the cultural beliefs and practices of the individual.

Biological Variations

Biological variations exist among particular ethnic or cultural groups. Physical differences affect assessment findings of individuals with varying skin color. In particular, the assessment of cyanosis, jaundice, and pallor is important in hospice/palliative care and must be evaluated based on individual characteristics. Of significance are the biological variations associated with drug metabolism and drug interaction. Drugs are metabolized in different ways and at different rates by persons of different races.[16, 26] Specific to hospice/palliative care, variations in the metabolism of psychotropic drugs and their side effect profile have been identified.[26, 27] In particular for pain management, the inability of some individuals to metabolize codeine is an important consideration in the clinical setting.[28]

Hospice and Palliative Care Issues Influenced by Culture

Issues that are of particular importance in hospice/palliative care are often influenced by cultural factors. Nutrition, decision making, pain management, and death and dying rituals are critical aspects of good hospice/palliative care. Assessing the influence of cultural beliefs on these aspects of care is essential. Knowledge about cultural groups' practices surrounding these aspects of care should be applied to the plan of care whenever individually appropriate.

Nutrition

The relationship between culture and food is complex. Food preferences and behaviors reflect the individual's and family's cultural heritage, lifestyle, socioeconomic status, religion, education, lifestyle, and nutritional requirements for age, gender, and body size.[29] The meaning of food is important in most societies. Across cultures, food is used in building or maintaining human relationships. The universal functions of food are well-known.[29, 30] Although there may be differences regarding essential nutritional needs, there is agreement that food is essential for life, to maintain body function, and to produce energy. Food is used in rituals, celebrations, and rites of passage to establish and maintain social and cultural relationships with families, friends, and others. It serves to assess social relationships or interpersonal closeness. A symbolic use of foods is to cope with emotional stresses, conflicts, or traumatic life events. It is also used to reward, influence, or punish the behavior of others. Food has economic and political implications, and influences the status of an individual or group. For centuries, food has been used to assess, treat, and prevent illness.

Dietary patterns of cultural groups need to be assessed and integrated into the plan of care. When working with patients and families to identify foods that affect symptoms, it is important to consider food practices that are culturally significant. For example, those individuals following cultural practices in the hot and cold theory believe that when an imbalance in hot and cold occurs, illness results. Offering hot foods to treat nausea, believed to be caused by eating too many cold foods, would be culturally acceptable. Some individuals may refuse team recommendations that violate hot/cold or yin/yang beliefs and practices.[29] Although it is impossible to suggest food choices based on stereotypical generalizations about cultures, asking about the significance of these practices to the individual is important in culturally competent care.

Hospice/palliative care issues surrounding food and fluids are culturally significant. In cultures that value food as a "life-sustaining" agent, withholding or withdrawing food or fluids may violate an individual's or family's beliefs. It may be important to ask the patient or family if involving a leader in their cultural or religious group may be helpful in making food and fluid decisions.[29, 31]

Decision Making

Over the past 25 years in the United States, ethical and legal considerations of decision making have focused on patient autonomy.[7, 32, 33] It is an overly narrow approach, based on Western medical practices. With the Patient Self-Determination Act (PSDA) of 1991, health care decision making shifted from the physician to the patient.[7] This act was the result of social change and the consumer rights movement in the early 1970s in the United States. It is based on the belief that the patient has an inherent right to information relevant to health care decision making. The assumption is that the patient wants control over the dying process. Advance directives were initiated as a result of the PSDA.[7, 33]

The four values that provide foundations for the PSDA and end-of-life decision making in America include patient autonomy, informed decision making, truth telling, and control over the dying process. This is the Euro-American vision of health care. It assumes that the individual, rather than the family or other social group, is the appropriate decision maker.[7, 32, 34] Many non-Euro-American cultures do not embrace this vision or these values. Their practices and beliefs should be honored and respected.

In many non-Euro-American cultures the concept of interdependence among family and community members is more valued than individual autonomy.[35] Families often plan and participate in all aspects of care. Many cultures are family-centered rather than individualistic, and would prefer that the family, rather than the patient, receive and process information. Autonomy may not be seen as empowering, but rather may seem burdensome to patients already too sick to make meaningful choices. It is critical that the hospice/palliative care team directly ask their patients, whether they, or their family, should receive information.

Some non-European cultures do not approve of full disclosure. This Western practice of blunt, truthful communication is seen as rude and disrespectful in some cultural groups.[36] These families prefer to receive threatening information and filter it before telling their loved ones. This practice is believed to encourage patients to maintain hope.[37]

Hospice/palliative care team members must consider the harm that may occur when the medical community violates cultural practices.[32] It may be helpful to explain the Euro-American perspective to enhance understanding and prevent needless suffering. Ersek and colleagues suggest ways to begin this discussion such as, "Your condition requires several decisions be made about your treatment. Is there someone, perhaps a family member, who you would like to be with you when we discuss these matters?" or, "How much of the information that needs to be discussed do you want to know?" or, "Would you feel more comfortable if I spoke primarily with (the designated person)?"[7]

It is essential for hospice/palliative care team members to be aware that ethical norms in the United States are guided by a Euro-American perspective and may not be appropriate in other cultures.[7]

Pain Management

Pain is a highly personal and subjective experience influenced by cultural learning.[38] "Pain is whatever the person says it is, and existing whenever the person says it does."[39] It is important to understand the meaning of pain to the individual and the cultural implications before initiating interventions.

Certain ethnic groups and cultures have strong beliefs about expressing pain and have expected pain behaviors. The individual reaction to pain may be influenced by cultural background.[38, 40] Bates and colleagues propose a biocultural model of pain suggesting that social learning from family and group membership can influence the psychological and physiological processing of pain, which then affects the perception and modulation of pain.[41]

Patterned attitudes of pain behaviors exist in every culture as demonstrated by Zoborowski's classic work.[42] Pain tolerance varies from person to person depending on numerous factors such as past experiences with pain, coping skills, motivation to endure pain, and energy level.[43] Western society places a high value on stoicism and high pain tolerance.[43]

Important implications for hospice/palliative care include culturally appropriate assessment of and interventions for pain. Recognize that one's own ethnocentric views of appropriate pain behaviors may affect the ability to assess pain in patients and families of different backgrounds. Team members' responses to the patient's expression of pain should be in an accepting, respectful manner.[25]

Assessment of pain can be identified using terms that describe pain intensity across most cultural groups. "Pain," "hurt," and "ache" are words commonly used by persons of different ethnic and educational backgrounds to describe pain.[43] Pain rating scales have been translated into numerous languages.[43] It is important to standardize the assessment and not rely on culturally laden pain indicators such as facial expression, body movement, and vocalization to assess pain.

Comprehensive pain management involves pharmacologic and nonpharmacologic interventions. Incorporating culturally appropriate complementary therapies may improve the ability to alleviate pain. Healing practices specific to cultures should be offered to patient and family.[40]

The assessment and management of pain in certain populations are important cultural considerations. In particular, the elderly and the cognitively impaired have unique needs. Studies have identified inadequate pain assessment in the elderly.[44, 45] Elders' not reporting pain may be a result of stoicism, fear that worsening pain means progression of disease, resignation to pain, or the desire to spare loved ones from worry.[46] Tools such as the discomfort scale may indicate pain to be present.[47]

Death Rituals in Mourning Practices

The meaning of death, and how it is recognized, acknowledged, and celebrated, varies among cultures.[48] The increasing diversity of the population requires increased knowledge about death rituals and mourning practices. Misunderstandings between hospice/palliative care team members and patients and families may cause unnecessary pain and suffering.[48] It is the responsibility of the team to learn about these rituals and weave them into a culturally meaningful context for the patient and family.

Most cultures have specific rituals that begin before death and may last for months or even years after death. It is important to identify families' wishes for attendance at the death, any special religious or ethnic practices that should be initiated at the time of death, and culturally appropriate care of the body after death. In some cultures, autopsies are acceptable. In others, there are strong prohibitions against the violation of the body.[49] In helping family members deal with death, the hospice/palliative care team must show respect for the family's cultural heritage and encourage the family to identify how they will commemorate the death of their loved one. DeSpelder et al. have determined important questions to ask about particular traditions (Table 13-4).[50]

During the dying experience and after death the major tasks of the grief process are universal regardless of the cultural differences.[51] These tasks are present in the varied rituals. The first is to accept the reality of the loss. The second task is to feel and experience the pain of grief associated with this loss.

TABLE 13-4   Family Questions Regarding Cultural Traditions in Dealing with Death

- What are the prescribed rituals for handling dying, the dead body, the disposal of the body, and rituals to commemorate loss?
- What are the group's beliefs about what happens after death?
- What do they believe about appropriate emotional expression and integration of a loss experience?
- What are the gender rules for handling the death?
- Are certain deaths particularly stigmatized or traumatic for the group?

DeSpelder, L. "Developing cultural competence." In *Living with Grief*, K. Doka and J. Davidson, eds., Philadelphia: Hospice Foundation of America, 1998, pp. 97–106.

If this pain is not worked through and expressed, it may lead to significant complications.[52] The third task is to begin to adjust to an environment without the deceased and to begin the transformation to new society and family roles. This transformation begins when it is apparent that the patient is not going to recover. This task takes time and may require years to complete. Finally, the fourth task is to withdraw emotional energy from the dead and focus energy on the living.[51]

Although the tasks associated with grieving are universal, it is important to recognize that cultures differ in public expression of grief. Expressions of grief could be misinterpreted as complicated grief if not recognized as within cultural norms. Some groups are more publicly open than others. Expectations of grief responses for men and women also differ.[49] Providing a safe environment, where permission is given to patients and families to express their grief according to their cultural practices, is critical in hospice/palliative care.[8]

Summary

Cultural considerations are an essential aspect of holistic hospice/palliative care. Cultural competence is not an end point. It is an ongoing process involving knowledge, attitudes, and skill. Striving for cultural competence leads to humane and effective interpersonal interactions that are the core for providing care to patients and families.[53]

Acquiring knowledge is a means for formulating questions necessary in learning about how a patient identifies with and expresses his or her cultural background. Knowledge serves as a guide to understanding the role of cultural values, beliefs, and practices for the individual.[52] Becoming aware of the way "I" am different from an individual, rather than the way that individual is different from "me" demonstrates a respect that transcends cultural limitations. Developing observational and listening skills contributes to an appreciation for persons of different backgrounds.

This chapter provides a framework for asking questions related to culturally significant phenomena (communication, space, social organization, time orientation, environmental control, and biological variations) and it emphasizes hospice/palliative care issues particularly influenced by culture. It is the hope of the author that readers will seek to learn about different cultures, recognize the impact of one's own cultural background on the ability to provide culturally appropriate care, and work to acquire the skills necessary for culturally competent care. It is in that process that "we come to understand the differences with our heads but our common humanity with our hearts."[54]

References

1. Giger, J., and Davidhizar, R., eds. *Transcultural Nursing; Assessment and Intervention,* 3rd ed., New York: Mosby, 1999.
2. Oncology Nursing Society, *Multicultural Outcomes: Guidelines for Cultural Competencies,* Pittsburgh, Pa.: Oncology Nursing Press, Inc., 1999.
3. Andrews, M. "Theoretical foundations of transcultural nursing." In *Transcultural Concepts of Nursing Care,* 3rd ed. M. Andrews and J. Boyle, eds. New York: Lippincott, 1999, pp. 1–22.
4. Leininger, M. "Quality of life from a transcultural nursing perspective." *Nursing Science Quarterly,* 7(1):22–28, 1994.
5. Doswell, W., and Erlen, J. "Multicultural issues and ethical concerns in the delivery of nursing care interventions." *Nursing Clinics of North America,* 33(2):353–361, 1998.
6. U.S. Bureau of the Census (2000). Current Population Reports, **www.government-guide.com/research_and_education**.
7. Ersek, M., Kagawa-Singer, M., Barnes, D., Blackhall, L., and Koenig, B. "Multicultural considerations in the use of advance directives." *Oncology Nursing Forum,* 25(10):1683–1701, 1998.
8. Showalter, S. "Looking through different eyes: Beyond cultural diversity." In *Living with Grief,* K. Doka and J. Davidson, eds. Washington D.C.: Hospice Foundation of America, 1998, pp. 71–82.
9. Pickett, M. "Cultural awareness in the context of terminal illness." *Cancer Nursing,* 16(2):102–106, 1993.
10. Davis, L., Dumas, R., Ferketich, S., Flaherty, Sr., M., et al. "AAN Expert Panel Report: Culturally Competent Health Care." *Nursing Outlook,* 40(6):277–283, 1992.
11. Zoucha, R. "The keys to culturally sensitive care." *American Journal of Nursing,* 100:24GG–24II, 2000.
12. Smith, L. "Concept analysis: Culture competence." *Journal of Cultural Diversity,* 5(1):4–10, 1998.
13. Lipson, J. "Culturally competent nursing care." *In Culture & Nursing Care: A Pocket Guide,* J. Lipson, S. Dibble, and P. Minarik, eds. San Francisco: UCSF Nursing Press, 1996, pp. 1–6.
14. Campinha-Bacote, J. *The Process of Cultural Competence: A Cultural Competence Model of Care,* Wyoming, OH: Transcultural C.A.R.E. Associates, 1991.
15. DeSpelder, L. "Developing cultural competence" In *Living with Grief,* K. Doka and J. Davidson, eds. Philadelphia: Hospice Foundation of America, 1998. pp. 97–106.
16. Andrews, M., and Herberg, P. "Transcultural nursing care." In *Transcultural Concepts of Nursing Care,* 3rd ed. M. Andrews and J. Boyle, eds. New York: Lippincott, 1999, pp. 23–77.
17. Talabere, R. "Meeting the challenge of culture care in nursing: Diversity, sensitivity, and congruence." *Journal of Cultural Diversity,* 3(2):53–61, 1996.
18. Lipson, J., and Meleis, A. "Culturally appropriate care: The case of immigrants." *Topics in Clinical Nursing,* 7(3):48–56, 1985.
19. Gostin, L., "Informed Consent, Cultural Sensitivity, and Respect for Persons." *Journal of the American Medical Association,* 274:844–845, 1995.
20. Hall, E. *The Silent Language.* New York: Doubleday, 1966.

21. Ferrell, B. "The family." In *Oxford Textbook of Palliative Medicine*, D. Doyle, G. Hanks, and N. MacDonald, eds. New York: Oxford University Press, Inc., 1998, pp. 909–917.

22. Goetschius. S. "Caring for families: The other patient in palliative care." In *Palliative Care Nursing: Quality Care to the End of Life*, M. Matzo and D. Sherman, eds. New York: Springer Publishing Co., Inc., 2001, pp. 245–274.

23. Andrews, M., and Hanson, P. "Religion, culture, and nursing." In *Transcultural Concepts of Nursing Care*, 3rd ed. M. Andrews and J. Boyle, eds. New York: Lippincott, 1999, pp. 378–443.

24. Campinha-Bacote, J. "Understanding the influence of culture." In *Comprehensive Psychiatric Nursing*, 5th ed., J. Haber, B. Krainovch-Miller, A. McMahon, and P. Hoskins, eds. New York: Mosby, 1997, pp. 76–90.

25. Juarez, G. "Culture and pain." *Quality of Life—A Nursing Challenge*, 4(4):86–94, 1997.

26. Lawson, W. "Racial and ethnic factors in psychiatric research." *Hospital and Community Psychiatry*, 37(1):50–54, 1986.

27. Glazer, W., Morgentsern, H., and Doucette, J. "Predicting the long-term risk of tardive dyskinesia in outpatients maintained on neuroleptic medications." *Journal of Clinical Psychiatry*, 54(4):133–139, 1993.

28. Sindrup, S., and Brosen, K. "The pharmacogenetics of codeine hypoanalgesia." *Pharmacogenetics*, 5(6):335–346, 1995.

29. Andrews, M. "Culture and nutrition." In *Transcultural Concepts of Nursing Care*, 3rd ed. M. Andrews and J. Boyle, eds. New York: Lippincott, 1999, pp. 341–377.

30. Leininger, M. *Transcultural Nursing Concepts, Theories, Research and Practices*, New York: McGraw-Hill, Inc., 1995.

31. Bodell, J., and Weng, M. "The Jewish patient and terminal dehydration: A hospice ethical dilemma." *American Journal of Hospice & Palliative Care*, 17(3): 185–188, 2000.

32. Blackhall, L., Murphy, S., Frank, G., Michel, V., and Azen, S. "Ethnicity and attitudes toward patient autonomy." *JAMA*, 274(10):820–825, 1995.

33. Koenig, B. "Cultural diversity in decision-making about care at the end of life." In *Approaching Death: Improving Care at the End of Life*, Committee on Care at the End of Life, M. Field and C. Cassel, eds., Division of Health Care Services, Institute of Medicine, Washington, D.C.: National Academy Press, 1997, pp. 363–382.

34. Hern, H., Koenig, B., Moore, L., and Marshall, P. "The difference culture can make in end-of-life decision-making." *Cambridge Quarterly of Health Care Ethics*, 7: 27–40, 1998.

35. Sherman, D. "Spiritually and culturally competent palliative care." In *Palliative Care Nursing: Quality Care to the End of Life*, M. Matzo and D. Sherman, eds., New York: Springer, 2001.

36. Carrese, J., and Rhodes, L. "Western bioethics on the Navajo reservation: Benefit or harm?" *JAMA*, 274(10):826–829, 1995.

37. Muller, J., and Desmond, B. "Ethical dilemmas in a cross-cultural context: A Chinese example." *Western Journal of Medicine*, 157:323–327, 1992.

38. Ludwig-Beymer, P. "Transcultural aspects of pain." In *Transcultural Concepts of Nursing Care*, 3rd ed., M. Andrews and J. Boyle, eds. New York: Lippincott, 1999, pp. 283–307.

39. McCaffrey M. *Nursing Practice Theories Related to Cognition, Bodily Pain, and Man-Environment Interactions.* Los Angeles: UCLA Student Store, 1968.

40. Fink, R., and Gates, R. "Pain assessment." In *Textbook of Palliative Nursing*, B. Ferrell, and N. Coyle, eds., New York: Oxford University Press, 2001, pp. 53–71.
41. Bates, M., Edwards, W., and Anderson, K. "Ethnocultural influences on variation in chronic pain perception." *Pain*, 52:101–112, 1993.
42. Zborowski, M. *People in Pain*. San-Francisco: Jossey-Bass, 1969.
43. Pasero C., Paice, J., and McCaffery, M. "Basic mechanisms underlying the causes and effects of pain." In *Pain: Clinical Manual*, 2nd ed., M. McCaffery and C. Pasero, eds., New York: Mosby, 1999, pp. 15–34.
44. Ferrell, B. "Overview of aging and pain." In *Pain in the Elderly*, B.A. Ferrell and B.R. Ferrell, eds., Seattle, WA: IASP Press, 1996, pp. 1–10.
45. Cleeland, C. "Undertreatment of cancer pain in elderly patients." *JAMA*, 279: 1914–1915, 1998.
46. Pasero, C., Reed, B., and McCaffrey, M. "Pain in the elderly." In *Pain: Clinical Manual*, 2nd ed., M. McCaffery and C. Pasero, eds., New York: Mosby, 1999, pp. 674–710.
47. Hurley, A., Volicer, B., Hanrahan, P., Houde, S., and Volicer, L. "Assessment of discomfort in advanced Alzheimer patients." *Research Nursing Health*, 15:369–377, 1992.
48. Kagawa-Singer, M. "The cultural context of death rituals and mourning practices." *ONF*, 25(10):1752–1763, 1998.
49. Ellis, R. "Multicultural grief counseling." In *Living with Grief*, K. Doka and J.Davidson, eds. Washington, D.C.: Hospice Foundation of America, 1998, pp. 249–260.
50. McGoldrick, M., Almeida, R., Hines, P., Rosen, E., Garcia-Preto, N., and Lee, E. "Mourning in different cultures." In *Living Beyond Loss*, F. Walsh and M. McGoldrick, eds., New York: W.W. Norton and Co., Inc., 1991, pp. 176–206.
51. Worden, J. *Grief Counseling and Grief Therapy*, 2nd ed., New York: Springer, 1991.
52. Cable, D. "Grief in the American culture." In *Living with Grief*, K. Doka and J. Davidson, eds. Washington, D.C.: Hospice Foundation of America, 1998, pp. 61–70.
53. Dienemann, J., ed. *Cultural Diversity in Nursing: Issues, Strategies, and Outcomes*, Washington D.C.: American Academy of Nursing, 1997.
54. Davidson, J. "Conclusion," In *Living with Grief*, K. Doka and J. Davidson, eds. Washington, D.C.: Hospice Foundation of America, 1998, pp. 285–288.

TABLE 13-5   Comparison of Diverse Religious Practices and Beliefs

	Hinduism	Islam	Judaism	Christianity	American Indian	Buddhism
Diet	vegetarian	no pork/ shellfish/ alcohol	no pork/ shellfish	no restrictions	regional traditional foods	vegetarian
Terminal care	modesty; cleanliness; maintain awareness; chanting; Ayurvedic medicine	modesty; ritual washing; do not prolong; daily prayers	do not prolong	varies: do not shorten; do not prolong	modesty; family caregivers: traditional healers	modesty; maintain awareness: meditation
DNR/advance directives	allowed/varies	no/varies	allowed	allowed/varies	no/varies	allowed
Drugs/blood	allowed/ may refuse pain medications	allowed	allowed	allowed Jehovah's Witness: refuse blood	allowed	may refuse pain medications
Autopsies	allowed	restricted	restricted	allowed	restricted	allowed
Organ donation	no position	allowed	restricted	allowed	restricted	no position
Death	priest: prayers	head facing east; family handles body; caretaker: use gloves	burial society prepares body; body not left alone; psalms and confession	last rite prayers; communion; confession	traditional rituals	family/teacher present; need time to allow spirit to leave
Burial	cremation; ashes in holy rivers	immediate burial; no embalmment	immediate burial; no embalmment	cremation/burial	cremation/burial	cremation/burial
Bereavement	reincarnation	grief counseling may be intrusive; resurrection	active mourning supported; 7 day, 30 day, 1 year rituals	resurrection; public grieving	pass into another reality; restricted; grief counseling may be intrusive	restrained; reincarnation

Table 13-5   **193**

TABLE 13-6   **Communication Style Differences**

Native American	Asian/Latino	European American	African American
speaks softly/slower	speaks softly	speaks loudly/to control listener	speaks with affect
indirect gaze when listening or speaking	avoidance of eye contact when listening or speaking to persons of higher status	greater eye contact when listening	direct, prolonged eye contact when speaking but less when listening
interjects less: seldom initiates communication	interjects less; seldom initiates communication	head nods; other nonverbal markers	interrupts when possible
delayed responsive style (silence)	mild responsive style	quick responsive style	quicker responsive style
low-keyed, indirect manner	low-keyed, indirect	objective; task-oriented	affective, emotional, interpersonal manner

Source: Sue, D. *Counseling the Culturally Different: Theory and Practice.* New York: John Wiley & Sons, 1990.

Palliation in Noncancer Disease

14

Brad Stuart, M.D.

Over the past hundred years, chronic illness has emerged as the major cause of death in the United States. In 1900, 75% of deaths resulted from acute causes related to trauma, infections, or complications of childbirth. The remaining quarter were due to chronic illness. By the year 2000, these proportions had reversed. Currently, 75% of all deaths are due to chronic illness. In turn, three quarters of those are from noncancer disease.[1]

These numbers will increase as the population ages. Mortality from chronic illness is age-related, and from 2000 to 2030, the over-65 population will double. Palliative care will play an increasingly important role in this setting, because it increases quality of care in late-stage disease, while helping to contain costs. Medicare now spends approximately 25% of its budget on less than 5% of its patients: those who are in the last year of life.

Almost half of the deaths from chronic illness are due to cardiovascular disease, chiefly congestive heart failure (CHF). This disease epitomizes the challenges that the U.S. health care system faces from chronic illness. About 5 million new cases of CHF are diagnosed in the United States each year. The five-year mortality rate of CHF is approximately 50%, which is worse than for some cancers. The annual national cost of treating CHF is more than $20 billion.[2]

CHF is the only cardiovascular diagnosis that is now increasing in incidence. The acute causes of cardiac death, mainly myocardial infarction (MI) and ventricular arrhythmias, are now treatable through coronary revascularization procedures such as bypass grafting and coronary artery angioplasty and stenting.[3] However, deaths from cardiovascular disease have not been prevented, just postponed.

Underlying coronary disease continues to progress in these cases, eventually progressing down the final common pathway of heart failure. Barring unforeseen therapeutic breakthroughs, cardiac epidemiologists foresee an epidemic of heart failure over the next several decades.[4] These patients experience lingering chronic illness, frequently with disabling symptoms such as breathlessness and chest pain. They are prime candidates for palliative care.

This chapter deals with the challenges of palliation in patients with CHF, as well as those with other common noncancer illnesses. These include advanced lung disease, dementia, and other organ failure, including chronic renal disease and liver failure.

The Challenge of Prognostic Uncertainty

Hospice, which in its early stages focused on pain and symptom management in cancer patients, is adapting slowly to the care of patients with noncancer disease. The primary challenge has been hospice's major eligibility requirement: that hospice enrollees be "terminal," defined as having a "prognosis of six months or less, assuming the disease runs its normal course." In cancer, determining whether the patient is terminal is relatively easy, because in its end stages cancer tends to cause obvious symptoms and signs such as loss of appetite and weight, fatigue, and pain. In contrast, noncancer patients decline more slowly, tend to be stable until an unpredictable exacerbation occurs, and usually have a higher level of function prior to death.[5] Therefore, it is often difficult to determine when a noncancer patient is terminal.

The relative responsiveness of noncancer disease to drug treatment is another complicating factor in determining when these patients might be nearing death. Cancer patients respond to "definitive therapy" (i.e., surgery, chemotherapy, and radiation) for only a period of time, and then these treatments tend to lose their disease-modifying potential. After that, even though the patient may undergo further definitive treatment, discontinuing it in favor of comfort care is a reasonable option. In noncancer disease, on the other hand, "active treatment" continues to be effective until very near death. Diuretics, for example, help CHF patients with pulmonary edema until the very end stages of disease, and intubation and mechanical ventilation can sustain even the sickest patient with chronic obstructive pulmonary disease (COPD) through many exacerbations. The clear distinction between "active treatment" and "comfort care" that often exists in cancer is rarely so clear in noncancer cases. In fact, "treatment" drugs like diuretics are essential to palliation in CHF, and opioids like morphine, usually considered "palliative," are actually effective in the treatment of dyspnea in chronic CHF cases.

Prognostic uncertainty makes it difficult to determine when noncancer patients are actually "dying."[6] This is why, although 60% of cancer patients now die in hospice, only about 15% of noncancer patients do. Prognostic uncertainty also reduces the length of stay in hospice programs. Currently, almost one third of new enrollees die before the end of their first week in hospice.[7] Although, strictly speaking, palliative care is not burdened with the same eligibility criteria as hospice, it still may not be applied until late in the disease trajectory. It is important to remember that symptom management, advance care planning, and psychosocial/spiritual support are appropriate regardless of apparent stage of disease.

Severity Indicators

Because prognosis is uncertain in noncancer disease, it is helpful to know indicators of severity that can help to determine which patients have end-stage illness. Whether or not these patients are actually near death, when their illness becomes sufficiently severe, their physical and psychosocial needs make them good candidates for a palliative approach. Severity indicators can also help with the cost/benefit analysis of palliative interventions. With limited staff and productivity considerations, palliative care programs need to begin care when it is most effective, and that is when disease is severe. The following criteria of advanced disease are adapted from those originally published by the National Hospice Organization.[8]

End-stage *heart disease* is usually manifested by heart failure. These patients are of two main types: those with *systolic failure*, whose left ventricle has become weakened and dilated, and those with heart failure and *preserved systolic function*, who have a small, poorly compliant (stiff) left ventricle that cannot tolerate pressure or volume stress and cause multiple episodes of "flash pulmonary edema" without ventricular enlargement.[9]

Patients can be said to have advanced systolic failure when they have reached New York Heart Association (NYHA) Class III or IV (see Table 14-1). That is, they become short of breath or have chest pain with minimal exertion, or they have these symptoms at rest.

Life expectancy decreases as patients with CHF progress through the NYHA classes. One-year mortality for Class II patients is 5–15%; for Class IV patients it is up to 70%.

Optimally, these patients should be treated with diuretics and angiotensin-converting enzyme (ACE) inhibitors or angiotensin-receptor blockers (ARBs). If therapy with these drugs is not optimal, it is difficult to tell whether the patient is end-stage or simply undertreated. Declining functional status is com-

TABLE 14-1 The New York Heart Association's Functional Classification of Heart Failure	
NYHA Class	**Symptoms**
I	Asymptomatic, or symptoms only with maximal exertion
II	Symptomatic with moderate exertion
III	Symptomatic with minimal exertion
IV	Symptomatic at rest

mon in late-stage heart failure, particularly when dyspnea is severe. If the results of echocardiography or coronary catheterization are available, an ejection fraction less than 20% indicates severe systolic dysfunction. Heart failure is advanced if patients continue to decline after hospitalization that involved invasive monitoring (with Swan-Ganz catheter). Any patient failing an inotropic infusion of dobutamine (Dobutrex®) or milrinone (Primacor®) should be considered for hospice evaluation or a primarily palliative approach.

Lung disease, including both obstructive types like COPD and chronic bronchitis, as well as restrictive disorders including pulmonary fibrosis and interstitial pneumonia, are considered advanced when patients have disabling dyspnea. Many of these patients have undergone multiple hospitalizations, often involving intubation and mechanical ventilation. Many have a blood gas deficit, with an arterial pO_2 below 60 on room air and pCO_2 above 50. If bronchospasm is present it is usually resistant to inhaled bronchodilators. If pulmonary function tests are available, forced expiratory volume in one second (FEV_1) is less than 10% of the predicted value for the patient's height and weight.

Dementia, including the Alzheimer and vascular types, are especially difficult diseases in which to determine prognosis. Even in cases of far-advanced dementia, where cognitive function is all but absent, patients may survive for years with meticulous and dedicated care. The dementing process is not fatal in itself; it is only when medical complications begin to occur that the patient can be said to be nearing the end of life. Indicators of severe dementia include loss of the ability to ambulate independently and loss of the ability to carry on a meaningful conversation. After patients have difficulty with walking and talking, the incidence of complications begins to increase. For instance, when patients become bedbound, the likelihood of pneumonia becomes much higher because aspiration of oral secretions is common, and because segmental atelectasis of the lung occurs from chronic hypoventilation. Other infections resulting in sepsis and death, particularly those of the urinary tract, may increase in incidence because of the use of indwelling catheters. As dementia becomes advanced, studies show that recurrent fever after a course of antibiotics predicts increased mortality even if the source of infection is not known.

Feeding tubes are commonly inserted because demented patients lose the ability to swallow, despite numerous recent studies documenting poor outcomes.[10, 11, 12] Weight loss despite a feeding tube indicates the need for a discussion with family and caregivers, because this may be the only sign of their increasing ambivalence about the feedings.

End-stage *liver disease* manifests as cirrhosis, which is the final common pathway for most of the diseases that cause hepatocellular necrosis, such as alcoholism and chronic hepatitis B and C. Ascites refractory to diuretics and encephalopathy resistant to lactulose and neomycin are often seen. Bleeding from esophageal varices is common, particularly if liver disease is so advanced that there is a shortage of liver-dependant clotting factors. This is reflected in elevation of prothrombin time (PT) or International Normalized Ratio (INR) in patients who are not taking warfarin (Coumadin®).

End-stage renal disease (ESRD) is usually treated with dialysis. Any patient who elects to discontinue dialysis should be offered the option of hospice. A small minority who began dialysis while they still had residual renal function, and who did not lose this while on dialysis due to progression of underlying renal disease, may survive beyond the usual several days to a week. For patients who have severe renal function abnormalities but who refuse dialysis, those with serum creatinine over 6.0, or creatinine clearance under 10 ml/min (15 ml/min for diabetics) experience increased short-term mortality.

Treatment Considerations

Palliation of symptoms in noncancer disease requires a working knowledge of the drugs used to treat these diseases, as well as expertise in the use of analgesics and sedatives. Excellent palliative care consists of a unified package of acute pharmacotherapy and medication for comfort, provided in a flexible manner. In noncancer disease, quality of care can suffer when patients are regarded as either "in active treatment" or "comfort care only."

Patients with late-stage chronic illness are best treated as "in transition" from predominately acute disease-modifying treatment toward care focused primarily on comfort, until hospice enrollment or an equivalent plan of care is achieved.[13] Separating treatment and palliation strategies is not optimal for many patients because:

- "Terminal illness" is difficult to define, so comfort care can be delayed if it is reserved only for those who are "dying."

- Many patients who undergo active treatment would prefer care oriented toward comfort, but their preferences are not assessed.

- Few patients receive the best of active and palliative treatment concurrently.

The treatment of CHF and COPD will be discussed in this chapter, both because these are the two most common noncancer diagnoses and because palliation in each requires skillful combinations of acute treatment pharmacotherapy with medications given for comfort.

Palliation of Advanced Heart Failure

Palliation seeks to preserve function and comfort. In CHF, this is best achieved by using drugs that primarily treat the disease, combined with others that primarily relieve symptoms. Once the pathophysiology of the disease and the pharmacodynamics of the drugs are understood, however, it becomes obvious that there is no meaningful distinction between "treatment" and "comfort" pharmacotherapy in CHF.

To understand the drug classes used to treat CHF, it is important to grasp the evolution of our understanding of cardiovascular physiology over the last several decades.[14] Until the 1970s, the cardiorenal model, in which the heart was visualized as a simple pump, regarded salt and water retention as the cause of failure. In this model, preload, or the volume of blood entering the heart, was the culprit that caused circulatory overload. Digoxin, which increases contractility to strengthen the "pump," and diuretics such as furosemide (Lasix®), which cause salt and water loss and thus decrease preload, were mainstays of drug therapy.

The hemodynamic model of the 1980s explained failing pump function by adding the concept of afterload, or the systemic blood pressure the heart must pump against. Reducing afterload was accomplished by adding vasodilators. ACE inhibitors, which were found to decrease peripheral vasoconstriction, were the most successful example.[15] However, even with optimal management of preload and afterload, CHF continued to progress.

Through the 1990s, the neurohormonal activation model became the accepted way of explaining why systolic heart failure progresses.[16] Two of the body's hormonal systems were found to be responsible for degeneration of left ventricular function: the renin-angiotensin-aldosterone (RAS) system and the sympathetic nervous system (SNS). Both evolved originally in all mammalian systems to preserve cardiac output in case of trauma or bleeding by increasing systemic blood pressure, heart rate, blood volume, and cardiac contractility. However, both are continuously "switched on" as the heart fails, and both lead to further progression of CHF by damaging the heart muscle through multiple physiologic pathways. This progressive damage leads to ventricular remodeling, which causes the left ventricle to weaken, stretch, and eventually assume a more spherical shape, which is much less effective as a pump than the normal elliptical (football-shaped) ventricular geometry. This further reduces cardiac output, which in turn further stimulates the RAS and SNS. A downward spiral ensues, which in its end stages results in severe and intractable ventricular failure.

Blocking the "switched on" RAS can be accomplished with ACE inhibitors, which slow the ventricular remodeling process (although they do not reverse it) and also reduce afterload. The ACE inhibitors first used in CHF include captopril and enalapril (Vasotec®); many others are now in use. Reducing an overly activated SNS requires beta-adrenergic blockers such as carvedilol (Coreg®).[17] Beta blockers were avoided in CHF until recently because they can reduce contractility and worsen heart failure symptoms. When they are used to reverse ventricular remodeling, they must be administered with close monitoring, and benefits of therapy can take months to occur. Beta blockers should be started in NYHA Stage I–III CHF. Although they have been shown to help patients with Stage IV disease, they must be used carefully because their risk/benefit ratio may not be as favorable. The risk/benefit ratio needs to balance the ability to lower blood pressure and treat angina with increased potential for bradycardia, dizziness, and increased interactions with other medications. Diuretics and ACE inhibitors, therefore, are more often regarded as drugs of both treatment and palliation.

Excellent palliation of symptoms in this disease requires providers to know how to assess and treat it. Subjective data gathered in any assessment should include questions about dyspnea on exertion, orthopnea (shortness of breath when lying flat), and paroxysmal nocturnal dyspnea (PND, or sudden onset of shortness of breath at night). Positive answers to any of these questions, particularly the latter two, may indicate fluid overload and the need for an increase in diuretic dose. Objective data should include at least the assessment of jugular venous distention (JVD) and lung sounds. Rales, or fine crackling sounds at the lung bases that progress further up the lung fields with further fluid overload, are important to follow in serial examinations. Sophisticated examiners will learn to evaluate for hepatojugular reflux (HJR). This is best assessed with the patient sitting upright or at about a 30 degree angle; pressure with the flat of the examining hand over the right upper quadrant of the abdomen produces elevation of the jugular venous meniscus in proportion to the degree of fluid overload. Edema of the lower legs is common in decompensated heart failure, but is a nonspecific sign. Other causes of leg edema, such as incompetent valves in the major veins of the legs, may also be responsible. Using elimination of leg edema as a clinical endpoint can result in dehydration and hypovolemia.

Monitoring of serial weights, done on the same scale each time, as well as heart rate and blood pressure monitoring, are also important. Postural vital signs should be checked in any patient complaining of lightheadedness, because the aggressive diuresis required to keep patients with advanced CHF in fluid balance may cause hypovolemia and postural hypotension, with attendant fall risk.

Diuretic management of fluid balance can only be optimal if salt balance is maintained as well. Patients with advanced CHF are very sensitive to even small increases in dietary sodium. Patients should be maintained on a no-added-salt diet, or even a 2 gm/day sodium intake, if possible. It is common for patients to want additional salt, because aldosterone production is often high in CHF, and this increases both thirst and appetite for salt. It is often helpful to tell patients that decreasing salt intake usually results in a considerable increase in comfort and reduced work of breathing. In addition, many providers personally check the cupboards and refrigerators of their CHF patients, because many are not aware of the high salt content of some foods, especially those that are commercially prepared and packaged. The addition of spironolactone (Aldactone®) to the diuretic regimen should be considered in all patients with advanced CHF,[18] because this drug blocks aldosterone production, and has been shown to benefit most of these patients. However, because spironolactone causes potassium retention, the dose of supplementary potassium used by most patients on loop diuretics should be reduced or even eliminated for a time. A serum potassium level can be checked after a week or so to ensure that hypokalemia, if it is present, can be treated by carefully reinstituting potassium supplements.

After fluid and salt balance is stabilized, other medications should be added to treat dyspnea. Opioids such as morphine (Roxanol®) are usually effective, and can be titrated upward until dyspnea is controlled. Opioids have physiologic effects that are specifically beneficial in CHF.[19] They lower sympathetic tone, decreasing the overactivity of the SNS that is universal in late-stage systolic CHF. This results in a decrease in oxygen consumption, as well as an increase in capacitance of the veins in the legs. The walls of these veins relax with morphine administration, so that the veins hold more venous blood, lowering the amount that returns to the heart through the vena cava to the left atrium. The net result is a decrease in preload, and a tendency toward stabilization of CHF. As a bonus, morphine and other opioids have a direct suppressive effect on centers in the midbrain that cause the subjective sensation of breathlessness. The sum total of all these effects is a reduction of dyspnea. Although there are few clinical studies of the effect of opioids in CHF, anecdotal experience in hospice shows that morphine may actually stabilize patients who appear near death from CHF, and may even lead to improvement. In some cases, patients who no longer responded to dobutamine infusions and were referred to hospice and started on morphine actually recovered enough to be discharged from hospice. This effect may be seen in certain patients with both systolic failure and preserved systolic function (diastolic dysfunction).

Sudden cardiac death is common in CHF; its incidence rises by a factor of five as soon as patients are diagnosed with heart failure.[20] Some authorities have stated that this makes a hospice or palliative approach impractical for CHF patients, because death is unpredictable and therefore it is impossible to determine when patients are "terminal."[21] However, sudden death occurs more often in NYHA Stage I–III patients than in those with very advanced disease. Most patients with Class IV disease die of pump failure, which is more predictable.

Palliation of Advanced Pulmonary Disease

Lung disease, especially COPD, is the fifth most common cause of death in the United States. Currently, 15 million patients are treated each year at an annual cost of $11 billion. Mortality from COPD increased over 50% from 1980 to the mid-1990s and continues to rise, chiefly because of an increase in the number of women smoking cigarettes.[22]

As in CHF, palliation of symptoms in advanced dyspnea is best accomplished through a rational combination of active treatment and symptom-relief approaches.[23] Classes of medications used include inhaled bronchodilators, corticosteroids, theophylline, and opioids and sedatives.

Inhaled bronchodilators fall into two classes: beta-agonist and cholinergic. Beta-agonist agents such as albuterol (Ventolin®, Proventil®) and their newer longer-acting counterparts such as salmeterol (Serevent®) and formoterol (Foradil®) have an effect on beta-adrenergic receptors opposite to that of beta blockers. Beta agonists stimulate beta-2 receptors, which results in bronchodi-lation. Older nonspecific drugs, as well as the body's own endogenously secreted beta agonists, epinephrine and norepinephrine, have a host of other effects, such as tachycardia and tremor, which are undesirable or even toxic. Beta-2 agonists can have these effects as well at the higher doses sometimes used by COPD patients, especially those with advanced disease and severe dys-pnea.

Beta-2 agonists have drawbacks in advanced COPD, particularly if they are used in excessive amounts. Although they work well in asthma, they do not produce as much bronchodilation in pure COPD.[24] Older patients achieve less bronchodilation, but as much or more toxicity. Arrhythmias, both supraven-tricular and ventricular, can be seen.[25] Systemic absorption causes toxic effects, especially tremor, at higher doses. In very severe COPD, where parts of the lung are not aerated, beta-2 agonists can cause pulmonary vasodilation, which allows blood to circulate through non-ventilated areas (ventilation-per-fusion mismatch).[26] This can result in a net decrease in oxygenation, the opposite of what is intended.

Cholinergic bronchodilators such as ipratropium (Atrovent®), on the other hand, reliably produce bronchodilation in COPD. There is lower sys-temic absorption than with beta-2 agonists, and few side effects are seen.[27] Cholinergics and beta-2 agonists are synergistic in COPD; bronchodilation is more pronounced when both are used together than with either used alone. Both agents are available in a fixed-dose mixture (Combivent®).[28]

Patients with advanced COPD commonly rely heavily on beta-2 inhalers, because the onset of action is quicker than with cholinergics. Toxicity some-times manifests in these patients as tachycardia, tremulousness, dyspnea, and anxiety. A useful therapeutic intervention is to increase the dose of ipra-tropium, while decreasing the beta-2 agonist. This approach can yield greater bronchodilation with less risk of toxicity.

Most end-stage COPD patients benefit from the addition of a spacer to their metered-dose inhaler (MDI). Their inspiratory volumes and pressures are often so low that the entire dose of medication cannot be inhaled in one breath. Most of it is deposited on the posterior pharynx, and then swallowed. Many elderly patients also have poor MDI mechanics; through lack of under-standing or physical disability they cannot coordinate triggering of the MDI with inspiration. Although spacers are adequate for most patients, a few will require nebulizers.[29] Proper assessment and administration of inhaled bron-chodilators can produce remarkable turnarounds for some patients who appear nearly moribund on initial evaluation.

Oral corticosteroids such as prednisone or dexamethasone (Decadron®) are routinely administered to patients with exacerbations of COPD. However, studies show that true bronchodilation results in only about 10–20% of cases.[30] No tests predict which patients will respond. Oral corticosteroids should never be stopped abruptly in patients who have been taking them continuously for more than a week or two, because over that time the pituitary-adrenal axis can become suppressed and patients cannot manufacture the endogenous corticosteroid necessary to maintain comfort. However, the decision to start and maintain a COPD patient on high doses of corticosteroids should be approached with caution unless there has been clear-cut benefit with prior administration of the drug. When patients are still functional (i.e., capable of independent ambulation) corticosteroids should be tapered over several weeks to avoid the muscle atrophy and osteoporosis often seen with long-term high-dose corticosteroids.

The use of theophylline (Theo-Dur® and others) is controversial. It results in little bronchodilation, but whatever beneficial effect the drug exerts is probably maximal at low serum levels. Higher levels are often associated with toxicity. Theophylline has been shown in the laboratory to strengthen respiratory muscles; a significant clinical effect is doubtful. The drug should probably not be used as primary therapy, but as an adjunct if necessary.[31]

Morphine and other opioids can be used with great benefit even in advanced COPD with carbon dioxide (CO_2) retention.[32] Morphine's reduction of oxygen consumption is particularly beneficial in patients with hypoxemia.[33] Its effect on the midbrain to reduce the sensation of dyspnea can produce profound relief for patients with even extreme shortness of breath. In addition, morphine reduces chemoreceptor sensitivity to CO_2, and it is elevation of pCO_2 even to a minimal degree that produces dyspnea in humans.[34] This is the reason that morphine has been thought to be contraindicated in COPD. Clinicians have long been taught that the reduction of "respiratory drive" resulting from the administration of opioids would cause apnea and death.[35] Many studies have shown, however, that morphine does not necessarily hasten death when it is used to relieve pain and dyspnea even in critically ill patients.[36, 37, 38] Morphine can be used safely and effectively if started at low doses (1–5 mg orally or sublingually every one to four hours), and titrated gradually to levels sufficient to relieve dyspnea. Anecdotal evidence indicates that relatively high doses can be tolerated as long as titration progresses slowly enough to allow the patient to adjust.[39] "Start low and go slow" is a reasonable approach to initiating opioids for dyspnea in COPD.

Even "weak opioids" can be effective for dyspnea. Cough suppressants containing codeine (Robitussin AC®) or hydrocodone (Hycodan®) are useful if patients, families, or physicians are "opiodophobic." Changing to immediate-release morphine may be accomplished once the benefits of opioids are apparent. Slow-release morphine preparations (MS-Contin®, Oramorph-SR®) may not be as effective. Inhaled morphine may be beneficial for dyspnea of COPD for patients who are already acquainted with mask ventilation.[40] However, inhaled morphine is rapidly absorbed systemically, and its site of action is probably the CNS and not the lung. Oral morphine is just as effective, and also easier to administer and less expensive.

Sedatives should not be used as primary therapy for dyspnea. Benzodiazepines, for instance, are commonly prescribed for breathless COPD patients, even though these drugs have never been found specifically to relieve dyspnea.[41] In addition, they can cause paradoxical agitation in elderly patients with dementia. The benefits of opioids for dyspnea, on the other hand, have been demonstrated. They should be used primarily, and titrated upward until dyspnea is controlled. Sedatives should be added only to manage anxiety that is not relieved by optimal doses of opioids.

Sedatives are useful adjuncts, however, as patients near the end of life. Delirium and agitation occur frequently as death nears, and sedatives can help patients as well as caregivers and family members by allowing them to obtain needed rest.[42] Hypoxemia is a major cause of agitation; assessment should be focused on reversible causes and treatment should maximize oxygenation. Opioids should be used to palliate obvious dyspnea. Unnecessary medications that can cause delirium should be withdrawn. If these measures fail to control agitation, neuroleptics such as haloperidol (Haldol®) or benzodiazepines such as lorazepam (Ativan®) can be administered orally, sublingually, or parenterally. Barbiturates such as pentobarbital (Nembutal®) may also be given orally, rectally, or transdermally.

Excessive respiratory secretions can be a problem near death. A healthy, well-hydrated adult can produce one to two liters of saliva per day. Oral secretions can be aspirated into the upper airways, particularly when patients who have lost the ability to swallow are kept in the supine position. Simple repositioning to the side often relieves the "death rattle," but if this is not possible, administration of sublingual atropine, widely available in the ophthalmologic 1% preparation, at 1–2 drops every 1–2 hours, may be effective. Alternatives are sublingual hyoscyamine (Levsin®), transdermal scopolamine (Transderm Scop®), or glycopyrrollate (Robinul®).

Summary

The aging population, increasing incidence of chronic illness, and necessity for cost containment all mandate a new approach for patients with advanced chronic illness. Palliative care can help these patients achieve comfort early in the disease process, and attain a higher quality of life even as it is coming to an end. These considerations are particularly important for patients with end-stage heart, lung, and other noncancer diagnoses. These diseases cause most deaths in the United States, even though patients afflicted with them appear "treatable" until the very end of life. Optimal outcomes can be achieved when providers recognize the late stages of disease, and combine the best of both active treatment and supportive care.

References

1. Hogan, C., Lynn, J., Gabel, J., Lunney, J., O'Mara, A., Wilkinson, A. *Medicare Beneficiaries' Costs and Use of Care in the Last Years of Life.* Washington, D.C.: Medicare Payment Advisory Commission (MedPAC), 2000.
2. Goff, D.C., Pandey, D.K., Chan, F.A., Ortiz, C., Nichaman, M.Z. "Congestive Heart Failure in the United States." *Arch Int Med* 2000;(160):197–202.

3. Hunink, M.G., Goldman, L., Tosteson, A.N., Mittleman, M.A., Goldman, P.A., Williams, L.W. "The Recent Decline in Mortality from Coronary Heart Disease, 1980–1990." *JAMA* 1997;(277):535–542.

4. Garg, R., Packer, M., Pitt, B., and Yusuf, S. "Heart Failure in the 1990s: Evolution of a Major Public Health Problem in Cardiovascular Medicine." *J Am Coll Cardiol* 1993;(22 Suppl A):3A–5A.

5. Teno, J.M., Weitzen, S., Fennell, M.L., and Mor, V. "Dying Trajectory in the Last Year of Life: Does Cancer Trajectory Fit Other Diseases?" *J Pall Med* 2001;(4):457–464.

6. Fox, E., Landrum-McNiff, K., Zhong, Z., Dawson, N.V., Wu, A.W., Lynn, J. "Evaluation of Prognostic Criteria for Determining Hospice Eligibility in Patients with Advanced Lung, Heart or Liver Disease." *JAMA* 1999;(282):1638–1645.

7. National Hospice and Palliative Care Organization. *Hospice Fact Sheet,* 2001.

8. Stuart, B., Alexander, C., Arenella, C., Connor, S., Herbst, L., Jones, D., Kinzbrunner, B., Rousseau, P. *Medical Guidelines for Determining Prognosis in Selected Noncancer Diseases,* 2nd Ed. Arlington, Va.: National Hospice Organization, 1996.

9. Marantz, P.R., Tobin, J.N., Wasserthal-Smoller, S., Steingart, R.M., Wexler, J.P., Budner, N., Rynes, T., Wohlfeiler, M., Cody, C., Buckley, S. "The Relationship Between Left Ventricular Systolic Function and Congestive Heart Failure Diagnosed by Clinical Criteria." *Circulation* 1988;(77):607–612.

10. Li, L. "Feeding Tubes in Patients with Severe Dementia." *Am Fam Physician* 2000 Apr. 15; 65(8): 1605–10, 1515.

11. Finucane, T.E., Christmas, C., and Travis, K. "Tube Feeding in Patients with Advanced Dementia: A Review of Evidence." *JAMA* 1999 Oct. 13; 282(14):1365–70.

12. Ciment, J. "Tube Feeding Bad for Patients with Dementia." *BMJ* 2 2000 Feb. 5; 320(723):33513.

13. Stuart, B. "Transition Management: A New Paradigm for Home Care of the Chronically Ill Near the End of Life." *Home Health Care Management and Practice,* in press. Sage Publications, LTD, London, U.K.

14. Mann, D.L. "Mechanisms and Models in Heart Failure: A Combinatorial Approach." *Circulation* 1999;(100):999–1008.

15. The Study of Left Ventricular Function (SOLVD) Investigators. "Effect of Enalapril on Survival in Patients with Reduced Left Ventricular Ejection Fractions and Congestive Heart Failure." *NEJM* 1991;(325):293–302.

16. Schreier, R.W., and Abraham, W.T. "Hormones and Hemodynamics in Heart Failure." *NEJM* 1999;(341):577–585.

17. Lombardini, W.L., Gilbert, E.M. "Carvedilol in the Failing Heart." *Clinical Cardiol* 2001;(24):757–766.

18. Cha, A.J., Malecha, S.E., and Judge, K.W. "Aldosterone: A New Appreciation of its Role in Heart Failure." *Pharmacotherapy* 2000;(20):1107–1115.

19. Zelis, R., Mansour, E.J., Capone, R.J., Mason, T. "The Cardiovascular Effects of Morphine: The Peripheral Capacitance and Resistance Vessels in Human Subjects." *J Clin Invest* 1974;(54):1247–1258.

20. Huikuri, H.V., Castellanos, A., Myerburg, R.J. "Sudden Death Due to Cardiac Arrhythmias." *NEJM* 2001;(345):1473–1482.

21. Lynn, J., Harrell, F. Jr, Cohn, F., Wagner, D., Connors, A.F. Jr. "Prognoses of Seriously Ill Hospitalized Patients on the Days Before Death: Implications for Patient Care and Public Policy." *New Horiz Crit Care* 1997;(5):56–61.

22. Viegi, G., Scognamiglio, A., Baldacci, S., Pistelli, F., and Carozzi, L. "Epidemiology of Chronic Obstructive Pulmonary Disease (COPD)." *Respiration* 2001;(68):4–19.

23. Chapman, K.R. "Therapeutic Approaches to Chronic Obstructive Pulmonary Disease: An Emerging Consensus." *Am J Med* 1996;(100 Suppl 1A):5S–10S.

24. Gross, N.J. "Ipratropium Bromide." *NEJM* 1988;(319):486–494.

25. Bouvy, M.L., Heerdink, E.R., de Bruin, M.L., Herings, R.M.C., Leufkens, H.G.M., and Hoes, A.W. "Use of Sympathomimetic Drugs Leads to Increased Risk of Hospitalization for Arrhythmias in Congestive Heart Failure." *Arch Int Med* 2000;(160): 2477–2480.

26. Cazzola, M., Imperatore, F., Salzillo, A., diPerna, F., Calderaro F, and Imperatore, A. "Cardiac Effects of Formoterol and Salmeterol in Patients Suffering from COPD with Preexisting Cardiac Arrhythmias and Hypoxemia." *Chest* 1998;(114):411–415.

27. Easton, P.A., Jadue, C., Dhingra, S., and Anthonisen, N.R. "A Comparison of the Bronchodilating Effects of a Beta-2 Adrenergic Agent (Albuterol) and an Anticholinergic Agent (Ipratropium Bromide), Given by Aerosol Alone or In Sequence." *NEJM* 1986;(315):735–739.

28. Petty, T.L. "The Combination of Ipratropium and Albuterol Is More Effective Than Either Agent Alone." *Chest* 1995;(5 Suppl):183S–186S.

29. Eiser, N., Angus, K., and McHale, S. "The Role of Domiciliary Nebulizers in Managing Patients with Severe COPD." *Resp Med* 2001;(95):265–274.

30. Callaghan, C.M., Dittus, R.S., and Katz, B.P. "Oral Corticosteroid Therapy for Patients with Stable Chronic Obstructive Pulmonary Disease." *Ann Int Med* 1991;(114): 216–223.

31. Jenne, J.W. "What Role Theophylline?" *Thorax* 1994;(49):97–100.

32. Wilson, W.C, Smedira, N.G., Fink, C., McDowell, J.A., Luce, J.M. "Ordering and Administration of Sedatives and Analgesics During the Withholding and Withdrawal of Life Support from Critically Ill Patients." *JAMA* 1992;(267):949–953.

33. Woodcock, A.A., Gross, E.R., Gellert, A., Shah, S., Johnson, M., and Geddes, D.M. "Effects of Dihydrocodeine, Alcohol, and Caffeine on Breathlessness and Exercise Tolerance in Patients with Chronic Obstructive Lung Disease and Normal Blood Gases." *NEJM* 1981;(305):1611–1616.

34. Manning, H.L., and Schwartzstein, R.M. "Pathophysiology of Dyspnea." *NEJM* 1995;(333): 1547–1553.

35. Weil, J.V., McCullough, R.E., Kline, J.S., Sodal, I.E. "Diminished Ventilatory Response to Hypoxia and Hypercapnia after Morphine in Normal Man." *NEJM* 1975;(292):1103–1106.

36. Wilson, W.C., Smedira, N.G., Fink, C., and McDowell, J.A., Luce, J.M. "Ordering and Administration of Sedatives and Analgesics During the Withholding and Withdrawing of Life Support from Critically Ill Patients." *JAMA* 1992;(267):949–953.

37. Bruera, E., Macmillan, K., Pither, J., and MacDonald, R.N. "Effects of Morphine on the Dyspnea of Terminal Cancer Patients." *J Pain Sympt Manage* 1990;(5):341–344.

38. Campbell, M.L., Bizek, K.S., and Thill, M. "Patient Responses During Rapid Terminal Weaning from Mechanical Ventilation: A Prospective Study." *Crit Care Med* 1999; (27):73–77.

39. Cohen, M.H., Anderson, A.J., Krasnow, S.H., Spagnolo, S.V., Citron, M.C., and Payne, M. "Continuous Intravenous Infusion of Morphine for Severe Dyspnea." *South Med J* 1991;(84):230–234.

40. Quelch, P.C., Faulkner, D.E., and Yun, J.W.S. "Nebulized Opioids in the Treatment of Dyspnea." *J Pall Care* 1997;(13):48–52.

41. Man, C.G.W., Hsu, K., Sproule, B.J. "Effects of Alprazolam on Exercise and Dyspnea in Patients with Chronic Obstructive Pulmonary Disease." *Chest* 1986;(90):832–836.

42. Ross, D.D., and Alexander, C.S. "Management of Common Symptoms in Terminally Ill Patients: Part II. Constipation, Delirium and Dyspnea." *Am Fam Physician* 2001;(64):1019–1026.

Brad Stuart is the Medical Director of Sutter VNA and Hospice.

Grief and Bereavement Issues in Hospice/Palliative Care

15

M. Murray Mayo, Ph.D.

Palliative and hospice care professionals by the nature of their work encounter grief- and bereavement-related issues across a wide range of clinical activities including assessment, treatment, systems intervention, case management, and consultation. Because of this, there is a need to keep current with ongoing developments in these areas. This chapter meets this objective by surveying the research literature to identify and report on recent developments in grief and bereavement within a palliative/hospice framework.

In this review of the research literature, the author attempts to position the discussion in terms of an end-of-life model proposed by Byock.[1] Byock's model offers health practitioners a paradigm of "dying well" that benefits not only the dying person but the family and friends as well. Consequently, the research developments reported are intended to support palliative/hospice care providers' efforts to work with such individuals on grief- and bereavement-related issues in order to find meaning and reconcile matters. A review of how the literature search was conducted and Byock's end-of-life model are provided.

Literature Review

Articles to be included in this review were identified by using search terms that referenced the clinical setting (palliative and/or hospice) and/or clinical issues (mourning, grief, and bereavement) of interest here. The search was conducted using databases known to index journals and conference proceedings reporting on research developments in this area, including Medline, CINAHL, Psychinfo, and Sociofile. In order to identify and report on current trends, only articles from 1998 to the present were included.

The literature search produced 146 articles meeting the time and content specifications noted above. Articles that featured pediatric populations, were not conducted in a palliative/hospice setting (i.e., palliative/hospice setting or issues were minor considerations), or did not focus on grief and bereavement issues were eliminated. The rationale for this was to ensure that this review provided insights and direction for the kinds of palliative/hospice care experiences that most clinical care providers were likely to encounter. These qualifications reduced the final sort to 33 articles. A review of the titles and content of these articles suggested that two major categories, grief/bereavement assessment and intervention, might be used to further organize a discussion of the results. Within each category, recent developments are reviewed along with some discussion of the literature referenced in the search articles themselves in order to provide a more detailed summary of the area. Following this review, results are then situated within Byock's model.

End-of-Life Model

As noted by Byock,[2] traditional health care and its allied fields are dominated by a clinical paradigm that is complete with its own set of distinct values and goals, such as the preservation of life, relief of suffering, and honesty in communication, to name a few. These values and goals have been applied across a wide range of patient populations and clinical settings. Within this health care culture, a problem-based approach or "medical model" has emerged as the conceptual framework guiding patient care. A central feature of this framework involves working with patients from their presenting problems to a diagnosis that denotes some treatment options.

Within palliative and hospice care settings, however, these same clinical values and goals are weighed differently. Preservation of life, for example, although still important is less compelling when a patient suffering from a life-limiting disease has entered a terminal phase. The primary focus should now shift from cure to care. Whether to initiate medical intervention is now viewed in terms of how it impacts the patient's immediate quality of life, not simply in terms of how a given regimen might manage or eradicate a disease and any related symptoms.

This shift in clinical care and focus is partly a result of a recent change in the trajectories of many chronic illnesses. Survival rates have improved tremendously as medical science has uncovered the causes of many diseases and identified new treatment options. Such advancements mean that many patients will face an extended course of treatment that includes periods of active symptoms and remission. A longer "dying" phase is often encountered. As a result, suffering becomes more prominent and a part of the patient's life.

The type of suffering of interest here is both physical and spiritual/existential. A core value of palliative and hospice care is symptom relief and pain management. As such, the problem-oriented approach to patient care is quite useful. Still, when physical suffering is held in check, patients as well as their families may face crises that are more psychological, social, or spiritual in nature. This type of suffering is often expressed as grief or bereavement, which is the central focus of this chapter. Although such suffering might be viewed as simply a clinical issue requiring some intervention from a problem-oriented approach, others have suggested different interpretations.

Silverman[3] has suggested that grief and bereavement be viewed as a normal life transition. From this perspective, grief is recognized as a normal part of everyone's life; like adolescence, it is uncomfortable sometimes, unremarkable on occasion, and every so often, awful. Silverman asks: "If we think of bereavement as a time of transition, what do people need to know in order to make this kind of shift?" (p. 5). Erikson,[4] a major 20th century psychologist/theorist, also views the end of life as just another one of life's stages when individuals must reconcile the choices they have made throughout their life. Individuals might experience despair or a sense of integrity, depending on the type of meaning they are able to attribute to their lives. What's important here is that these writers see grief and bereavement as a normal transition or opportunity to grow rather than a problem for the medical team to resolve.

Byock[2] notes that viewing the end of life and suffering from this perspective signals that a different model for patient care may be appropriate here. That is, palliative and hospice care may be more akin to pediatric practice where the practitioner pays attention to the patient's social and emotional developments as well as physical concerns. Additionally, both disciplines see the family and non-related close friends as the unit of care rather than focusing exclusively on the patient. Consequently, both disciplines may work with others in the social network to affect the patient's health and well-being. For example, the pediatrician might provide supportive counseling and guidance to parents by discussing how to work with a child entering the "terrible twos." In palliative and hospice care, nurses might provide the family with a description of impending physical, emotional, and social changes (e.g., withdrawal or lack of appetite) that the patient will be experiencing as the end of life approaches.

In order to provide care in this manner, palliative and hospice care professionals need to recognize suffering (in the form of grief and bereavement) and what growth opportunities it may afford the patient. Although almost all palliative and hospice care workers have witnessed the various forms that grief and bereavement can take, many may not be as familiar with the various types of growth opportunities available during this time. Byock[1] has identified a number of areas where the palliative/hospice care professional might assist the patient to grow and find meaning. The search for meaning near the end of life is partly a result of the patient having to forgo a number of roles (e.g., colleague, parent, sports participant) that were once central to his or her identity. This list includes:

- Sense of completion with worldly affairs
- Sense of completion in relationships with community

- Sense of meaning about one's individual life
- Experienced love of self
- Experienced love of others
- Sense of completion in relationships with family and friends
- Acceptance of the finality of life—of one's existence as an individual
- Sense of a new self beyond personal loss
- Sense of meaning about life in general
- Surrender to the transcendent, to the unknown—"letting go"

It is not necessary for patients to examine each of these areas. Some might find that allowing themselves to experience the love of others is all that is needed to create or restore some meaning and order in their lives. The goal here is to develop a sense of closure or resolution. How individuals arrive at this goal will vary. Byock[1, 28, 32] and others suggest some techniques that health care professionals might use to encourage end-of-life development for interested patients. These include storytelling, life review, and reframing problems to embrace a larger context. Any of these techniques or others might be used to help the patient seek forgiveness, extend affirmation to others or oneself, or reinterpret life events. By developing a sense of closure or resolution, the patient may find meaning and identity at a time when his or her connection to the world seems to be slipping away. In these cases, patients report being at peace or even at times exhilarated as they experience life and others anew.

To emphasize this point further, Byock contrasts the "good death" to "dying well." A good death conjures up images of a sudden, painless demise. Dying well suggests that some preparation and work may be necessary in order to realize this ending state. This work may be initiated by palliative and hospice care professionals using grief and bereavement as indicators where patients and/or significant others might focus on to realize some renewed meaning or identity.

The process of dying well is really about living life fully while dying. If one views grief and bereavement as normal transitions of life, then the palliative and hospice practitioners can help the patient and family focus on opportunities for diminishing the suffering.

Search Results

Grief and Bereavement Assessment Issues

The terms "grief" and "bereavement" are often used interchangeably. Technically, "grief is defined as a response to a loss, while bereavement refers specifically to that period of time following a death when survivors experience patterns of grieving."[5] Given that grief is something that can occur during bereavement, it is understandable that the two terms are often intertwined.

In their review of some of the classic works regarding loss, grief, and bereavement, Lev and McCorkle[5] attempt to better delineate these terms as well as highlight some of the intricacies surrounding this area of study. Grief, according to Parkes,[6, 7] is seen not as a single response but rather as a series of phases one encounters. In the alarm phase, actual physical visceral distress is felt. As this phase subsides, a more emotionally based set of reactions occurs including anger, depression, guilt, and anxiety. For most, these emotional reactions dissipate over time and the final, third stage of recovery begins. During this final stage, individuals adjust to the changes, with some going on to find new meanings and identities in their lives. Like grief, bereavement is also looked upon as a multifaceted process. Bereavement can be considered "a holistic response to loss that usually includes physical, psychological, and behavioral responses."[5]

Although some conceptual understanding of terms might be useful here, we find that within palliative and hospice care settings grief and bereavement work can be much more complicated. Grief, for example, can follow any number of actual and/or perceived losses or failures (e.g., plans put indefinitely on hold, reduced functioning, death, or failure to reach some desired level of care) experienced by the patient or family. A vivid example of this is found in an article by Whitney[8] that describes the many added responsibilities and pressures experienced by families who have a loved one with Alzheimer's type dementia. Due to the slow progression of the disease and the unremitting social/psychological deterioration it brings, the family and patient endure myriad losses. Some of these losses are public and readily acknowledged. Other losses are symbolic or private and catch the person and others off guard.

Although Alzheimer's demonstrates that grief can result from a wide range of losses, it also underscores the fact that grief as well as bereavement is not limited to the patient and immediate family or friends. Given the extended trajectory of this and other chronic diseases, there is time for the patient to develop a "surrogate" family consisting of staff, volunteers, and fellow nursing home residents.[9] As a result, palliative and hospice care workers need to monitor and evaluate the grief and bereavement status of all those who know and work with the patient. Kavanaugh[10] describes one nursing home program where families, residents, staff, and others can meet with a psychologist in a group forum to discuss their losses and the various emotional issues they are facing.

Despite our best efforts to assess and anticipate grief and bereavement, a number of other factors can interfere. First, individuals may not react in the ways we would predict following some traumatic event. Lev and McCorkle,[5] for example, observed that mothers who were very emotional while caring for a child with leukemia were relatively calm following their deaths. Second, grief can also be difficult to assess in patients who have problems communicating. Read[11] notes that palliative care patients with learning disabilities, for example, have problems communicating effectively and in reciprocal ways. They can adopt a number of compensatory strategies (e.g., avoiding difficult situations or topics, pretending to understand) to ease "communication distress."[12] In such cases, the palliative/hospice care team must rely on nonverbal communication, significant others, and learning disability specialists (e.g., community learning disability nurse) to assess and subsequently respond to grief and related issues. Working with learning disabled patients highlights the fact that palliative/hospice care providers at times must rely on others to help diagnose and respond to grief and bereavement problems. This is true also of other conditions that hamper patient communications such as dementias and cerebral-vascular disorders.

Finally, recognizing and understanding grief can be trying in the face of difficult topics that come up during the course of treatment. Holmes[13] noted that providing food and hydration to the dying is filled with many biological, emotional, and sociological meanings and losses. Professionals and families alike can be caught up in trying to promote patient well-being and comfort while at the same time trying to gauge life expectancy. Such a delicate balancing act is weighted with hope, despair, and grief for those charged with deciding the patient's fate. Hooks and Daly[14] also describe this dilemma in their case review of a family that experienced guilt for not assisting their loved one in suicide. Whitney[8] notes, for example, that family members may experience strong feelings of guilt because of having to make a critical care decision (e.g., cessation of IV antibiotics or hydration) for the patient with dementia. These studies point out the fact that grief can pervade any course of treatment selected and may complicate bereavement as a result.

Not only is the current assessment of grief and bereavement a challenge, predicting its course is also tricky. Survivors will vary in terms of the length of the bereavement period as well as in terms of the type and severity of complications they will encounter. A few will deteriorate as grief takes on more pathological forms (i.e., suicidal ideation, inability to function). Walsh-Burke[15] provides some guidance here in terms of identifying factors associated with more involved episodes of grief and bereavement. In a review of the research literature, Walsh-Burke[15] discusses a host of client (preexisting psychiatric disorder, unresolved loss, age), situational (relationship to deceased, excessive dependency, traumatic death), and environmental (limited social support, financial difficulties) factors that palliative and hospice care providers might want to consider when assessing a patient or family member.

Some caution is needed, however, not to overact and misinterpret any one factor or report as indicative of complications. Barbato and colleagues[16] note that the incidence of parapsychological events (e.g., sensing a presence of the deceased, visual or auditory hallucinations) is relatively common and often subsides within the year following a loss.[17] These researchers recommend validating the experience and using it as a means to aid grieving, not simply viewing it as a signal of some psychological disorder.

In sum, this discussion gives some indication of the intricacy that can be involved in detecting grief and bereavement and projecting its course. As important as detection is, it is equally important to understand how to respond to patients and family members in these situations. The first impulse is to relieve suffering, a primary goal in palliative and hospice care settings. Other treatment options are also available if we consider that symptoms like suffering have meanings beyond those attributed by the prevailing biomedical and cultural systems. Lobchuk and Stymeist[18] note that the family culture also applies norms and values to interpret what symptoms mean. Those palliative/hospice care providers that decipher these meanings may find pleas for help as well as requests to consider some life issues in greater detail. Moraes says it well when he states, "The act of dying is unique to each of us and may reflect his or her whole life experience. It is up to the hospice team to unravel the puzzle and symbolic meanings of each person's biography."[28]

When loss has left the patient or family member with some void of meaning or identity, palliative/hospice care providers may find Byock's[1] framework a useful tool for understanding the nature of grief as well as how bereavement may unfold. For example, a suffering patient may reveal reluctance and sorrow surrounding having to let go of some cherished roles. A survivor's sorrow at difficulty adjusting following some loss might signal that he or she is trying to make some sense out of life in general. These and other themes described by Byock may help the palliative/hospice care provider to pull together the various and often discrepant symptoms found in grieving and bereaved individuals in order to plan some intervention effort.

Grief and Bereavement Intervention Issues

In palliative/hospice care, transdisciplinary teams have been assembled to help respond to the wide range of issues encountered by the patient and family members. Practitioners from medicine, nursing, spiritual care, social work, and expressive/occupational therapies as well as volunteers all interact with the patient and family to provide holistic care. The blend is both comprehensive and synergistic. Prior to the patient's death, any number of these team members may become involved with a given case. Team members meet regularly to discuss how to care for the patient and family. During these transdisciplinary team meetings as well as planned interventions, team members must be able to identify and differentiate their concerns and attitudes from those of the patient and family members. By doing so, the practitioner is better able to attend to the matters of highest priority to the patient and family and promote dignity and closure.[19]

In the literature, we find a variety of interventions for both patients entering the dying phase and family members following the death. Central to many of these interventions is the notion of promoting communication among family members as well as with the patient.[20, 21, 22] To begin, the palliative/hospice care professional needs to identify where concerns or fears lie by inviting questions from the patient and family members.[23] Parkes notes that "experience in the field of palliative care suggests that people seldom ask questions unless they are prepared for the possible answers they may receive."[24] By supplying information in manageable pieces the patient and family are better able to internalize matters in order to cope with current and impending events. Indeed, a study by McCorkle and colleagues suggests that the survivors' post-death grief can be reduced by advance practice nursing interventions during the dying phase.[25]

In addition to responding to questions and supplying factual information, interventions can address more emotional and personal areas as well. The issue of hope, for example, was cited in a number of articles reviewed and represents an interesting challenge to patients, family members, and practitioners. Bowman[26] reports that, "The hoping person is fully aware of the harshness and losses of life. . . . Hope is a sense of possibility. . . in despair and in trouble."[27] Finding and maintaining a realistic sense of hope is often a daily struggle for those delivering as well as receiving palliative and hospice care.

Hope holds out the possibility that something new can be had in spite of impending losses and life's end. Two articles were found that noted how expressive therapies were used to create hope or a sense of possibility and to discover and share new meanings about the patient and family members' present difficulties. Moraes states "their understanding of the meaning of life can be shared and processed by others who are involved in their final stage of life. Thus the arts may enable a new beginning for the people left behind."[28] The author worked with a family, for example, where a music therapist was able to relieve a dying woman's distress by turning her final thoughts into a song to leave to her three-year-old daughter. The patient described all her thoughts and wishes to the music therapist, who wrote music to accompany the words. The song was taped for the patient's daughter.

Bowman noted how poetry could provide patients and survivors with the necessary words to express the grief that they were experiencing: "Poems tell stories; poems recount ideas; but poems embody feeling. Because emotion is illogical . . . the poem exists to say the unsayable."[26] Bowman encourages practitioners to use a number of literary resources to provoke feelings or thoughts about one's own story. An example of such a literary device is provided here.

> *Just when you seem to yourself*
> *Nothing but a flimsy web*
> *Of questions, you are given*
> *The question of others to hold*
> *In the emptiness of your hands,*
> *Songbird eggs that can still hatch*
> *If you keep them warm . . .*
> *You are given the questions of others*
> *As if they were answers*
> *To all you ask. Yes, perhaps*
> *This gift is your answer.*[29]

After the patient's death, a host of interventions with family members may be appropriate, including cognitive and action-oriented coping strategies, relaxation training programs, grief counseling, support groups, and therapeutic relationships with bereavement specialists. Keep in mind, however, that although grief and bereavement are difficult transitions, they are a normal part of life, so many family members do fine with minimal assistance. Muller reports that only 30% actually seek counseling following a loss, with 10% requiring further intervention from medical/psychological professionals.[30]

Gray notes that the purpose of group interventions is ". . . to help resolve the conflicts of separation, facilitate the completion of grief tasks, provide a social support system and give permission to mourn."[31] For interventions that focus on the family unit, Kissane and colleagues recommend improving relationships among members and ignoring overall family functioning, both of which are seen as positively impacting psychological outcomes and bereavement experiences.[32] Still, it must be recognized that any therapeutic intervention offered before or following the patient's death may be disrupted by any of the client, situational, and environmental risk factors reported on earlier by Walsh-Burke.[15] In addition, palliative/hospice care workers may be reluctant to intervene, fearing they might uncover larger issues than they are prepared or have the time to address. Despite these obstacles, it is important for us to remember that the time spent listening to and validating the patient's feelings and uniqueness is useful and appreciated by the patient and family.

We must keep in mind, however, that the kind of grief and bereavement work described here cannot occur unless we ". . . keep patients comfortable and alert so that they may participate in activities that are important to them."[5] Even then, grief and bereavement work must build on the interests and concerns of the patient and family members while always keeping in mind their respective capacities and limitations. Doing so, according to control theory, helps maintain a sense of order in life and mitigates psychological distress and depression.[33] Rahman provides an example of this in an article describing how occupational therapy can "empower patients to feel like they still have some sense of control, even in the process of letting go."[34] Within this context, grief and bereavement work is often cyclical, providing support when needed, offering information and encouragement during periods of growth and transcendence. Kissane's work helps us keep in mind throughout all of this that the goal of palliative/hospice care is to aid individuals to live fully while dying by "approaching their fate with courageous awareness and acceptance."[35]

Byock[1] provides us with a some leads on where practitioners might help patients and others to look for new meanings and identities in order to realize this opportunity for closure at the end of life. Remember, however, that this existential search may itself engender distress along the way and give rise to demoralization or psychiatric disorders in some cases when new meanings and identities are not readily forthcoming. Kissane[35] outlines a number of complicating factors that might predispose someone to a crisis here and also provides direction to palliative/hospice care workers on how to manage the patient and family's efforts to respond to a given existential challenge. These challenges are seen as a foundation of the developmental model outlined by Byock[1] and key issues surrounding grief and bereavement work within palliative and hospice care settings.

Future Directions and Conclusions

Historically, palliative and hospice care has largely been based on anecdotal data and reports. Recently, there has been a call for researchers to provide more evidence-based practice to guide the development and refinement of clinical assessment and care within palliative and hospice care.[36, 37, 38, 39] This same research mandate applies to the study of grief and bereavement. The literature search here turned up several studies that investigated grief and bereavement outcomes and related issues including gender differences,[40] length of hospice stay,[41] caregiver concerns,[42] anticipatory grief,[43] and factors associated with bereavement prognosis.[44]

As this evidence-based literature develops, it may be important to keep in mind the purpose and goal of palliative and hospice care intervention with respect to grief and bereavement. Doing so should impact the kinds of outcomes studied. If grief and bereavement are complicated, symptom management may be important to keep the patient and family members functioning. If we believe that the end-of-life represents opportunities for growth and development, then the successful negotiation of this life transition becomes our goal.

References

1. Byock, I. "The Nature of Suffering and the Nature of Opportunity at the End of Life." *Clinics in Geriatric Medicine*, 12(2):237–252, 1996.
2. Byock, I. "Conceptual Models and the Outcomes of Caring." *Journal of Pain and Symptom Management*, 17(2):83–92, 1999.
3. Silverman, P. R. "Living with Grief, Rebuilding a World." *Innovations in End-of-Life Care*, 3(3):www.edc.org/lastacts, 2001.
4. Erikson, E. *Identity and the Life Cycle.* New York: W. W. Norton & Co., 1994.
5. Lev, E. L., and McCorkle, R. "Loss, Grief, and Bereavement in Family Members of Cancer Patients." *Seminars in Oncology Nursing*, 14(2):145–151, 1998.
6. Parkes, C. M. *Bereavement: Studies of Grief in Adult Life.* New York: International Universities Press, 1972.
7. Parkes, C. M. "Bereavement." *British Journal of Psychiatry*, 146:11–17, 1985.
8. Whitney, P. J. "Role of Hospice in Alzheimer's Care." *Provider*, 25(9):87, 89–91, 1999.
9. Maher, L. A. "Dignified Departures." *Contemporary Longterm Care*, 23(12):24–29, 2000.
10. Kavanaugh, K. M. "Illinois Nursing Homes Develop Successful Programs to Promote Comfort During End-of-Life Care." *Balance*, 5(1):19–21, 2001.
11. Read, S. "The Palliative Care Needs of People with Learning Disabilities." *British Journal of Community Nursing*, 3(7):356–361, 1998.

12. Ambalu, S. "Communication." In J. O'Hara, A. Sperlinger, eds. *Adults with Learning Disabilities: A Practical Approach for Health Professionals*. Chichester, United Kingdom: John Wiley & Sons, 1997.
13. Holmes, S. "The Challenge of Providing Nutritional Support to the Dying." *International Journal of Palliative Nursing*, 4(1):26–31, 1998.
14. Hooks, J., and Daly, B. J. "Hastening Death." *American Journal of Nursing*, 100(5):56–63, 2000.
15. Walsh-Burke, K. "Matching Bereavement Services to Level of Need." *The Hospice Journal*, 15(1):77–86, 2000.
16. Barbato, M., Blunden, C., Reid, K., Irwin, H., and Rodriguez, P. "Parapsychological Phenomena Near the Time of Death." *Journal of Palliative Care*, 15(2):30–37, 1999.
17. Datson, S. L., and Marwit, S. J. "Personality Constructs and Perceived Presence of Deceased Loved Ones." *Death Studies*, 21:131–146, 1997.
18. Lobchuk, M. M., Stymeist, D. "Symptoms as Meaningful 'Family Culture' Symbols in Palliative Care." *Journal of Palliative Care*, 15(4):24–31, 1999.
19. Nardi, D. A., Ornelas, F., Wright, M., and Chrispell, R. "Clergy and Social Workers' Attitudes Towards Death and Palliative Care in an Acute Care Setting." *International Journal of Palliative Nursing*, 7(1):30–36, 2001.
20. Hockley, J. "Psychosocial Aspects in Palliative Care." *Acta Oncologica*, 39(8): 905–910, 2000.
21. McGrath, P., Yates, P., Clinton, M., and Hart, G. "'What Should I Say?': Qualitative Findings on Dilemmas in Palliative Care Nursing." *The Hospice Journal*, 14(2):17–33, 1999.
22. Legrand, M., and Gomas, J. "Being Present at the Last Moments of Life." *European Journal of Palliative Care*, 5(6):191–194, 1998.
23. Kavanaugh, K. M. "Meeting the Psychosocial Needs of Terminally Ill Patients." *Balance*, 2(6):7–9, 1998.
24. Parkes, C. M. "Coping with Loss: Consequences and Implications for Care." *International Journal of Palliative Nursing*, 5(5):250–254, 1999.
25. McCorkle, R., Robinson, L., Nuamah, I., Lev, E., Benoliel, J. "The Effects of Home Nursing Care for Patients during Terminal Illness on the Bereaved's Psychological Distress." *Nursing Research*, 47:2–10, 1997.
26. Bowman, T. "Literary Resources for Bereavement." *The Hospice Journal*, 14(1):39–54, 1999.
27. Fairchild, R. W. *Finding Hope Again: A Pastor's Guide to Counseling Depressed Persons*. San Francisco: Harper Row, 1980.
28. Moraes, P. "Empathy Creativity and the Arts in Palliative Care." *European Journal of Palliative Care*, 6(3):99–102, 1999.
29. Levertov, D. "A Gift." In *Sands of the Well*, New York: New Directions Books, 1996.
30. Muller, M. "The Role of Bereavement Counselling in Hospice Work." *European Journal of Palliative Care*, 7(1):29–32, 2000.
31. Gray, S. W., Zide, M. R., and Wilker, H. "Using the Solution Focused Brief Therapy Model with Bereavement Groups in Rural Communities: Resiliency at Its Best." *The Hospice Journal*, 15(3):13–30, 2000.
32. Kissane, D. W., Bloch, S., MeKenzie, M., McDowal, A. C., and Nitzan, R. "Family Grief Therapy: A Preliminary Account of a New Model to Promote Healthy Family Functioning During Palliative Care and Bereavement." *Psycho-Oncology*, 7:14–25, 1998.

33. Redding, S. "Control Theory in Dying: What Do We Know?" *American Journal of Hospice & Palliative Care*, 17(3):204–208, 2000.
34. Rahman, H. "Journey of Providing Care in Hospice: Perspectives of Occupational Therapists." *Qualitative Health Research*, 10(6):806–818, 2000.
35. Kissane, D. W. "Psychospiritual and Existential Distress." *Australian Family Physician*, 29(11):1022–1025, 2000.
36. Mak, J. M. H., and Clinton, M. "Promoting a Good Death: An Agenda for Outcomes Research—A Review of the Literature." *Nursing Ethics*, 6(2):97–106, 1999.
37. Field, M. J., and Cassel, C. K. (eds). "Approaching Death: Improving Care at the End of Life." Washington D.C.: Committee on Care at the End of Life: Institute of Medicine, National Academy Press, 1997.
38. Byock, I. "Completing the Continuum of Cancer Care: Integrating Life-Prolongation and Palliation." *CA: A Cancer Journal for Clinicians*, 50(2):123–132, 2000.
39. Wilkes, L. "Palliative Care Nursing Research Trends from 1987–1996." *International Journal of Palliative Nursing*, 4(3):128–134, 1998.
40. Quigley, D. G., and Schatz, M. "Men and Woman and Their Responses in Spousal Bereavement." *The Hospice Journal*, 14(2):65–78, 1999.
41. Gilbar, O. "Length of Cancer Patients' Stay at a Hospice: Does it Affect Psychological Adjustment to the Loss of the Spouse?" *Journal of Palliative Care*, 14(4):16–20, 1998.
42. Stajduhar, K. I., and Davies, B. "Palliative Care at Home: Reflections on HIV/AIDS Family Caregiving Experiences." *Journal of Palliative Care*, 14(2):14–22, 1998.
43. Chapman, K. J., and Pepler, C. "Coping, Hope, and Anticipatory Grief in Family Members in Palliative Home Care." *Cancer Nursing*, 21(4): 226–234, 1998.
44. Kelly, B., Edwards, P., Synott, R., Neil, C., Baillie, R., and Battistutta, D. "Predictors of Bereavement Outcome for Family Carers of Cancer Patients." *Psycho-Oncology*, 8:237–249, 1999.

Care of the Patient as Death Approaches in the Hospice/Palliative Care Setting

16

Walter B. Forman, MD, FACP, CMD
Denice Kopchak Sheehan, MSN, RN

As death approaches for the patient and their family, the health care professional is often asked about changes that can occur as the person's illness progresses to the final stage. Unfortunately, very few health care workers in this era have actually been taught about dealing with this time in a person's life cycle. In this chapter we will outline what is known about this period, some of the major signs and symptoms, and the management of these symptoms. There are several good articles on the subject.[1, 2, 3] In addition, Chapter 20 contains an excellent listing of web site resources that address issues confronted by the health care provider, the patient, and the patient's family.

General Issues

The National Hospice and Palliative Care Organization has compiled the following statistics.[4] In the year 2000, 2,400,000 individuals died in the United States from a variety of causes, including accidents, homicides, and other unnatural causes. Furthermore, 600,000 (or 40%) were active in a hospice program. Note that this 40% represents all persons that die in the United States, regardless of age group or cause of death. However, over 82% of hospice care is delivered to people over 65 years old who are enrolled in Medicare. Thus, the majority of hospice care is delivered in what would be considered the older age group. These people have their own unique medical needs and the hospice professional should be very familiar with them, as addressed in other areas of this book.

In examining the Medicare hospice data, 55% of care recipients were women and 45% were men. Eighty-two percent of hospice patients were Caucasian, 8% African American, and 2% Hispanic. It is of some concern that the greatest percentage of recipients were Caucasian, whereas only a handful at best were Native Americans. Why this imbalance exists is unclear. However, access to hospice care is a prominent feature. The place of death greatly influences the quality and quantity of care. As opposed to earlier data, which indicated that over 75% of people died in a hospital, in the year 2000 the number of people dying in hospitals has decreased to approximately 50%. The remainder of individuals died at home (25%) or in a long-term care facility (25%). In regards to deaths that occurred in the hospice setting, 56% died at home, 19% in a long-term care facility, 12% in an inpatient hospice, and only 7% in a hospital.

For those of us working in a hospice setting these data are both encouraging and daunting. They are encouraging because death in the hospital is becoming less frequent, which allows the dying person to be near their families and in familiar surroundings. They are daunting because treatment of the dying person is now becoming the responsibility of the hospice professional.

When a patient enters the stage called dying the hospice professional must address a series of clinical signs and symptoms that need to be treated with both "medical" and "nonmedical" or nontraditional therapies. Of great importance to the interdisciplinary hospice/palliative care team is the opportunity to continue their involvement as the person and their family reach this stage. The introduction of an unfamiliar institution at this time can be very difficult, causing discontinuity of care with new health care professionals and confusion when the surroundings have not been part of the dying persons experience.

Symptoms at the End of Life

Most of the symptoms that the patient will have are related to the underlying illness that brought them to the hospice program. Examples might include the lack of pain in a person with obstructive pulmonary disease as opposed to severe dyspnea, which will need hospice attention. Debilitating pain related to bony metastasis will trouble people with metastatic bone involvement from carcinoma of the breast or prostate.

Much of the data related to symptoms at the end of life have been collected from people dying of cancer. Although this information will be reviewed as a major issue in this chapter, the reader should be aware that there is a plethora of new information about symptoms in noncancer terminal illnesses.[5, 6]

Tools to Evaluate Symptoms at the End of Life

The reader will find many tools designed to evaluate symptoms during this stage in a person's life. However, many of these tools evaluate quality of care and/or the quality of life, as opposed to determining what physical or mental symptoms are interfering with living at the end of life. For example, in an excellent review, Volcier and colleagues demonstrated that three tools they developed could be used for "investigating the effectiveness of interventions at the end of life"[7] and could improve quality of care during this time period.

A different approach to this problem has been carried out by Emanuel and colleagues.[8] They have proposed a new tool that evaluates four dimensions of end-of-life care. This tool both addresses the issues of the person who is dying and that person's family. This tool, known as the "Needs Near the End of Life Care Screening Tool," seems to overcome many of the limitations of earlier instruments by addressing symptoms, as well as other parameters. A mnemonic (*NEST: N*—social needs; *E*—existential; *S*—symptoms; and *T*—therapeutic) has been developed to make the instrument more user friendly. Future work will determine its usefulness. For now, we can say that a great deal of work is needed in the area of symptom assessment at the end of life.

Symptoms

Others in this book have addressed symptoms that occur in people who have advanced illness. In this chapter we will address only those symptoms that are a problem in the last week of life, and in particular the last 48 hours.

The SUPPORT study, which was conducted in the intensive care units of several teaching hospitals, demonstrated that during the last three days of life pain was the major symptom in 50% of 1400 patients.[9] However, other studies have shown that fatigue, not pain, is the major complaint of individuals at the end of life.[10] Other problems faced by patients during the last week of life include sleepiness (57%) and generalized weakness (44%). Pain is reported to be a major symptom in only about one third of patients.

Another symptom that becomes more apparent at this time of life is shortness of breath (dyspnea). Dyspnea, or the sensation of inability to "catch one's breath," increases as death approaches and is a complaint of 20–78% of people.[11] This symptom is most prominent in people with cancer of the lung and nonmalignant pulmonary disease. In a study by Coyle, 44 different symptoms were noted in the last 4 weeks of life. Individuals had from one to nine of these symptoms.[12] In Lichter's study of 200 terminally ill people, noisy respirations were the most common symptom (56%), with urinary dysfunction (53%), pain (51%), and agitation (42%) the next most common.[13] Fentafridda et al. noted the most common symptoms to be dyspnea (52%) and pain (49%).[14] Delirium, which was also a problem, occurred in 17% of patients. Another factor that interfered with a peaceful death was restlessness or terminal angst.

Respiratory Problems

Of the respiratory problems that occur at this time the most difficult for the patient and family are dyspnea and the "death rattle."

Dyspnea

Although we think of oxygen for the treatment of dyspnea, at the end of life oxygen alone might be insufficient to relieve this symptom. For many people the use of a fan that is placed in front of an open window and directed at the person might be sufficient and could prevent the use of tubes and such that accompany the use of oxygen.

Two classes of agents also may be useful. For those patients who are suffering from anxiety as a cause of their dyspnea, an antianxiety medication might be needed. The medication that has been found to be most useful is a short-acting benzodiazepine. Lorazepam, which does not need to undergo hepatic metabolism, can be used sublingually at 0.5 to 1.0 mg/4 hours. A subcutaneous infusion of midazolam can be employed at the rate of 10 to 50 mg/24 hours. Morphine remains a useful agent in this situation. It can be prescribed in its short-acting formulation beginning with a rate of 5 mg/4 hours either PO, SL, or by rectal suppository.

Death Rattle

The death rattle usually occurs during the last 12 hours of life. It is very disconcerting to the family, although the patient is usually unaware of this symptom. Thus, this is a symptom that must be controlled so that the family will not be upset that their loved one is "drowning." Because this illness is related to pooling of secretions in the pharynx, positioning of the head can be very useful. The person's head can be elevated by the use of pillows, or if the person is in a mechanical bed the head can be elevated to 45 degrees. If this does not bring immediate relief, the use of medication is indicated.

Anticholinergics are the mainstay of therapy. Scopolamine can be applied as a postauricular patch (1.5 mg/patch) that can be changed every two to three days.[15] However, this therapy is slow in onset. A more rapid agent, glycopyrollate, is an excellent medication for this situation. It can be given as an oral (sublingual) medication 0.1 mg/6 hours or subcutaneously at a dose of 1 to 2 mg/24 hours.

Pain

This symptom should be controlled with little difficulty by the hospice professional. A variety of routes are available. The most commonly used route is sublingual, for example, a morphine IR solution of 20 mg/ml given at appropriate intervals. The dose is based on whether the person is receiving opioids. The dosing is calculated from the formula for "rescue dosing." Calculate 25–50% of the total daily dose of the opioid and give that dosage every four hours depending on the pain status of the person.

The subcutaneous route can be very useful in relieving pain. Here, knowledge of the various potencies of the opioid agonists is important. Hydromorphone is approximately seven times more potent than oxycodone or morphine. Thus, in choosing an opioid, hydromorphone might be of benefit because it mitigates volume concerns.

Delirium

Loss of the ability to communicate in an understandable manner can be of concern for both the person and his or her family. Delirium is characterized by confusion and disorientation in regards to time, place, or person that can wax and wane over hours or days. For a more complete definition and discussion, see the article by Stoutz.[16] Delirium has been reported to occur in 70 to 90% of patients near death.[17]

Treatment varies depending on the etiology of the delirium. In patients who are in the terminal part of their lives, the process of diagnosis and specific treatment might be too strenuous or intrusive. Thus, we will only outline general treatment regimens.

In some situations the delirium is easily controlled by providing light or music in the room, or by having the family present.[18] If the situation is associated with agitation, then medications might be indicated. The medication of choice is the "gold standard" is butyrophenone (haloperidol). This drug can be given orally (1–5 mg/8 hours) or as a subcutaneous infusion (5–10 mg/24 hours). If this medication is counterindicated, the use of midazolam, as a bolus injection of 10–20 mg intravenously over 15–20 minutes with a continuous subcutaneous infusion of 25–50 mg/24 hours, is also an effective regimen in this clinical situation.

Terminal Angst

This symptom of thrashing, restlessness, crying out, and general unrest is another syndrome that produces distress in the person and his or her family. If the person is able to communicate, which is often not possible, the social worker or spiritual counselor can attempt to ascertain the cause of the angst. Angst in this setting is usually caused by the person's unresolved personal business. Unfortunately, when this syndrome is encountered the person often is no longer able to participate in life review. Thus, continuous sedation might be the only therapy that can be employed. Choices of medications include phenobarbital, lorazepam, or midazolam. The hospice professional should become comfortable in the use of this therapy, if it needs to be utilized. And of course, the introduction of this therapy should be discussed with the family as well as the interdisciplinary hospice team.

Miscellaneous Symptoms

Other acute emergencies at the end of life include hemorrhage from gastrointestinal sources or from eroding malignancies such as head and neck carcinomas; urinary retention from drugs or obstructive malignancies; and seizure disorders. Please refer to the work of Dickerson and Wrede-Seaman for detailed discussions of these disorders.[19, 20]

General Treatment Planning

The interaction among the hospice/palliative care interdisciplinary team, the patient, and the patient's family requires planning in order to bring closure with a minimum of psychological trauma to all involved. Twycross and Lichter provide a review of this work in the *Oxford Textbook of Palliative Medicine*.[21] Here we will highlight several management issues from the point of view of the hospice/palliative care team.

Of major concern to all is the question "Is the end near?" The interdisciplinary team should be prepared to deal with this situation. The team member who has been most involved with the family should act as the discussion leader. It is of major concern that the family receives only one message. The remainder of the team then can be supportive to the family, as well as to the spokesperson. The spiritual counselor may play an important role in these discussions. Hopefully, much of the care at this time in the patient's life will occur at home. The team needs to make certain not only that psychological issues are addressed but also that preparations are in place if emergency pharmacological therapy is required. An "emergency kit," as outlined by LeGrand et al., is the most satisfactory solution.[22] Durable medical equipment, such as oxygen and towels, also should be easily available in order to respond to an emergency.

Summary

The hospice/palliative care team has an important role in end-of-life care. This chapter outlines the role they can play and offers some suggestions as to the needs of the family and the patient. Each of the members has an important task in providing for a peaceful death. This can be done in a very professional manner. When it is accomplished, the dignity of the person can be maintained without an added burden to their loved ones.

References

1. Maher, E. J. "How long have I got doctor?" *Eur J Cancer* 3:283–284, 1994.
2. Maltoni-Pirovano, M., Nanni, O. et al. Prognostic factors in terminal cancer patients. *Eur J Palliat Care* 1:122–125, 1994.
3. Chang, V. T. Thaler, H. T., Polyak, T. A. et al. Quality of life and survival. The role of multidimensional symptom assessment. *Cancer* 83:173–179, 1998.
4. NHPCO Facts and Figures. Update December 10, 2001. Alexandria, Va.: The National Hospice and Palliative Care Organization.
5. Iwashyna, T. J., and Christakis, N. A. Signs of death. *J Pall Care* 4:451–452, 2002.
6. Abrahams, J. L., and Hansen-Flaschen, J. Hospice care for patients with advanced lung disease. *Chest* 121:220–229, 2002.
7. Volicer, L., Hurley, A. C., and Blasi, Z. V. Scales for evaluation of end of life care in dementia. *Alz Dis Assoc Disord* 15:194–200, 2001.
8. Emanuel, L. L., Alpert, H. R., and Emanuel, E. E. Concise screening questions for clinical assessments of terminal care: The needs for the end-of-life care-screening tool. *J Pall Med* 4:465–474, 2002.
9. The SUPPORT study investigators: A controlled trial to improve care for seriously ill hospitalized patients. *JAMA* 274:1591–1598, 1995.
10. Ward, A. W. M. Terminal care in malignant disease. *Soc Sci Med* 8:413–420, 1974.
11. Heyse-Moore, L. H. How much of a problem is dyspnea in advanced cancer? *Pall Med* 5:20–26, 1991.
12. Coyle, N., Adelhardt, J., Foley, K. M., and Portenoy, R. K. Charter of terminal illness in the advanced cancer patient: Pain and other symptoms during the last four weeks of life. *J Pain Sympt Manage* 5:83–93, 1990.
13. Litcher, L., and Hunt, E. The last 48 hours of life. *J Palliative Care* 6:7–15, 1990.
14. Fentafridda, V., Ripamomonti, C., de Conno, F., et al. Symptom prevalence and control during cancer patients' last days of life. *J Pall Care* 6:7–11, 1990.
15. Dawson, H. R. The use of transdermal scopolamine in the control of the death rattle. *J Pall Care* 5:31–33, 1989.
16. DE Stoutz, N. D., and Stiefel, F., Poutenoy, R. K., and Bruera, E., eds. Assessment and management of reversible delirium. In *Topics in Palliative Care*. Volume 1. p. 21–43. Oxford University Press, 1997.
17. Lipowski, Z. L. *Delirium: Acute Confusional States.* New York: Oxford University Press, 1990.
18. Moments Musicaux: Music Therapy. A thematic issue and companion CD-ROM. *J Palliative Care* 17:135–188, 2000.
19. Dickerson, E. D., Benedetti, C., Davis, M. P. et al. in *Palliative Care Pocket Consultant.* Upper Arlington, Oh.: Ohio Hospice Organization 43:221, 2001.
20. Wrede-Seaman, L. in *Symptom Management Algorithms: A Handbook for Palliative Care.* Yakima, WA.: Intellicard, 2000.
21. Twycross, R. G., and Lichter, I. The terminal phase. In Doyle, D., Hanks, G., and Macdonald, N. eds. *Oxford Textbook of Palliative Medicine.* Oxford: Oxford University Press, 1993.
22. LeGrand, S. B., Tropiano, P., Marx, J. D., et al. Dying at home: Emergency medications for terminal symptoms. *Am J Hosp Palliat Care* 18:421–423, 2001.

Death Education and Family Support 17

Diana Longaway

End-of-life care, hospice care, is a celebration of life. Every individual is treated with respect and dignity, with special attention given to pain control and other comfort-giving measures. The amount of ongoing support that can be provided to the patient and other family members months before a patient dies is enormous. In spite of this fact, many referrals continue to be made in the final weeks, days, and hours of life, when family systems are already stressed and fractured from worry and fatigue.

Definition of Terms

In order to accomplish the goals of this chapter it is appropriate to review key terms:

- *Death* as defined by the *Psychiatric Dictionary* is:

  Cessation of life, physical and mental; total and permanent cessation of the functions or vital actions of an organism.[1]

- *Education* is defined by *The Living Webster Encyclopedic Dictionary of the English Language* as:

  The process of educating, teaching or training; a part of or a stage in this training; the learning or development which results from this process of teaching or training.[2]

- The final term in this chapter is *family*, which possesses a complex dynamic different from the traditional connotation of the term. As defined by *A Dictionary of the Social Sciences*, a family can be any of the following:

  Biological family made up of a man, a woman, and children.

- *Nuclear family* would echo the previous description, but would allow for the adoption of children as well.
- *Extended family* encompasses other individuals added through marriage and incorporating the families of the newly acquired family member.[3]

In addition, society today also is composed of single parents who were never married, whose spouse died, or who are divorced. There are also other family situations to consider such as same sex marriages; significant other relationships, where partners are not legally married; and communal living systems.[4]

With such a wide variety of family systems, it is incumbent upon those in the position of professional service, especially in the discussion of terminal illness, to be informed and sensitive to this diversity. Every person is uniquely important. Their feelings, needs, and belief systems should be treated with understanding and respect. Accurate management of medical systems is required by the Joint Commission on Accreditation of Healthcare Organizations (JCAHO), so organizations must employ or have available trained translators to assist with patient communication, and must also develop effective ethnically sensitive in-service education. Staff members will benefit by providing appropriate care for minority patients whose needs are often complex.[5]

Hospice Interdisciplinary Team

Hospice interdisciplinary teams are made up of a group of professionals and volunteers, including:

•Doctors	•Social Workers	•Physical Therapists
•Nurses	•Chaplains	•Occupational Therapists
•Home Health Aides	•Counselors	•Dieticians
•Art Therapists	•Volunteers	•Music Thanatologists

These individuals are trained to work gently and effectively with patients and their families, no matter where they are in their process of acceptance, rejection, or denial of the terminal diagnosis. Hospice team members work together to support the patient and family on physical, emotional, social, and spiritual levels. The team seeks to control pain, problem solve, and model appropriate behaviors to empower the patients and their support system to act for themselves whenever possible. It is important that in many situations the family and patient be made aware that they have choices and can select a course of action best suited to themselves. Ongoing education of the patient and family becomes an important function of the team. A team goal of great importance is to develop good coping skills among family members whenever possible so that they will be as ready as possible to meet the forthcoming challenges of declining health matters as they occur.[6]

Breaking Bad News

When a life-threatening condition needs to be disclosed to an individual and family, great care and empathy must be employed by health care professionals. Preparation for presenting news of a terminal diagnosis has, traditionally, not been stressed within the programs of most medical or nursing schools. Little attention is focused on the personal feelings, past history, and needs of the health care provider as an individual. Many people have experienced trauma around issues of illness, grief, and loss in their personal lives that has never been addressed or expressed. It would be much more humane to provide physicians and nurses with an emotional support system or outside requirement that would compel them to acquire assistance in working through their own problems around these highly charged issues. In this way, they can better care for themselves before they complete training and come face to face with suffering individuals who deserve the highest and best efforts that they have to offer.

Without this training, it is not surprising that many physicians feel uncomfortable acquainting their patients and their families with devastating news that will change their lives. Although it seems clear that more attention needs to be paid to this part of medical education, it is possible for these physicians to be supported by interdisciplinary team members. When support is present for both the family and the physician, difficult news can be handled more comfortably and effectively for all concerned.[7]

The following is a creative reenactment of such an encounter.

What the physician says:

> Your test results were not encouraging. (Pause) Unfortunately, your condition is terminal. (Pause) Hospice care could be helpful to you and your family in the weeks and months ahead, and I recommend it. With your approval, I will make a referral to hospice today. They will call you to arrange a time to come out and explain in detail the services that they can provide. (Pause) I will be happy to answer any questions that you may have.

The person receiving this news has just been told something that is unacceptable and unthinkable. The doctor says that I am going to die! It is normal that somewhere inside, the patient is replaying what he or she has just been told, often with distortion, anger, and disbelief. Frequently, a silent internal dialogue is raging within the patient, which might resemble the following:

> Can it really be true? Is the doctor saying that I can't be cured?
>
> I am going to die? It must be a mistake!
>
> Why me? What will happen to my family?
>
> I don't smoke, drink, or take drugs. How could this happen?
>
> This cannot be happening.
>
> This is a terrible dream and I must wake up. We have two children to raise.
>
> What will happen to our home?

It is not until this moment that many people begin to give serious thought to their own mortality. Usually, they are in no way prepared financially, emotionally, or spiritually for such news. Life as they and their family have known it will never be the same again. Most often the family is experiencing the same emotions and is overwhelmed by this information.

In most cases, the individuals must be made aware of the medical findings and the physician has the responsibility of making recommendations and keeping the flame of hope alive.[7] In some cultures the person with the terminal diagnosis is not to be told. The family acts in the best interests of the individual.[8]

When Do We Begin to Die?

R. A. Kalish addressed this question in *Death, Grief and Caring Relationships* as follows: ". . . subjectively . . . my dying begins when I learn that I have a condition that will eventually cause my death."[9]

When discussing the reaction of family and friends to the news of a terminal diagnosis, Kalish goes on to say that, ". . . my dying begins when you learn that I have this condition."[9]

It is at this point, when the worst news possible is being struggled with by the patient and everyone in the family unit, that the hospice team is introduced and charged with providing palliative care. In spite of the fact that hospice has been a recognized and funded provider of health care in the United States since the mid-1980s, many people are not aware of the program and its multiple benefits.

Window of Time

When meeting a family who is trying to understand and come to terms with a terminal diagnosis for one of its members, it is useful to help them see that for some reason they have been given a window of time to do many of the things that need doing. Knowing that someone has time left to live is very different than suddenly being informed that someone in your family has been killed in an accident. Although having a window of time is not easy, it at least allows the patient, the family, and friends to have an opportunity to prepare themselves for the changes to come. The terminal individual has a chance to experience where he or she has been and to ponder what is to come. During this window of time the family unit is provided a chance to reflect upon the past and begin to lay plans for the future.

Advance Directives

One of the first tasks faced by members of the hospice team is addressing the need for the patient and family to decide on the right actions for the patient should he or she become unable to indicate his or her wishes on health care matters. Advance directives and the Do Not Resuscitate/Do Not Intubate (DNR/DNI) forms act to protect the patient, because they can dictate what they want or do not want to happen should they be unable to act for themselves. Selecting an individual who has the trust of the patient to be listed as having the durable power of attorney (DPA) centers control of future actions in the hands of the patient and the DPA. By attending to these matters in the beginning, the hospice team can work to educate the family and avoid much confusion in times of later crisis. Note that in some Native American cultures the concept of advance directives is not appropriate; other solutions are being developed.

Types of Support

Nursing Support

The hospice nurse is a highly trained, experienced professional who possesses superior knowledge of pain medications and their side effects. Individuals who enter hospice nursing are comfortable offering end-of-life care and are sensitive to the needs of the families as well as to the needs of their patients. The nurse is often the case manager in charge of a particular group of patients. The role of the nurse is to work closely with the referring hospice agency and physicians and the interdisciplinary team on patient-related matters.

In many places hospice nurses are trained by the Office of the Medical Examiner to pronounce the time of death, thus circumventing the need for the police or any other authority to be called. The nurse often is the person who places the call to the mortuary chosen by the family. He or she will prepare the body for viewing while still in the home or facility, if appropriate to family traditions. In many circumstances, the nurse will also disconnect the medical equipment and call for it to be removed as soon as possible. After the patient dies, the nurse is legally responsible for the disposal of unused medicines. This is done with a witness present who is asked to sign a statement reporting that he or she can attest that all narcotic medications were counted, recorded, and destroyed.

Emotional Support

It is important for the family to continue to function as they normally would. Although everyone on the hospice team is a good listener, the social worker and chaplain in particular are available to counsel and encourage the family unit to function as normally as possible: visit, cry, tell stories, watch movies, listen to music, and maximize the everyday events that now take on greater importance due to the limit on time set by the terminal diagnosis. Each hospice team member has a role to provide in giving emotional support for the patient and the family.

Both patients and caregivers have need of support from the hospice team members. Being a caregiver is one of the most demanding tasks that anyone can undertake. The responsibilities are constant—twenty-four hours a day, seven days a week—with the hospice nurses always available to help. Keeping the caregiver safe and healthy becomes a major concern of the hospice team.[10]

Support of the Children

It is absolutely necessary to be honest with children about illness and death. The information provided should reflect the child's developmental level. Children are very smart and have a tendency to absorb bits of information from conversations they overhear adults having and often put the pieces together in such a manner that they create a monster of giant proportions that the parents have no knowledge of.[11] Different age groups in childhood have tendencies to blame themselves for imagined wrongs that they have done that resulted in sickness or death of another family member. If a sibling is the hospice patient, the parents would be wise to consult with the social worker about obtaining outside counseling for their other children.[12] Some school systems are very involved and can supply counselors to assist students who are undergoing heavy stress caused by illness, issues of grief, loss, and death at home.

Spiritual Support

In hospice and palliative care, not only physical pain is addressed, but attention must also be focused on spiritual and emotional pain. There is a difference between organized religion and spiritual belief, even though organized religion can have great spirituality. Frequently, individuals pull away from the religious traditions of their childhood and either stop going to services, try other belief systems, or just stop dealing with the subject of religion in general.

Many individuals, who proclaim they are atheists or agnostics when they are first being served by the hospice team, during the course of their involvement with the hospice team decide to speak with a chaplain. Hospice chaplaincy is gentle, loving, forgiving, and non-denominational.[13] Many times the chaplain will become a regular visitor; often the request is made to reconnect the patient with clergy of a belief system that has not been thought about in years. Sometimes when a special connection is made between the chaplain and the family, he or she is asked to perform the memorial ceremony when the patient dies. It is necessary for the team members to be aware of changing spiritual needs, with appropriate referrals being made.

Social Work Support

The social worker plays an important role by providing referrals, resources, insurance assistance, and assistance with financial affairs. Applications for financial assistance can be completed and turned in for processing. Assistance and direction can be given so that wills can be written, property sold or deeded, and titles on vehicles transferred. Outside legal assistance can be suggested wherever appropriate along with resources for home repairs, both of which can often be supplied for little money if the need is great. Grief and loss counseling of patient and family also is often provided by the social worker.[8]

Bereavement Support

It is important to be of aware of and have training in dealing with issues surrounding death because women and men in diverse cultures have very different grieving patterns. For example, in the Anglo world women are free to express their emotions and gain sympathy and support. Men have been trained from birth to submerge their true feelings so as to appear manly. Children and teenagers also require special training when illness, grief, loss, and death become part of the fabric of their lives. They all may be experiencing some of the five phases of dying made famous by Elisabeth Kübler-Ross in her 1969 book, *On Death and Dying*.[14] How and if these phases emerge will be very different for each individual; however, they can serve the clinician well as a general template for assessing where an individual is in the emotional process. Depression often goes untreated by the physician in a patient with a terminal diagnosis. The following guide will have a variety of applications, depending upon various age groups:

- *Denial* can be especially strong in a younger person who feels cheated and outraged by being denied many more years of life. An older person may be tired of being sick and more accepting of a terminal diagnosis, but not always.

- *Anger* often accompanies an inner dialogue that revolves around thoughts of the diagnosis being unfair. Not me, not now, not ready are commonly expressed themes.

- *Bargaining* often involves speaking with God and trying to make a deal, such as becoming an organ donor or leaving one's body to science. Family-related events also come into play here—graduations, marriages, and new births are all reasons for the necessity of prolonged life.

- *Depression* reflects much inner processing and when extreme can be helped with medications. It is important to provide support, as appropriate, to the depressed individual, whether it be the patient, spouse, or other family member.

- Acceptance can sometimes be noted when a quiet peace develops within and around the patient. Some people have a special lightness and calm when they have worked through their issues and attained the level of acceptance.

It should be noted that patients and their families can vary greatly in their feelings and acceptance of death. Often those left as survivors have great difficulty accepting the changes forced on them by the death of the patient. Hospice bereavement services are designed to remain in touch with surviving family members and supply needed individual counseling, group therapy, and outside referrals as appropriate.

Every hospice is charged by the federal government to provide a bereavement group that is available for at least one year to members of deceased patients' families. Many hospice bereavement groups are open to the general public at no charge. Hospice bereavement departments keep in touch by phone and through the mail with the family member for at least one year. Memorial services are held once or twice each year, and all bereaved family members are invited. It is not uncommon for individuals to come for bereavement support thinking they need assistance because of a recent loss, when in reality they are suffering from cumulative grief from multiple deaths. The current loss may necessitate that time at long last be taken to address the significant losses of the past. Others, who had long periods of time to prepare for the death of someone special, may experience a shorter period of mourning after the death because of their prolonged period of anticipatory grief. Individual counseling is available with referrals to other therapists being made when grief is noted to be destructive or in any way abnormal.[15]

Travel and Quality of Life

Travel can increase the quality of life and is possible for hospice patients when they have the approval and support of their physician. Relatives can come to visit, and whenever possible, hospice patients are encouraged to travel wherever they would like to go. The hospice team can assist patients with preparation for local camping trips, outings, and trips to malls and museums within several hours drive of home. Hospice teams thrive on assisting patients in accomplishing their goals. This is possible because of a network of over 3200 hospices across the country, which can be called on to be available to traveling patients in their areas. Pertinent information is faxed to them along with the name of the family and the address and phone number of where the individual will be staying while in the area. The traveling hospice individual is given the name and phone number of the hospice to call while he or she is away from home. In some cases, it is necessary to have medical equipment (i.e., oxygen or a wheelchair) set up and waiting before the individual arrives.

Funeral/Memorial Planning

This is an area that has changed greatly in the past century. The importance of ritual declined as the pomp and expense of funerals increased. The Victorian concept of ritual was alive and well in America at the dawn of the 20th century. Obituary sections of the newspaper were banded in black, as was personal stationery sent out by bereaved family members. Men often wore black armbands, and women family members wore dark attire for a prescribed period of time. A black wreath was placed on the front door of the family home to announce to one and all that those inside were experiencing a state of mourning. Considerations and respect were extended by society at large to those who had suffered a loss. In some areas funeral directors would come to help out with arrangements in the home.[16]

Until the middle of the 20th century, whole families lived together or near to one another. The young were aware of and present every day with their elder family members. When illness required that the family provide care for the individual, it was done as a matter of course, with the children often being of assistance in small ways to the ailing family member.

When death occurred, it was no surprise and the body was washed and laid out at home for viewing prior to burial. Some belief systems furnished additional people to assist with preparations of the body before burial, with attention paid to ceremony and custom. Family planning and attention were part of every action pertaining to the care of and burial of the expired family member. Illness and death were viewed as normal parts of life. Funeral services were usually solemn. However, they were sometimes followed by a gathering of family and friends that could, in some traditions, become boisterous and rowdy. Spiritual beliefs influenced the actions of the family and friends. The departed individual was often thought to be in a much more agreeable and idyllic place. Other belief systems were more somber in nature and threatened punishment and damnation.

In contrast, present generations of Americans are generally in denial of death and loss, and place a great emphasis on youth, material success, sex, and accomplishment. The subjects of old age, illness, and death are shut away in the hidden corners of the mind because they are considered morbid. Older family members are often viewed as an inconvenience, so placing them in nursing facilities has become an acceptable action, particularly as more and more women have had to leave their homes in order to assist in supporting their families.[17]

Individuals who are able to provide time to become caregivers for ailing relatives and friends often find this period of caring difficult but rewarding. The built-in demands, fatigue, and bittersweet reality can serve to become a time of personal growth. Individuals are honored and proud to be of service to someone they love. It allows for testing of the self, reviewing of priorities, provides time to value life more fully, and gives meaning to being alive.[18]

Today it is often helpful for the hospice social worker and/or chaplain to assist with the planning of the funeral/memorial ceremony. Ritual is important for those who are alive. The countless funerals in New York City following the World Trade Center attack for the firefighters and police had a solemn ritualistic importance that was moving and meaningful for all concerned. First-hand knowledge of the individual was not necessary in order to be deeply touched by the honor, ceremony, and respect that was accorded to their passing.

Families can benefit from the experience of hospice team members in the case of military burial. Papers such as those issued for an honorable discharge need to be in readiness at the time of death in order for proper burial procedures to be followed.

Individual reactions to what happens to the body vary greatly—some family members know exactly what they want, including the coffin model, whereas others refuse to take an active part in decision making, insisting that other family members must make all of the arrangements. Although funerals are traditional, they can be very expensive, especially for families of limited means. Cremation can become a more acceptable choice. It is frequently employed when cost is a major factor. Most cities have cremation societies that are willing to work with families in advance or at the time of death. Indigent burial is offered by many communities when the deceased is financially poor. The social worker can work with officials in the county where the patient lives in advance of the death so that a plan is in place that will permit a dignified burial. It is important to remember that memorial ceremonies can take place anytime and anywhere deemed appropriate by those who wish to remember and honor the deceased. After the person has died, there is ample time, in most cases, to develop a plan, time, and place for the memorial service.

Summary

National attention has begun to focus on issues of aging, illness, and dying as the Baby Boom generation approaches their elder years. The media has begun to explore the topic to educate the public on end-of-life issues, providing programs such as the Bill Moyers series, *Death in America*, which aired in the fall of 2000. This outstanding series interviewed individuals who were in the process of dealing with real end-of-life issues and demonstrated the wide-ranging benefits of hospice care.

Americans are now living with public threats involving anthrax and the possibility of future terrorist acts within the borders of the United States. Many people are reviewing their priorities, asking questions, and making changes wherever appropriate in their lives. Professional societies like the American Psychological Association (APA) are sponsoring conferences on end-of-life issues. Powerful groups such as the Alliance for Healthcare Reform and the Partnership for Caring are striving to educate the Congress and Senate on these vital end-of-life issues.

The Last Acts Campaign, a national coalition to improve care and caring near the end of life, has been mobilized, and notables such as former First Lady Rosalyn Carter are taking an active role in making information and help readily available to the American public. Medical centers are beginning to focus attention on pain as the fifth vital sign in patient care and new instruments that measure quality of life are being developed.[19]

The Medicare Care Improvement Act (S. 1589 and H.R. 3188) introduced in the House and Senate by Senator John Rockefeller and Representative Pete Stark, is focused on expanding Medicare benefits to improve conditions for the chronically ill. At the present time the House is scheduling committee hearings on the use of OxyContin® in the treatment of pain.

It is clear that a great distance has been traveled in health care and patient education. There is a long way to go to ensure that people are kept free of pain so that they and their families can experience comfort, peace, and a sense of dignity right up to the end of their lives. Perhaps Elisabeth Kübler-Ross expressed it best when she said that everyone has the right to "live until we die."[12]

References

1. Hinsie, L. E., Campbell, R. J. *Psychiatric Dictionary*, New York: Oxford University Press, 1960.

2. *The Living Webster Encyclopedic Dictionary of the English Language*, Chicago: Columbia University Press, 1963.

3. Gould, J., Kolb, W. L. *A Dictionary of the Social Sciences*, New York: MacMillan Publishing Co., Inc., 1964.

4. Chase, D. *Dying at Home with Hospice*. St. Louis: C.V. Mosby Company, 1986.

5. Irish, D. P., Landquist, K. F., and Nelson, V. J. *Ethnic Variations in Dying, Death and Grief*. Philadelphia, PA: Taylor and Francis Publishers, 1993.

6. Wentzel, K. B. *Hospice Means Hope*. Boston: Charles River Books, 1981.

7. Byock, I. *Dying Well*. New York: The Berkley Publishing Group, 1997.

8. Parry, J. K., Ryan, A. S. *A Cross-Culture Look at Death, Dying and Religion*. Chicago: Nelson-Hall Publishers, 1995.

9. Kalish, R. A. *Death, Grief, and Caring Relationships*. Monterey, Ca.: Brooks/Cole, 1985.

10. Collett, M. *At Home with Dying*. Boston: Shambhala Publications, 1997.

11. Krementz, J. *How it Feels When a Parent Dies*. New York: Alfred A. Knopf, 1994.

12. Kübler-Ross, E. *To Live Until We Say Goodbye*. Englewood Cliffs, NJ: Prentice-Hall Inc., 1978.

13. Remen, R. N. *Kitchen Table Wisdom*. New York: Riverhead Books, 1996.

14. Kübler-Ross, E. *On Death & Dying*. New York: Macmillan, 1969.

15. Rando, T. A. *Treatment of Complicated Mourning*. Champaign, Ill.: Research Press, 1993.

16. Habenstein, R. W., Lamers, W. M. *The History of American Funeral Directing*. Milwaukee, Wis.: Bultin Printers, Inc., 1962.

17. Irion, P. E. *The Funeral: Vestige or Value?* Nashville, Tenn.: Parthenon Press, 1966.

18. Rando, T. A. *Grief, Dying and Death*. Champaign, Ill.: Research Press Company, 1984.

19. Clark, D. *The Future for Palliative Care*. Philadelphia: Oxford University Press, 1993.

For Further Reading

Callanan, M., and Kelly, P. *Final Gifts*. New York: Simon & Schuster, Inc., 1992.

Doka, K.J., and Davidson, J. *Living with Grief When Illness Is Prolonged*. Bristol, PA: Taylor & Francis, 1997.

Gill, D. *Quest, The Life of Kübler-Ross*. New York: Harper Row, 1980.

Kalish, R.A. *Death, Grief and Caring Relationships*. Monterey, Ca.: Brooks/Cole, 1985.

Kessler, D. *The Rights of the Dying*. London: Ebury Press, Random House UK, 1997.

Kübler-Ross, E. *Living with Death and Dying*. New York: MacMillan Publishing Company, 1981.

Kubler-Ross, E. *On Children and Death*. New York: MacMillan Publishing Company, 1983.

Kübler-Ross, E. *Questions and Answers on Death and Dying*, New York: Macmillan Publishing Company, 1974.

Levine, S. *Healing Into Life and Death*. New York: Anchor Books, Doubleday, 1987.

Mitford, J. *The American Way of Death*. New York: Fawcett Crest, 1979.

Munley, A. *The Hospice Alternative*. New York: Basic Books Inc., 1983.

Rinpoche, S. *The Tibetan Book of Living and Dying*. San Francisco: Harper, 1992.

Saunders, C. *Beyond the Horizon*. London: Darton, Longman and Todd, 1990.

Shepard, M. *Someone You Love Is Dying*. New York: Crown Publishers, 1975.

Staudbacher, C. *Men and Grief*. Oakland, Ca.: New Harbinger Publications, Inc., 1991.

Waters, E. B., and Goodman, J. *Empowering Older Adults*. San Francisco: Jossey-Bass Publishers, 1990.

Wentzel, K.B. *To Those Who Need It Most, Hospice Means Hope*. Boston: Charles River Books, 1981.

Solving Issues in Hospice/Palliative Care through the Use of Case Problems

18

Walter B. Forman, MD, FACP, CMD

In this chapter the reader is introduced to actual problems that we as hospice/palliative care professionals have encountered. This chapter provides several exercises in hospice/palliative care problem solving. There are four cases, each concerning a different clinical issue. Each should be studied and the questions answered *before* looking up the "correct" answers in the back of each case. This is important because it will allow you to problem solve, review the answers, and then be able to critique your responses. Remember, it's the process of problem solving in hospice/palliative care and not just the correct answer that is important. You might even have a different answer to the problem than the one we supplied. If so, please let us know!

Now for the first case. Good luck.

Case Problem I: Is This Person Eligible for the Hospice Medicare Benefit?

Mr. H, a 67-year-old, self-employed long distance trucker, is bothered by his failing memory. He has not been receiving medical attention for this problem, because he refuses to discuss his memory loss. During a thorough history, he does state that the memory problem interferes with his work. He offers as an example that he constantly is getting lost when he attempts to negotiate cross-country deliveries. His past medical history includes:

- Hypertension, for which he is taking medications
- Chronic obstructive lung disease secondary to a 55-year, pack-a-day history of cigarette smoking
- Benign prostatic hypertrophy resulting in frequent nocturia

His family noted the memory problem at home because he forgets grand-childrens' names and gets lost going from the shopping center to home. They want him to retire from truck driving.

He comes to you for evaluation. You note that he is not as carefully groomed as when you last saw him. He complains of incontinence of bladder. A Folstein's Mini Mental Status Examination (MMSE) reveals a score of 19/30. He agrees to have the family sit in on the discussion concerning his health care.

Before you meet with the family, you do the following:

- Review Buckman's Six Steps for breaking bad news
- Determine who should be present at the family conference. Who decides? How do you determine if the "decision maker" is at the meeting?
- Determine which members of the health care team should be present and outline their roles in this conversation

During the meeting, the family asks about hospice care. You review with them Mr. H's eligibility for hospice care by discussing the FAST (Functional Assessment Staging) and applying the data to Mr. H's situation. You then discuss which of the FAST factors determine his hospice eligibility.

The family would like you to outline:

a. The services and the other items such as cost of hospice care that apply in this situation

b. How each member of the hospice/palliative care team will interact with them

c. Explain and offer examples of a DNR/DNI form and how it applies in your state

Issues

Issues that need to be addressed include whether he is eligible and agrees to hospice care.

So, please discuss:

1. How often should the aide visit and what should he do when he comes to the house?

2. The chaplain wants to know something about the person and family. He might ask for what information?

3. Describe the role of the nurse in the care of this person.

4. In reviewing the medication list, the pharmacist wants to alter and change some medications in order to be more hospice appropriate.

What medications that Mr. H might receive would be paid by the hospice Medicare benefit? Please list six such medications.

5. Please list at least four issues that are of concern to the social worker in this matter.

Answers

In his book *How to Break Bad News: A Guide for Health Care Professionals*, Robert Buckman outlines six steps. They are:

1. Getting started
2. Finding out how much the patient knows
3. Finding out how much the patient wants to know
4. Sharing the information
5. Responding to the patient's feelings
6. Planning and follow through

We would suggest that you review this information, as there is much information that is valuable and can be utilized in presenting the information to Mr. H and his family.

It is important that you, as the initial contact with Mr. H and his family, are able to determine who should be present for the initial discussions. Again, we refer to Buckman for advice in this matter. Your choices could include professionals who will be involved in his hospice care, such as the nurse, social worker, or chaplain. These professionals form the backbone of the hospice program.

The information concerning the FAST stage is outlined in *Medical Guidelines for Determining Prognosis in Selected Non-cancer Diseases*, published by The National Hospice and Palliative Care Organization. This is an important publication to have at the ready for your program or for your own information. Mr. H is able to speak and ambulate, is incontinent of urine, and has a low MMSE. In order to be eligible under the dementia classification the person must be in the FAST stage 7(C) range. Mr. H does not make this classification and therefore is not hospice eligible using the guidelines. The staging of all people is critical in order for your program to be in compliance with national standards.

You should be familiar with the services hospice can provide. As to reimbursement, it is on a per diem reimbursement and not based on cost of care. What is the reimbursement per diem for hospice care in your area? The cost of care beyond what is related to hospice care is funded by whatever mechanism the person has previously used. You should discuss this issue with a hospice team member who has this information in your program.

The four team members who are the major part of the IDT are:

- Nurse. Case manager.
- Social worker.
- Spiritual counselor.
- Physician.

Who has power of attorney, if the person is incompetent or unable to speak? Know the laws in your area of practice and in your state.

There are many documents that assist people in creating a living will. One such document is the Five Wishes, which can be obtained using the address in the references.

Finally, the health care worker should ask all the people they encounter in their practice what they wish to happen to them if they are unable to speak for themselves.

References

1. 5 Wishes: *www.agingwithdignity.org*
2. SUPPORT: A controlled trial to improve care for seriously ill hospitalized patients. *JAMA* 274:1591–1598, 1995.
3. *Palliative Care Ethics: A Good Companion.* Eds. Randall, F., and Downie, R. S. Oxford University Press, 1996.
4. *Culture and Nursing Care: A Pocket Guide.* Eds. Lipson, J. G., Dibble, S. L., and Minarik, P. A. San Francisco: UCSF Nursing Press, 1997.

Case Problem II: Planning for the Future

Ms. M is a 55-year-old woman who is the executive director of a bank. She is widowed and lives alone. Her three adult children live close to her. Ms. M underwent biopsy of a breast mass last week. The biopsy report showed it to be malignant. This office visit is to discuss with her the approach to the treatment of illness. Ms. M, when asked what she understands about her illness, states that she must first get "her affairs in order" before she can begin to discuss treatment. She asks about a living will and a durable power of attorney for health care. Your first thought is to refer her to her legal advisor. You give her copies of a variety of living wills and powers of attorney for health care for her to read and then proceed to explain to her the variety of medical decisions that must be made.

Issues

You need to be aware of what these documents contain and how they apply in your area. Please outline how you would obtain this information before attempting to undertake this discussion.

How would you begin a conversation about living wills? Each of us in the field of palliative care should be aware of the information needed to carry on this conversation. Please answer the question from your discipline's point of view.

How much of this information that Ms. M will gather should be part of the medical record? Who is responsible for placing that information in her chart (office and/or hospital)? Do you have a method that would indicate that the information is available in time of an emergency?

Answers

This exercise has many choices and most need to be considered according to your area of practice. The rules vary by state in regard to the need to have these documents. There is a federal mandate that requires all institutions that receive Medicare reimbursement to ask patients if they would like to complete an advance directive as they are admitted to the institution. This law was part of the Medicare Act in 1996 and is known as the Stark Amendment. You should be familiar with this law.

In the state you practice, look up the laws regarding these documents.

Case Problem III: Pain in the Person with Cancer

Mr. A, a 92-year-old retired physicist, is living alone in a retirement center. He has no living family members. Three months ago weight loss and night sweats led to the diagnosis of cancer of the colon, Stage D. He is receiving chemo/radiotherapy with severe episodes of nausea, emesis, diarrhea, and sore throat. In your office today he notes a new symptom: pain in his back, aching in character, severe in nature that is keeping him awake, and is not relieved with topical heat, cold, or oral acetaminophen.

Issues

1. What steps are needed to define this person's pain?
2. How would you "rate" this person's pain? Does his age interfere with the rating?
3. What would you anticipate finding on physical examination related to the pain?
4. What laboratory examinations, including radiographic studies, would you employ to determine the etiology of this person's pain?

5. While you are evaluating this person's pain, you should begin treatment based on the data you currently have available. List three different approaches for therapy such as drugs, physical methods, and alternative methods.

Answers

In Chapters 11 and 12, the reader will find the tools necessary to assess the pain that this person is experiencing. Remember that pain is what the person with the pain says that it is, not what the observer thinks it might be. The important issues in evaluation include the nature of the pain, the character of the pain, the amount of the pain, and what brings relief. Rating the information can also be found in the chapters cited. Age, sex, and ethnic background are all important issues to keep in mind when rating pain. In the references we list some articles that apply to this issue. Physical examination of pain is by definition a somewhat problematic issue. This type of pain could be related to the onset of Zoster, in which case one might find a rash or spinal cord compression. In the latter situation, one could expect changes in sensation to pin prick or light touch in the area affected. In Mr. A, we have not defined where in his back he is having pain. A key component of any pain evaluation is to clearly note the area in which the pain is occurring.

Appropriate examination should include plain radiographs of the area in question, isotope scanning of his skeleton, or an MRI of the vertebral column. We would suggest that when in doubt about spinal cord compression syndrome, the health care provider should employ the MRI in order to have as accurate an assessment as possible. If treatment begins early in the course of spinal cord compression the onset of paralysis might be prevented. Treatment is directed at control of the symptoms. So, please do not wait for the diagnosis. The physical examination is critical. Treat with medication or physical means that address the problem. If Zoster is the cause, an antiviral agent and pain medication are important. On the other hand, if the pain was caused by spinal cord compression, corticosteroids and/or radiation therapy must be utilized. If his pain were due to bone involvement, an NSAID would be important to initiate therapy. Usually, individuals with bony metastasis causing pain will also need to have opioid therapy initiated.

References

1. Mannix, K., Ahmedzia, S. H., Anderson, H., et al. Using bisphosphonates to control the pain of bone metastasis: Evidence-based guidelines for palliative care. *Pall Med* 14:455–463, 2000.
2. *Cancer Pain Management.* Eds. McGuire, D. B., Henke-Yarbo, C., and Ferrell, B. R. Boston: Jones and Bartlett, Inc., 1995.
3. *Handbook of Palliative Care in Cancer.* Eds. Waller, A., and Caroline, N. L. Woodburn, MA: Butterworth-Heinemann, 2000, pp. 301–309.

Case Problem IV: A Person with Bowel Obstruction

Ms. T, a 79-year-old retired postal clerk, has been treated for three years for Stage 4 carcinoma of the ovary. During this cycle of chemotherapy her ascites is increasing. Her stomach is compressed by the cancer. As a result, she can eat only small bits of food or half a glass of fluid. Early satiety and emesis have caused her to lose 15 pounds in the past month. Emesis that was initially treated has returned. She notes that in association with the emesis she has cramping abdominal pain and anorexia and has been unable to have a bowel movement for the past five days. She does not wish a surgical consultation but requests a hospice referral.

Issues

1. At the initial joint home visit, the doctor and nurse examine her abdomen. Please cite the findings that one could expect in this situation.

2. What role should the social worker have in regard to the need for assistance with her living conditions?

3. Using the data obtained, the hospice team meets and begins therapy aimed at comfort measures. Outline the therapy that best suits this person's present condition.

4. After several days of marked relief of her pain she notes a new severe right upper-quadrant pain. It is described as 9/10, constant, and without radiation. The pain is so severe that it makes her want to hold her breath in order to relieve the symptom.

5. What might be causing the new abdominal pain? Outline your diagnostic evaluation and therapy for this problem.

6. How can the hospice chaplain assist in her care at this point?

7. Is she a candidate for a respite admission?

Answers

Ms. T has probably developed an obstruction of her large intestine caused by the ovarian carcinoma. Physical examination should demonstrate what one would expect to find: distention; generalized tenderness during palpation, without masses; tympany at percussion; and high pitched, infrequent bowel sounds on auscultation. Rectal examination, a must in a person with abdominal pain, is noncontributory in this case to assisting with the diagnosis. Bowel obstruction is referred to in Chapter 10 and further information can be found in Reference 3.

Therapy is aimed at control of the pain, emesis, and relaxation of the distended bowel. This is best treated with the use of a continuous subcutaneous infusion of haloperidol (nausea), morphine (pain), octreotide (bowel disten-sion), and scopolamine (secretions). The formulation of this preparation might include 5 mg haloperidol, 25 mg of morphine, 500 ugms octreotide, and 2 mg scopolamine in 100 mg of normal saline, to be infused subcuta-neously over a 24-hour period.

The role of the social worker and spiritual adviser is discussed in Chapter 2. In this situation the individual needs both psychological support to address the issues she is facing in regards to the fatal complication of her illness and assistance with activities of daily living. Independent activities of daily living are also compromised.

A new cause of abdominal pain is investigated by physical examination. Note that the liver is very tender, which in this situation indicates an intrahe-patic hemorrhage caused by the metastatic deposit. Other laboratory examina-tion is limited to obtaining a hematocrit. Although useful, scans and other laboratory evaluations are of little use in this clinical situation because of the person's debilitated state. At this point a corticosteroid is added to the subcu-taneous infusion. Although the person's pain is relieved, the chaplain discov-ers that she is frightened to remain at home. Thus, respite care is arranged.

References

1. *Palliative Care Pocket Companion.* 1999. Eds. Dickerson, E. D., Benedetti, C., Davis, M. P., et al. Upper Arlington, Ohio: Ohio Hospice Organization.
2. www.palliativedrugs.com
3. Muir, J. C., and vonGunten, C. F. Antisecretory agents in gastrointestinal obstruc-tion. *Cl Geri Med.* 16:327–334, 2000.
4. Moore, B. Social work in palliative care in *Oxford Textbook of Palliative Medicine, First Edition.* Eds. Doyle, D., Hanks, G. W. C., and MacDonald, N. Oxford University Press, 1993.

Further Reading

Buckman, Robert. *How to Break Bad News: A Guide for Health Care Professionals.* Baltimore, MD: Johns Hopkins Press, 1992.

Folstein, K. C., Folstein, S. E. & McHugh, P. R. Mini-mental state: A practical method for grading the cognitive state of patients for the clinician. *J of Psych. Research,* 12:323–329, 1975.

Johanson, G. A., Johanson, I. V. Chapter 4: The Care Team in *Hospice and Palliative Care: Concepts and Practice.* Eds. Sheehan, D. C. and Forman, W. B. Sudbury, MA: Jones and Bartlett Publishers, 1995.

Medical Guidelines for Determining Prognosis in Selected Non-cancer Diseases. Arlington, VA, The National Hospice and Palliative Care Organization, 1995.

Reisberg, B. Functional Assessment Staging (FAST). *Psychopharmo Bull.* 24:653–659, 1988.

U.S. Department of Health and Human Services. *Medicare: Hospice Manual.* Washington, DC: U.S. Dept. of Commerce National Technical Information Service, 1992.

Volciers, L., & Hurley, A. *Hospice Care for Patients with Advanced Progressive Dementia.* New York: Springer Publishing Co, 1998.

The Information Superhighway and Palliative Care

19

Dennis Pacl, MD

Technological advancement grows at an exponential rate. Nowhere is this statement more evident than in the innovations in data processing and telecommunications occurring over the last decade, culminating in the potential for a virtual society via personal computers and the Internet. How quickly can we as health care professionals adapt to the new technology? This chapter will identify ways to stay on top of information resources and gain familiarity with the tools that allow access to resources that might improve the care we provide to our patients and families dealing with life-limiting illness.

Informatics and the Electronic Medical Record

Informatics in health care refers to the management of information. As with other businesses, these information systems first grew out of a need to handle financial data. This focus on financial systems as informatics led to a large delay in gaining access to clinically useful information in a health care information system. Eventually the need for sharing clinical data led to the development of the Internet, which in its infancy was used solely by scientists and researchers at large private institutions and government agencies. After powerful desktop computers became widely available, the Internet exploded to become the ubiquitous information medium that we are familiar with today.

The electronic medical record and remote consultation through telemedicine hook-ups have become realities. The penetration of these tools throughout health care is now a given. Thus, it is now only a matter of where the information is needed and whether we possess the competency to access it. With competency comes the power of where to use the information. Much of the recent development in informatics arises from the underground of Internet entrepreneurship, driven from a practical utility rather than a financial need. The "what" (Internet) and "when" (anytime you have online access) have been solved and the "where" is no longer restricted to researchers in some government laboratory, or hospital billing offices. The natural extension of unfettered access to clinical information online is toward a paperless office. Billing and coding systems, once the domain of hospitals and physician offices, are downloadable to a handheld computer. Detailed patient information can be entered using a simple template. If not for the durable equipment and the examination room space needed, we may not even need to have an office at all. The Windows operating system for your desktop, the Palm operating system for the handheld, and readily available and affordable hardware give us the power to redefine our place of business.

The Electronic "Curbside Consult"

As a health professional, real-time access to information resources is invaluable. Also needed is collegial interaction for clinical problem solving. Thus, our requirements for information systems and the Internet are much broader and more rigorous than those of most other professions. A "curbside consult" on the Internet offers a rich expertise by virtue of universal access to the Internet, twenty-four-hour accessibility, and a format most expedient to meet our needs. No appointment is necessary. How do we get information that we need wherever we may be? How do we find and deliver the information to those who need it the most, our patients? Even the best hospital information systems alone cannot assist the clinician with all of the information needed for decision making. Even with access to all manner of medical record data, including diagnostic and imaging studies, utilization data, consultant reports, demographics, and procedure consents, the provider may still seek collegial advice from a trusted source.

The up side of having access to "curbside consults" is leafing through online medical texts in the palm of your hand and searching the Internet from a personal computer. The down side is that the Internet remains an underground operation and patients may be getting consults of their own, unable to make the proper distinctions to find reliable information. Therefore, it is incumbent upon all practitioners to know how to get the best information to help guide clinical decision making.

The future may make the electronic house call the norm. Telemedicine hook-ups will become standard practice, especially in rural areas, due to cost-effective remote sensing devices and imaging tools. Relatively sophisticated monitoring could be done in the home. Most data entry will be through handheld devices performed at the bedside in real time. IT (information technology) is no longer just for the hospital. Palliative care supports patient-directed terminal care in the home. With the advances in information technology, a home care system may bring with it the trappings of institutional-type terminal care and the sophisticated monitoring that goes with it.

Security and Privacy

Security and privacy considerations are challenges for medical informatics. Utmost respect for individual privacy is paramount. Any medical information that has personal identifiers must conform with the Health Insurance Portability and Accountability Act (HIPAA, 1996). HIPAA seeks to help guarantee privacy and confidentiality of patient medical records when information is transmitted electronically (i.e., fax, e-mail, personal data assistants).

Health Information on the Internet

One aspect of the practice of medicine that has improved dramatically with the advent of sophisticated information technology is our ability to refer patients to potential sources of support specific to their immediate needs. It is increasingly likely that our patients and colleagues possess a home PC and a Web browser so they can visit a wide array of support services. Providers have to become familiar with the pearls and pitfalls of health information on the Internet in order to competently advise patients. Ideally, a basic familiarity with a few of the more reliable resources will meet the needs of a majority of patients. Although an exhaustive list of reputable Web sites would be outdated sooner than it could be printed (see the appendix to this chapter for a list of Web resources current at the time of publication), a few ground rules exist for evaluating health-related information on the Internet.

The least common denominator for any information resource is it reliability. Credible Web sites routinely undergo editorial review and update content information to keep the material relevant and timely for a target audience. Unfortunately, the editorial policy may not be readily apparent or may be unavailable to viewers. In the absence of such, one can look for several revealing signs: clinical citations embedded in the text, author identification, authors who are qualified health professionals, the site's policy regarding advertising, and reputable sponsors. Nonprofit sites or governmental agencies are less likely to be subject to the influence of sponsors. The single most important factor for considering the reputability of Internet health information is whether it is sponsored by a reputable organization. A reputable organization will constantly be updating medical information due to the changes in medical knowledge.

Assessing Web Sites for Utility and Reliability

Useful information need not be limited to the National Institutes of Health (**www.nih.gov**) or large reliable medical centers. On the contrary, many Web sites have disease-specific information, such as the Alzheimer's Association (**www.alz.org**), the American Cancer Society (**www.cancer.org**), and the American Heart Association (**www.americanheart.org**). A brief look at the mission statement, accessed by clicking an "about us" button or link, can help in establishing the premise of the information in the Web site. Looking at the mission statement and the site map are two quick steps that will help assess the utility of a Web site without wasting much time.

In order to ascertain accountability for the posted information, review the Web site for endorsements or awards from professional societies or trade groups. Have they achieved a quality endorsement from an Internet rating service? The most widely respected rating for health information sites is the HON Code, which was created by the nonprofit Health On the Net Foundation at **www.hon.ch**. This approval rating is useful because the editors at HON review Web sites regularly to assure that compliance with qualifying criteria is being maintained. Therefore, you have reasonable assurance that the Web site resource has an obligation and is accountable for maintaining compliance with the qualifying criteria. Another item to watch for on Web sites is when statistical information is cited, it should indicate the source. If you can't find out where the numbers came from, then the conclusions drawn from them must be questioned.

The primary responsibility of our information gatekeeping is assuring the reliability of the source, accountability for the information provided, and that the needs of the patient/family can be met. Train your patients to consider the source in both content and reliability (see the section in the appendix entitled "Resources for Patients and Caregivers").

Internet Resources for the Palliative Care Professional

As clinicians who care for patients with advanced life-limiting illness, we will encounter difficult challenges in our ability to achieve adequate relief of severe symptoms. The Internet can provide primary access to needed interdisciplinary expertise and information. In addition, it is important for the palliative care provider to remain current with the literature; new drugs; alternate routes of drug delivery; innovative, off-label use indications; and developing standards of care. Here, too, we have a powerful tool with the Internet. The development of discussion boards, online chat rooms, live Webcasts, and listservs offer a variety of ways to stay abreast of practice trends and professional interests (see the section in the appendix entitled "Resources for the Health Care Professionals"). Seeking the "curbside consult" becomes infinitely easier, while at the same time the breadth of expertise on "professionals only" Web sites is often well beyond that which is available in your community.

When utilizing discussion boards or online chats, caution is again prudent and necessary. Consideration of the source is paramount; critical appraisal of the response to your questions is even more important. One can quickly get bogged down with anecdote. Readers are encouraged to familiarize themselves with the IICN (Inter-Institutional Collaborating Network) at Growth

House (**www.Growthhouse.org**), an example of a Web site that has gone through a painstaking process over several years to ensure the quality and freshness of its content. Growth House, a nonprofit independent Web site, has cultivated an active base of professional users through a restricted registration process limited to health professionals. The moderation and editorial board are drawn from recognized experts in a variety of disciplines and professional interests. It is important to be familiar with a "gold standard" Web site such as Growth House, by which you can better compare other similar professional interest Web sites. Providers should consider participating online as often as possible to remain current. Register on at least one general medical site like Physicians' Online (**www.pol.net**), Medscape (**www.medscape.com**), or Web MD (**www.Webmd.com**). Then seek out a variety of professional interest sites such as Growth House or the American Academy of Hospice and Palliative Medicine (**www.aahpm.org**). Keep in mind that commercial sites like WebMD and Physicians' Online have advertising banners that will definitely slow the transfer rates of Web pages, and sponsors may also influence content.

Handheld Computers: Distance Insensitive Computing

Not unlike pagers and cellular phones, the handheld computer has quickly become indispensable, making day planners, notebooks, and file cards obsolete and inconvenient. Referred to as handhelds, palm tops, personal information managers (PIMs), or personal data assistants (PDAs), these devices give you tremendous computing power for quick and easy reference.

One of the many advantages to such a device is the ability to directly input information via the operating system of the PDA or through your home or office personal computer (PC). Industry-standard operating systems (OS) such as the Palm OS or Microsoft Windows OS have a high degree of compatibility that allows for a generous variety of software programs. Applications like electronic billing and coding, clinical records, and reference materials complete with high-resolution illustrations are legion.

Most PDA applications are written for the Palm OS; likewise software programmers write desktop applications for Windows OS. The true value of the compatibility between PDA and PC is realized through the process of *synchronization* of the PDA with your PC. During synchronization, each OS updates the memory of the other machine with any changed information. The synchronization procedure creates redundancy between the two system memories, adding protection for the most valuable information, such as schedule, contacts, and business or patient information. Many PDAs have the capacity to transfer collected data, in the form of 4 to 8 megabyte chips. This large chip capacity allows for storage of large files such as medical texts, and keeps the demands on device memory to a minimum and available for other application usage.

As mentioned, the number of useful applications for a PDA are legion. The Palm OS can operate the applications shown in Table 19-1. Some Web sites specific to PDA applications that the author has found helpful are listed in Table 19-2. The reader is encouraged to explore the wide variety of applications for PDAs and assess this utility for individual usage needs.

TABLE 19-1 Handheld Electronic Applications
Scheduler
Note pad
To do list
Professional and personal contacts
Expense report
Calculator
Drug information
Standard medical text
Individual patient data

TABLE 19-2 Useful PDA Web Sites

Download.com (www.download.com)	ePocrates (www.epocrates.com)	PDAMD (www.pdamd.com)
Offers general computing resources and shareware software downloads for a wide variety of business and leisure applications.	A free palmtop drug listing with prescribing information. A free antibiotic prescribing guide is also available.	A proprietary site offering handhelds and software for health professionals.

Clinical Implications

Consumer access to the information now available on the Internet has redefined the physician–patient relationship. Palliative care and palliative medicine professionals will experience a variety of changes in demand patterns caused by increased consumer knowledge. The patient and family have a wider array of health care options without even leaving home. Future directions might include a telemedicine link between the patient/family and the interdisciplinary group, as defined in the conditions of participation of the Medicare Hospice Benefit (MHB). An electronic therapeutic presence has the potential to increase the level of sophistication in home services so that they parallel a clinic or outpatient service.

Summary

The Information Superhighway is already here and available for integration and support of the ongoing development of palliative care professionals. Future clinical effectiveness will be influenced by the willingness to adapt to new technology; "early adapters" are already on the leading edge. Where will the consumer turn if we cannot respond effectively? If we can't answer this question, how can we be informed partners and professional guides for families requesting supportive services? Embracing the potential of the Internet and its related technology is becoming an integral part of palliative care.

Appendix

Resources and Educational Initiatives in Palliative Care

Since the first edition there has been a wonderful explosion of resources, training programs, and interest in end-of-life care. So we have chosen to include in this edition references that will allow the reader to delve into the subject of end-of–life care using Web-based resources. We hope that you will find a variety of resources in this listing that can be used both at the beginning of your learning about hospice/palliative care and as you move along the journey that deals with this relatively new and fascinating subject.

We recognize that this is by no means an exhaustive list, nor is there any endorsement intended of these sites by the author or publisher. This appendix is merely for informational purposes only. These resources should be evaluated in the manner outlined earlier in this chapter. This is a small sampling of sites we have found useful in the past. Many of these sites carry "link" pages that can direct you to information specific to your needs or the needs of patients and caregivers. We strongly recommend that you familiarize yourself with the Growth House Inter-Institutional Collaborative Network (IICN), where you can link to many of the resources listed below.

Resources for Health Care Professionals

Education for Physicians on End-of-Life Care (EPEC)
The EPEC Project
www.epec.net

AACN End of Life Nursing Education Consortium (ELNEC)
www.aacn.nche.edu/ELNEC

Guidelines for End-of-Life Care in Nursing Homes: Principles and Recommendations (click on Policies, Position Papers)
John A. Hartford Foundation Institute for Geriatric Nursing
www.hartfordign.org

Improving Palliative Care for Cancer
Editors: K. M. Foley and H. Gelband
National Academy Press, Washington, D.C.
www.nap.edu

Partnership for Caring
www.partnershipforcaring.org

Center to Improve Care of the Dying (George Washington University)
www.gwu.edu/~cicd

Growth House
www.growthhouse.org

Growth House Inter-Institutional Collaborative Network
www.growthhouse.org/iicn.html

Last Acts
www.lastacts.org

The New Mexico Rural Hospice Network
hsc.unm.edu/nmruralhospice

The Five Wishes
www.agingwithdignity.org/5wishes.html

Family Caregiver Alliance
www.caregiver.org

National Institute on Aging
Resource Directory for Older People
www.nia.nih.gov/health/resource/rd2001.htm

American College of Physicians
Home Guide for Advanced Cancer Patients
www.acponline.org/public/h_care/contents.htm

The National Institutes of Health
www.nih.gov/

The National Academy of Sciences—Institute of Medicine
www.iom.edu/

British Medical Journal
www.bmj.com/cgi/collection/palliative_medicine

Resources for Patients and Caregivers

The Five Wishes
www. agingwithdignity.org/5wishes.html

Family Caregiver Alliance
www.caregiver.org

National Institute on Aging
Resource Directory for Older People
www.nia.nih.gov/health/resource/rd2001.htm

American College of Physicians
Home Guides for Advanced Cancer Patients
www.acponline.org/public/h_care/contents.htm

The National Institutes of Health
www.nih.gov

The National Academy of Sciences—Institute of Medicine
www.iom.edu

Partnership for Caring: America's Voices for the Dying
www.partnershipforcaring.org

Americans for Better Care of the Dying
www.abcd-caring.org

Organizations in Palliative Care/Palliative Medicine

These groups have particular interest in end-of-life care and are easily accessible. You can search them very easily and obtain much information.

American Academy of Hospice and Palliative Medicine
www.aahpm.org

American Society of Law, Medicine, and Ethics
www.painandthelaw.org

Hospice and Palliative Nurses Association
www.hpna.org

Edmonton Regional Palliative Care Program
www.palliative.org

Palliative Drugs
www.palliativedrugs.com

Americans for Better Care of the Dying
www.abcd-caring.org

Center to Improve Care of the Dying (George Washington University)
www.gwu.edu/~cicd/

National Hospice and Palliative Care Organization
www.nhpco.org

The National Institutes of Health
www.nih.gov

The National Academy of Sciences—Institute of Medicine
www.iom.edu

Academic Programs

Medical College of Wisconsin Palliative Medicine Program
www.mcw.edu/pallmed

The Center to Advance Palliative Care
www.capcmssm.org

The End-of-Life Physician Education Resource Center (EPERC)
www.eperc.mcw.edu

Community Resources for Hospice/Palliative Care Patients

20

N. Elizabeth Eutsler

Since the beginning of time, every culture has established specific roles related to the care of the dying and to the mourning process. In the past, if a person became ill, family and friends took care of all of his or her needs because this large extended family, usually in close geographical proximity, had no other choice. Death was usually quick.

The Industrial Revolution and subsequent movement of families from small farming communities to cities radically changed the roles of family and friends when caring for the dying patient. Now people outside the family, and often located far from the dying patient, came to be in charge of his or her care. Both the dying patient and the family have specific needs and the community can provide resources to help meet those needs.

When considering resources for the palliative/hospice care patient, the provider must always look at the needs of the total person. The provider caring for the dying patient and his or her family should consider Maslow's "hierarchy of needs" (see Further Reading) as a means to assess the immediate and long-term needs of the patient. If the basic needs of the terminal patient are not met, the patient and family will face additional stress. Often medical professionals believe that as long as the patient is getting the best available medical care, all the patient has to deal with is the psychological stages of dying, which have been most eloquently defined by Elisabeth Kübler-Ross in her book *On Death and Dying*. Understanding and accepting these stages become much more difficult if the person does not have the money or resources to acquire food, housing, utilities, and transportation.

The first level of Maslow's hierarchy consists of *physical survival needs*, which include water, food, and sleep. In our society this necessity can translate into simply knowing where the person is to reside, what he will have to eat and drink, and how he will stay warm in the winter and cool in the summer. The person must have adequate finances to pay for these needs or family or friends who can provide for them. The provider should inquire about where the patient is living and how he is supporting himself. If the patient is retired, the provider should assess his income, including any significant assets he might have. This brief assessment will help define which resources may be made available. If the patient is under 65 years old, the provider must ask whether the person has worked five out of the last ten years. If so, he may be eligible for Social Security Disability. Similarly, the provider should ask whether the patient, male or female, has served in the armed forces, because this may make the patient eligible for a Department of Veteran's Affairs Non-Service or Service Connected Pension.

The second level in the hierarchy of needs is *safety*. A patient who is dying should be in a place where he or she is out of danger. Often the hospital staff is introduced to dying patients who have been brought in by Adult Protective Services because they were living in states of self-neglect. Other safety issues revolve around the patient's ability to perform her own activities of daily living. Often these issues can be resolved through the ordering of appropriate durable medical equipment. A bedside commode in the patient's room can reduce the likelihood of falls on a long trip to the bathroom. Likewise, a wheelchair can reduce the risk of falls when a patient ventures out of the home.

The third level is *belonging*, being accepted as oneself. Usually "belonging" means with family, but it can also involve close friends and religious communities. Again, the family and friends should be the primary resources for the dying, but the provider cannot assume that all patients have close friends or relatives to care for them in their last days. If family and friends are not available, then society must care for them. A frequently used resource is nursing home placement from either home or hospital. In larger communities, inpatient hospice services may be available. These services can be associated with particular diseases, such as AIDS, where people may have limited "traditional" family support.

The fourth level is the *ego*, the need to have the approval of others and to have appropriate recognition. Many patients need to "settle" with family before dying. An important part of the dying process is to close the issues that may have caused pain to either the dying patient or to members of the family. This is the time to finish family business such as writing wills and trusts, if that has not been done. The medical staff is often asked to help with family and legal issues. Another concern, indeed a major stressor, for the dying patient may involve a personal or family pet. The provider's knowledge of local animal shelters or rescue groups for particular breeds will make placement easier for the patient.

The top of the hierarchy is *self-actualization*. Patients with terminal illnesses often have time to "put their lives in order" and come to terms with their own lives. Confirmation of this stage can be accomplished by talking to competent professionals in mental health, spiritual guides, pastors, or medical staff.

Many resources are available for assistance in meeting these needs. The first resource is *family*. The Family Leave Act allows most family members to take up to 12 weeks of unpaid, job-protected leave per year to care for a dying family member. This act is helpful if the caregiver has enough vacation time, but it can create additional strain when he does not have the vacation time to provide care to the dying family member. Medical staff is often asked to write letters on behalf of the patient and family. Through family meetings, the provider can evaluate the needs of the patient and family if they choose to care for the dying at home. If the family does not have the financial, emotional, or physical resources to care for the terminally ill patient, then an alternative plan must be devised. The plan could include a nursing home placement or an in-patient hospice placement. Medicaid waiver programs may help pay family or friends to care for the dying patient.

Most *towns and cities* have resource directories that address various social services. The United Way (**www.national.unitedway.org**), Councils of Churches (**www.ncccusa.org**), Agencies on Aging (**www.aoa.gov**), and others have excellent local directories. Churches and religious groups have long assisted their members with volunteers, food, and money. They also provide spiritual support throughout the dying process.

Each *state* has Health and Human Services directories of assistance programs. States can assist low-income patients with money, food stamps, and housing. Through Institutional Medicaid, states can help fund nursing home placements when families cannot care for their dying members or when the patient has no family. The local Adult Protective Services is another resource for patients who appear to be dying alone or in a setting of self-neglect. Each state is mandated to have an Adult Protective Services program to assist those who are abused or neglected and may find themselves in a life-threatening situation.

The *federal government* has many resources available for the palliative care patient. Since the late 1980s, home hospice care has become an alternative for terminal patients who wish to die at home. Although a licensed hospice agency is not a federal agency, they generally receive most of their funding from the federal Medicare program, which covers most of the expenses associated with home hospice. This is the best source for obtaining comprehensive care for the dying patient with a good support system at home. To verify whether benefits are currently available, the provider can check with the Social Security Administration either by phone at 1-800-772-1213 or on the Internet at **www.pueblo.gsa.gov/cic_text/fed_prog/hospice/hospice.htm**.

The federal government has several programs to financially assist people once they become disabled. The provider can help the family or patient apply for Social Security Disability and Supplemental Security Income at the onset of any life-threatening disease. Many people will not apply for disability because they believe they will be denied. Another common misconception is that one has to be 62 years old to apply for Social Security. A visit to the Social Security Administration Web site at **www.ssa.gov** will help both the provider and the patient when beginning the application process. Social Security expedites applications for the terminally ill.

The Department of Veteran's Affairs is also a major resource for eligible veterans and sometimes their dependents. This organization provides medical and psychological care for the patient as well as financial and burial assistance. The Web site **www.va.gov** provides an overview of benefits and locations for services for burial, compensation, health services.

There are literally thousands of *volunteer and non-profit organizations* set up to assist nearly every conceivable group. The Internet can be used for information and the identification of these resources. Estimates indicate that nearly 75% of U.S. households have access to the Internet. Patients, families, and health care professionals can access hundreds of sites that can assist with information. Each disease and condition may have several Web sites, listservs, and chat rooms. Medical staff should familiarize themselves with these diagnosis-related Internet sites to understand what many patients are using to educate themselves about their condition. A partial list of these sites for patients and health care professionals can be found at the end of Chapter 20.

Burial options for the disposition of the body are the final issue that the health care provider may be asked about. State and local laws differ widely throughout the United States. The medical organization should provide the family with a list of mortuaries and direct services companies that can assist the family after the patient has died. Many people have burial insurance. Although many people believe that Social Security will pay for the burial, at this time they will pay only $255 to the widow or surviving children for this service, considerably less than the actual cost. Families of deceased veterans who can prove their service can be buried at a national cemetery. They may also be eligible for a VA payment for burial if they have a VA Compensation of Pension.

The staff caring for the dying must always be aware that different cultures may have different burial customs, procedures, and laws. In an area with a large Native American population, it is not unusual for the family to come to the morgue and take their loved one home in their own vehicle for burial in a traditional manner.

Social Workers

An excellent resource for the health care professional working in palliative care is a competent social worker with a strong background in the community. The following two case studies, using fictitious names, demonstrate how the "problems" of the dying patient can be addressed by the medical staff and the community.

Using Multiple Agencies to Solve a "Simple Request"

Mr. Martinez came to the hospital with a diagnosis of metastatic lung cancer. He was to receive therapy but began a gradual decline and the therapy was postponed. In an early interview, he told the social worker that he had a wife in Mexico and that she would be coming to visit him soon. He said that she was working with the Immigration and Naturalization Service (INS) and that he did not need any help with her INS or visa issues. Shortly after this conversation he was transferred to the palliative care unit at the hospital. He asked for his wife but was unable to say her name. The name he had given to the admitting clerk was that of his first wife, whom he had divorced decades earlier. The social worker called the referring oncologist's office and learned they had no reference to a wife but did have a next of kin listed as his son John, who lived near a mining town in another state. The social worker went to the Internet and searched for a John Martinez in the named state and found one listing near a known mining town. She called and left a message asking if he were the son of Mr. Martinez and if so to call back. He called back later saying he knew his father had remarried but had never met his wife. He gave the social worker his sister's phone number in case his sister might know where the stepmother was. She too did not know anything about her father's latest marriage, but said that she was willing to help out in any way she could, though she lived nearly 2000 miles away.

Knowing time was short for Mr. Martinez, the social worker called the police department of the small town where he lived. The dispatcher said that he was new to town but that Officer Joe had lived there a long time and he might know where the wife was. She was transferred to the officer who said, "Of course I know Martinez. How's he doing?" When told why the social worker was trying to locate the man's wife, he said that he did not know her but thought she was in Mexico. He said that he would post the information at city hall and knew that something would come up.

An hour later, Mr. Martinez' minister called the social worker and said that he knew Mr. Martinez was married to a Mexican woman, but that he did not know her name or where she lived. He said that he would try to help find her. The next morning, the mayor/ambulance driver for the town called with a message for the social worker. The social worker was directed to the INS office at the US – Mexico border where Mrs. Martinez was waiting for verification of her husband's condition. A medical statement was faxed to the INS and Mrs. Martinez, along with her mother, received a two-week visa to visit her husband. She arrived later that day to a very pleased husband. He remained lucid for a couple of days before passing away.

Mrs. Martinez came with very little money, having had to borrow funds for the 300-mile bus ride to the hospital. She was given enough money from a special hospital fund to buy food for herself and her mother, but it was obvious that she needed a way to get home and a way to have her husband's body cared for. Through an interpreter, she said that Mr. Martinez had told her he wanted to be cremated, but she was afraid the children would object. The social worker contacted both children and received permission for the cremation. Now the problem was to arrange for the cremation and lodging for the weekend. The social worker contacted a local Catholic charity, which graciously agreed to pay for two nights' lodging. A local veteran's service organization was contacted, and they bought two one-way bus tickets back to the border town. Then the social worker contacted a direct service company that agreed to cremate the patient at a price the wife and family could pay. Mr. Martinez died on a Saturday with his wife and mother-in-law at his side. Afterward, his wife checked into a motel, her husband's body was cremated, and his ashes were delivered to his wife. His wife and mother were taken to the bus station and returned to Mexico one day before her visa expired.

The Town That Came to the Rescue: Traditional Care for the Dying

Mr. Wilson came to the Veteran's Affairs Medical Center and was diagnosed with acute leukemia. He had been working as an independent trucker. He had his own equipment and had been the sole supporter of his wife and two children. He was devastated that he was not able to work and that he had no way of paying his bills. The social worker assisted him with applications for Social Security Disability and VA Non-Service Connected Pension. There was discussion with the patient and his wife about selling the business, which the wife did while her husband was being treated. He had an extended stay in the hospital as the result of therapy and his wife left for home to care for the minor children. When, after two cycles of chemotherapy, Mr. Wilson decided not to continue treatment, he told the social worker of all the help he and his family had received. He said that the little town of about 400 held bake sales, car washes, and other fund-raising events to help him and his family. He said that a local café donated one day's receipts to his family. Through the kindness of the entire community the Wilsons could continue living without the constant worry of where the next meal would come from or how the utilities would be paid. The money raised by the community kept the family out of debt until his federal benefits began.

Mr. Wilson made it clear that he did not fear death. He said that his faith has helped him through the dying process. His only concern toward the end of his life was that his family would be cared for. He had conferred with his pastor and planned his funeral. He said that it would be the most joyous funeral ever held. Three days before he died, Mrs. Wilson called the social worker asking what to do about her husband who was in a great deal of pain that was not being adequately addressed by the hospice agency. The worker consulted with a physician who indicated the patient should go the nearest hospital (90 miles away) if his current care was not adequate. The wife said her husband would not go that day because their daughter was a homecoming queen candidate and he wanted to be with her at the football game. She said that she would call the hospice nurse again for advice.

The following week, the wife called the social worker to inform her that Mr. Wilson had died quietly the night before. She said that he was so happy when he walked his daughter to the stage on the football field. Her son and the local Emergency Medical Technicians were all there to help if he needed assistance on the field. The daughter, though only a sophomore, was elected homecoming queen, making her father the happiest man in the state.

The above two cases illustrate that community resources are essential partners in the interdisciplinary team care of a dying patient. Similar to the needs of a developing child, it takes a village to support the journey of a dying member of a community.

Further Reading

Federal Benefits for Veterans and Dependents. Veterans Affairs Pamphlet 80-01-1. Department of Veterans Affairs, Washington, D.C.

Kübler-Ross, E. *On Death and Dying*, New York: Macmillan, 1969.

Lauria, M. M., Clark, E. J., Hermann, J. F., Stearns, N. M. *Social Work in Oncology: Supporting Survivors, Families and Caregivers*. Atlanta, Georgia: American Cancer Society, 2001.

Maslow, A. *Motivation and Personality*, 3rd Ed., New York: Harper and Row, 1987.

Parry, J. K. *Social Work Theory and the Practice with the Terminally Ill.* 2nd Ed., The Haworth Press, 2001.

Index

A

ABCDE approach to pain, 151, 152, 152t
Abraham, W. T., 200
Abrahams, J. L., 222
Abuse, verbal, from patient, 124-125
Acceptance, of death, 235
Accountability, of health care providers, 1
ACCP/SCCM Consensus Panel, 93
ACE inhibitors, 197, 200
Acetaminophen (Tylenol), 162-163, 164, 166
Activism, social, 13
Acute care, 49-50
Aday, L., 70, 82
Addiction, 90, 150, 151
Adelhardt, J., 223
Adjuvant medications, 173-174
Admission criteria for hospice, 37, 37t. *See also* Hospice, eligibility for; Medicare, eligibility for
Adult Protective Services program, 263
Advance directives, 1, 110, 185, 232-233, 244-245
types of, 113-114
Advil (ibuprofen, Motrin), 164, 166
African Americans, 177, 178, 221
Agency for Health Care Policy and Research, 90, 143
Agency for Healthcare Research and Quality, 143
Agitation, 205, 223, 225
Ahmedzia, S. H., 246
AIDS patients, 6, 51, 54, 89
Airway obstruction, treatment for, 136
Albuterol (Proventil), 202-203
Aldactone (spironalactone), 201

Aldosterone, 201
Aldridge, D., 28
Alexander, C. S., 197, 205
Alliance for Healthcare Reform, 238
Allodynia, 145
Almeida, R., 187
Alpert, H. R., 223
Alternative medicine, for pain, 152-153
Alzheimer disease, 54, 198, 213
Alzheimer's Association, 253-254
Ambalu, S., 214
Amenta, M., 20
American Academy of Hospice and Palliative Medicine, 255
American Cancer Society, 254
American College of Physicians Health and Public Policy Committee, 96
American Geriatrics Society, 58
American Heart Association, 254
American Medical Association, 93, 96
American Pain Society, 62, 96, 150
American Psychological Association, 238
American Thoracic Society, 93
American Way of Death, The (Mitford), 1
Amitriptyline (Elavil), 172
Analgesics, 161-175. *See* Medications, for pain
Ancient civilizations, 8-9
Anderson, A. J., 204
Anderson, H., 246
Anderson, K., 186
Andrews, M., 177, 178, 180, 182, 183, 184, 185
Anemia, 130-131, 133
Anesthesia, discovery of, 3, 9
Anger, at prognosis, 235
Angst, terminal, 225. *See also* Anxiety

S